JOHN C. BAER, M.D.

International Ophthalmology Clinics

International Ophthalmology Clinics (ISSN 0020-8167) (ISBN 0-316-45652-7). Published quarterly by Little, Brown and Company, 34 Beacon Street, Boston, Massachusetts 02108-1493. Send address changes and subscription orders to Little, Brown and Company, Subscription Department, PO Box 2033, Langhorne, PA 19047-9480; (800) 628-4221. Subscription rates per year: personal subscription, U.S. and possessions, $86; foreign (includes Mexico), $111; Canada, $98, PLEASE ADD 7% CANADIAN GST FOR ALL CANADIAN SUBSCRIPTIONS (Registration No. R128537917); institutional, U.S., $105; foreign, $137; Canada, $116. Special rates for students, interns and residents per year: U.S., $58; foreign, $80; Canada, $69. Single copies: $31 for subscribers, $39 for nonsubscribers. In Japan please contact our exclusive agent: Medsi, 1-2-13 Yushima, Bunkyo-ku, Tokyo 113, Japan. Subscription rates per year in Japan: individual, ¥24,200; institutional, ¥28,400 (air cargo service only). Second-class postage paid at Boston, Massachusetts, and at additional mailing offices.

Postmaster: Send address changes to International Ophthalmology Clinics, PO Box 2033, Langhorne, PA 19047-9480.

International Ophthalmology Clinics is indexed in Index Medicus, Current Contents/Clinical Practice, Excerpta Medica, and Current Awareness in Biological Sciences.

International Ophthalmology Clinics

Volume 32
Number 1
Winter 1992

Pediatric Ophthalmology

EDITED BY

Frederick A. Jakobiec, M.D.

*Massachusetts Eye and Ear Infirmary and
Harvard Medical School, Boston,
Massachusetts*

AND

Dimitri Azar, M.D.

*Wilmer Ophthalmological Institute,
The Johns Hopkins University Hospital, and
Bayview Eye Center, Baltimore, Maryland*

Little, Brown and Company
BOSTON

Editors

Gilbert Smolin, M.D.
F.I. Proctor Foundation, San Francisco
Department of Ophthalmology,
University of California, San Francisco
Medical Center

Mitchell H. Friedlaender, M.D.
Division of Ophthalmology,
Scripps Clinic and Research Foundation,
La Jolla, California

Editorial Office
931 West San Bruno Avenue
San Bruno, CA 94066

Publisher
Little, Brown and Company, Boston, Massachusetts

Publishing Staff

Publisher
Lynne Herndon

Managing Editor
Sherri Frank

Sales and Marketing Manager
Anne Orens

Production Manager
Fredda Purgalin

Contents

Contributing Authors

Dimitri Azar, M.D., EDITOR
Wilmer Ophthalmological Institute at
   The Johns Hopkins University Hospital *and*
Bayview Eye Center,
Baltimore, MD
Address correspondence to:
Wilmer Ophthalmological Institute
Maumenee-327
The Johns Hopkins University Hospital
600 N. Wolfe Street
Baltimore, MD 21205

Dr. Azar was Chief Resident at the Massachusetts Eye and Ear Infirmary during the initial phases of this project.

Frederick A. Jakobiec, M.D., EDITOR
Department of Ophthalmology
Massachusetts Eye and Ear Infirmary
243 Charles Street
Boston, MA 02114

Eddy Anglade, M.D.
Department of Ophthalmology
Massachusetts Eye and Ear Infirmary
243 Charles Street
Boston, MA 02114

Martin Arkin, M.D., Ph.D.
Department of Ophthalmology
Massachusetts Eye and Ear Infirmary
243 Charles Street
Boston, MA 02114

John C. Baer, M.D.
University of Maryland
22 South Green Street
Baltimore, MD 21201

Ann M. Bajart, M.D.
Ophthalmic Consultants of Boston
50 Staniford Street
Boston, MA 02114-2517

Eliot L. Berson, M.D.
Berman-Gund Laboratory
Massachusetts Eye and Ear Infirmary
243 Charles Street
Boston, MA 02114

Paul R. Cotran, M.D.
Department of Ophthalmology
Massachusetts Eye and Ear Infirmary
243 Charles Street
Boston, MA 02114

Donald S. Fong, M.D.
Department of Ophthalmology
Massachusetts Eye and Ear Infirmary
243 Charles Street
Boston, MA 02114

C. Stephen Foster, M.D.
Department of Ophthalmology
Massachusetts Eye and Ear Infirmary
243 Charles Street
Boston, MA 02114

Anthony Fraioli, M.D.
Department of Ophthalmology
Massachusetts Eye and Ear Infirmary
243 Charles Street
Boston, MA 02114

Anne Fulton, M.D.
The Children's Hospital Medical Center
300 Longwood Avenue
Boston, MA 02115

Cynthia Grosskreutz, M.D., Ph.D.
Department of Ophthalmology
Massachusetts Eye and Ear Infirmary
243 Charles Street
Boston, MA 02114

Ramzi K. Hemady, M.D.
University of Maryland
Baltimore, MD
Address correspondence to:
20 Wendsworth Bridge
Lutherville, MD 21093

David G. Hunter, M.D., Ph.D.
The Wilmer Ophthalmological Institute, B1-35
The Johns Hopkins Hospital
600 N. Wolfe Street
Baltimore, MD 21205

Vera O. Kowal, M.D.
Department of Ophthalmology
Massachusetts Eye and Ear Infirmary
243 Charles Street
Boston, MA 02114

Jeffrey C. Lamkin, M.D.
Department of Ophthalmology
Massachusetts Eye and Ear Infirmary
243 Charles Street
Boston, MA 02114

Leonard A. Levin, M.D., Ph.D.
Department of Ophthalmology
Massachusetts Eye and Ear Infirmary
243 Charles Street
Boston, MA 02114

M. Lisa McHam, M.D.
Department of Ophthalmology
Massachusetts Eye and Ear Infirmary
243 Charles Street
Boston, MA 02114

Craig A. McKeown, M.D.
Pediatric Ophthalmology
Massachusetts Eye and Ear Infirmary
243 Charles Street
Boston, MA 02114

Monte D. Mills, M.D.
Department of Ophthalmology
Massachusetts Eye and Ear Infirmary
243 Charles Street
Boston, MA 02114

Shizuo Mukai, M.D.
Department of Ophthalmology
Massachusetts Eye and Ear Infirmary
243 Charles Street
Boston, MA 02114

Samuel E. Navon, M.D., Ph.D.
Department of Ophthalmology
Massachusetts Eye and Ear Infirmary
243 Charles Street
Boston, MA 02114

Annabelle A. Okada, M.D.
Department of Ophthalmology
Massachusetts Eye and Ear Infirmary
243 Charles Street
Boston, MA 02114

Elias Reichel, M.D.
Berman-Gund Laboratory
Massachusetts Eye and Ear Infirmary
243 Charles Street
Boston, MA 02114

Richard M. Robb, M.D.
Department of Ophthalmology
The Children's Hospital Medical Center
300 Longwood Avenue
Boston, MA 02115

Lois B. H. Smith, M.D., Ph.D.
Department of Ophthalmology
The Children's Hospital Medical Center
300 Longwood Avenue
Boston, MA 02115

Nicholas J. Volpe, M.D.
Department of Ophthalmology
Massachusetts Eye and Ear Infirmary
243 Charles Street
Boston, MA 02114

In the Summer 1991 issue of International Ophthalmology Clinics (*Volume 31, Number 3,* Systemic Associations of Ocular Disorders), *Dr. F. Rodney Eve's degrees were not listed completely. His correct degrees are as follows:*

F. Rodney Eve, M.D., F.R.C.S.(C.), F.C.Ophth.

The Editors apologize for this omission.

Preface

On Saturday, January 26, 1991, under the guidance of faculty preceptors, the residents of the Massachusetts Eye and Ear Infirmary gave a course entitled "Pediatric Ophthalmology." A 360-page syllabus was distributed at the course, and it was quite apparent that with a little more work, a project worthy of publication was in the making. Dr. Gilbert Smolin reviewed the syllabus and gave the green light to proceed with preparation of the final manuscripts and illustrations. As the initial coordinators of the residents' program, we served as editors for this special issue of *International Ophthalmology Clinics*. We are pleased to announce that the residents' course, with a different overarching theme each time, is now a standard biannual offering among the educational programs at the Infirmary.

This issue begins with a paper on how to estimate visual acuity in the preverbal child. Following that is a discussion of theories and recent experimental work regarding ocular growth and its regulation, which is also inextricably intertwined with some features of amblyopia. Rather than presenting updates on all aspects of strabismus, articles that concentrate on Duane's and Brown's syndromes have been included.

Papers on anterior segment disorders of the eye encompass corneal opacities, neonatal conjunctivitis, Kawasaki syndrome, and cataracts in the pediatric age group. Representative posterior ocular disorders have a focus on posterior uveitis, retinal degenerations, albinism, and retinopathy of prematurity.

Finally, an analysis of orbital diseases concentrates on an overview of the most common primary tumors of the orbital soft tissues and on ways to distinguish optic nerve meningioma from glioma. The concluding article takes up the controversial issue of immunosuppressive therapy for corticostcriod-resistant uveitis associated with juvenile rheumatoid arthritis.

It is our hope that the topics covered in this issue of *International Ophthalmology Clinics* will prove valuable to general ophthalmologists, pediatric ophthalmologists, and pediatricians.

Frederick A. Jakobiec
Dimitri Azar

Can This Baby See?: Estimation of Visual Acuity in the Preverbal Child

Jeffrey C. Lamkin, M.D.

Most tests for visual function require a voluntary, subjective, usually verbal response. As such, these tests presume an alert, cooperative, verbal patient who is capable not only of resolving the stimulus but also of recognizing it, interpreting it correctly, and reacting as directed by the examiner [1]. In adults, the sequence occurs rapidly without conscious effort. In children, these skills do not develop simultaneously; thus, standard acuity tests are not appropriate for preverbal or impaired children. Before the 1970s, little attention was given to the visual capabilities of neonates, infants, and toddlers. In fact, the limitations in assessing visual function in preverbal children led to the widely held, naive belief that visual acuity did not reach adult levels until the age of 5 years (coincidentally, paralleling linguistic development).

Now, the importance of reliable visual testing in preverbal children is more fully appreciated. Why is quantifying visual function in children important? First, reliable visual screening permits early, efficient detection of preventable or treatable causes of visual loss. This inherent assumption in the adult ophthalmic population is even more important in the very young child. "Sensitive periods" for visual development have been proved to exist in both animals and humans, representing the developmental windows during which the visual system is most responsive to both insult and therapy [2]. Visual acuity testing is critical in detecting vision-limiting conditions, as well as for monitoring response to therapy. The study of visual development may yield clues to development in other neurological systems. Some studies indicate that neonatal visual function may be a significant independent predictor of future mental performance [3]. Thus, accurate assessment of vision takes on systemic implications as well.

In adults, acuity is the most routinely tested visual function and is considered most representative of global ocular function. Visual acuity represents an estimate of spatial resolution capabilities at high or maximal contrast. Of course, acuity is only a part of complete visual function. Many

1

other levels of visual function are important for daily life, including contrast sensitivity, color vision, stereopsis, peripheral visual field function, and motion detection. Since we live in an increasingly literate world, acuity remains the standard for assessing overall visual performance, and this chapter will concentrate on the findings of various methods of assessing *visual acuity*. Still, the modalities to be discussed have been used to assess the other visual processing systems, and these will be reviewed briefly also.

■ Visual Acuity

Definitions and Concepts

A full review of the definitions and nature of visual acuity is beyond the scope of this chapter, but excellent source materials are available [4]. *Visual acuity* may be defined as "the spatial limit of visual discrimination"; its measurement requires determination of a threshold in which the variable is spatial dimension. Important subdivisions in types of acuity are best differentiated on the basis of the criteria set for the response of the observer, including the following:

1. The presence or absence of a single object ("minimum visible," so-called detection acuity)
2. The presence or absence, or internal arrangement of identifying features, of a visible target ("minimum resolvable," so-called resolution acuity)
3. The discrimination and description of familiar stimuli from competing familiar stimuli ("minimum recognizable," so-called recognition acuity)
4. The *relative* location of visible features ("spatial minimum discriminable," so-called hyperacuity)

A full discussion of the various subtypes of acuity is found elsewhere [4]. Detection acuity tests are actually tests of contrast threshold; the other acuity subdivisions do require the eye to discriminate spatially. Resolution acuity (minimum resolvable) may be evaluated with gratings (see below) or with patterned targets such as the illiterate E or Landolt C (Fig 1). Recognition acuity (minimum recognizable) is a refinement of resolution acuity,

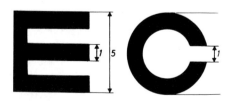

Figure 1 *Snellen E and Landolt C tests for resolution acuity. (Reprinted with permission from DeLaey [1].)*

adding the task of recognizing and naming familiar targets, often from within a group of other familiar targets. This has the advantage of avoiding binary decisions, reducing the likelihood of correct responses by chance, and optimizing information transfer between patient and examiner.

A variety of methods have been used to determine the minimum angle of resolution. They share the feature of enlargement or reduction of the target object to the threshold size at which the required judgment can be made correctly for an arbitrary percentage of trials (typically between 50 and 75%). Normal subjects can correctly distinguish (resolve) targets that vary in the position of critical elements (gaps or squares) whose angular subtense at the retina is 30 to 60 seconds (½ to 1 minute of arc). Commonly, the overall dimension of the target is five times that of the critical element (see Fig 1).

Optical Gratings

Typical acuity tests based on the principles just described require a certain level of verbal and motor sophistication that renders them useless for the very young child. The modalities discussed in this chapter utilize stimuli and procedures unbound by these limitations. Typically, the stimuli consist of repetitive gratings of predictable, mathematically precise luminance variations (Fig 2). Luminance variations create the striped appearance and can be generated by square-wave or sinusoidal mathematics. Both minutes of arc (arcmin, square-wave) and cycles per degree (cpd, sinusoidal) are units of spatial frequency. Square-wave gratings of 1 arcmin are considered visually (not mathematically) equivalent to sinusoidal gratings of 30 cpd. Snellen acuity equivalents can be derived, since the 20/20 images have critical elements whose basic spatial frequency is 1 arcmin (30 cpd) at the appropriate test distance. Thus, square-wave gratings of 1 arcmin are equivalent to sinusoidal frequencies of 30 cpd and Snellen letters of the 20/20 line. Figure 3 provides a chart for converting one to another of the three different spatial frequency units. *In exploring the various techniques used to estimate visual acuity in the preverbal child, it is critical to understand that*

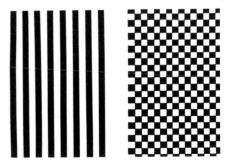

Figure 2 *Optical grating.*

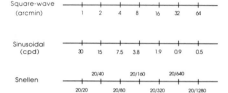

Figure 3 *Conversion table for spatial frequency units.*

these conversions do not imply that grating frequencies are identical to Snellen frequencies. The nature of the targets is inherently different. The only feature they share is their basic spatial frequency. The differences between the stimuli are as important in analyzing acuity testing results as are their similarities.

■ Test Methods

Three basic methods for estimating visual acuity in the preverbal or impaired child have gained acceptance over the past two to three decades. This chapter will concentrate on the modalities of optokinetic nystagmus (OKN), preferential looking tests (PLT), and visual evoked potentials (VEP). Each has clinical advantages and disadvantages and has found meaningful use in pediatric ophthalmology and neurology. The tests routinely used for preverbal or impaired children are sometimes referred to as *objective measurements* since they require no self-measured response from the subject. The tests do, however, require subjective participation by an examiner. The studies to be cited have gone to great lengths to eradicate the examiner's bias from the test results. The potential for subjective bias is important to remember when applying the tests in an uncontrolled setting (e.g., a busy clinic). It can be used to advantage, as will be discussed, to streamline the tests to make them more useful, efficient, and universally applicable.

Optokinetic Nystagmus

Background and Literature Review OKN has the distinction of being the first tool to be recognized as potentially useful in estimating visual acuity. Ohm's original technique [5], described in 1922, stimulated OKN with a suprathreshold grating drum. Small objects (graded balls) were then placed between the drum and the subject. Suppression of OKN implied ability to detect the interposed object. Ohm used the technique in adults with acceptable results; it has yet to be applied to infants or children. It is a *detection* acuity test and, as such, gives little information about resolution or recognition acuity, which are the standards for comparison with larger populations and studies. Gorman [6] brought OKN into modern use by creating a canopy of moving stripes that rotated above a supine infant. Acuity was measured as the finest grating that elicited a visible OKN response binocularly. Dayton and co-workers [7] used electrooculography (EOG) measurements to detect OKN responses more reliably near threshold. In an attempt to make the measurements easier and more practical, Catford and Oliver [8] developed a lightweight, portable, hand-held apparatus with moving dots to elicit an OKN-like eye movement. Although their results correlated well with Snellen acuity in normal adult eyes, the correlation broke down in eyes with measurable visual loss. Their apparatus routinely obtained falsely high acuity values in diseased eyes.

Agreement among various OKN studies of healthy preverbal children is good (Fig 4) [9]. Gratings of spatial frequency equal to Snellen 20/20 elicit detectable OKN by 20 to 30 months of age. Studies using EOG yield better acuities at any age and 20/20 OKN acuity within the first 12 to 18 months [7]. Since most clinical settings do not permit routine EOG measurement, the more conservative data are more applicable for screening purposes. (The EOG study of Dayton's group [7] also used hand-drawn gratings, which probably contained imperfections and low-frequency noise, thus systematically overestimating acuity.)

Applications of OKN   The primary use of OKN in the clinical setting is as a rapid screen for the gross integrity of the visual system [10]. Some investigators have used OKN to follow normal development from the neonatal period, as well as to follow acuity improvement after cataract surgery with optical correction [11].

Advantages and Disadvantages of OKN   OKN targets range in size and convenience. Most of the clinically useful targets are accessible and portable. The trade-off for the convenience is loss of detailed acuity information, as well as difficulties in ensuring that the visual world of the subject is entirely filled and that interest is maintained on the target. A certain level of alertness and attention is required on the part of the subject, but testing time is generally short. The targets themselves must be of uniform width and have uniform space-average luminance; the quality of the targets must be high enough so that incidental disturbances in the grating pattern do not contribute low-frequency stimuli that might elicit a response

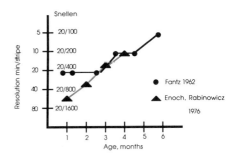

Figure 4   *Optokinetic nystagmus acuities in healthy infants.*

where there would otherwise be none. The speed of presentation and illumination are intertest variables that may be difficult to control. The responses themselves, by nature, become more difficult to detect as the threshold is approached. Even experienced observers may have difficulty pinpointing exactly the target size at which the last real response is made. EOG measurements address this problem, but this technique is not practical for most clinical settings. The greatest limitation in OKN testing is that the response is not dependent solely on afferent visual processing. The absence of a response to a moving OKN target may reflect merely the child's preferential interest in other elements in the environment. More importantly, a positive OKN response requires an intact oculomotor system, from pursuit centers to saccade centers to brainstem to cranial nerves to extraocular muscles. Disturbances anywhere in this complex chain will result in abnormal OKN responses despite intact afferent visual processing. Conversely, intact OKN responses have been elicited from infants with no visual cortex, implying extrageniculate or subcortical pursuit systems, or both [12].

Even in healthy infants, direct comparison of OKN and Snellen acuities is not appropriate, because the stimuli used in OKN testing are inherently different from Snellen letters. To equate vertical stripes moving in a horizontal plane to recognition of familiar forms is specious. Moreover, since targets are moving, temporal visual processing (the *ambient* processing system) is involved interactively with the spatial processing system (the *focal* system). Thus, OKN responses yield information essentially different from Snellen acuity.

OKN testing remains clinically useful as a primary screen for basic visual behavior but is not routinely used for reliable quantitative visual assessment.

Preferential Looking Tests

Background and Literature Review Fantz [13] is generally credited as the first to recognize and utilize the principle of preferential looking. He observed that infants will demonstrate a greater tendency to fixate a pattern stimulus than a homogeneous field. This assumption is broadened to include the inference that patterns too small to be resolved will be fixated with a frequency similar to a homogeneous alternative. Fantz's procedure places an infant in a test chamber exposed to a pair of stimuli—black and white stripes of a given width (spatial frequency) versus a gray field of matched space-averaged luminance—for 20 seconds. The positions of the stimuli are reversed, and another 20-second exposure is performed. An observer watches the infant and scores the number of fixations for each stimulus, as well as the duration of fixation. Fantz estimated acuity by selecting the spatial frequency of the stripe that was fixed longer than the homogeneous field by 75% of the infants at a given age. His method has

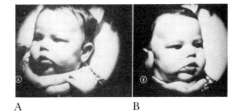

Figure 5 *Examples of fixation preference behaviors: (A) right and (B) left.*   A   B

been used reproducibly with increasing refinement but has attendant statistical considerations and bias.

These limitations prompted Teller and colleagues [14] to develop a modified version with greater power and reliability. Their two-alternative, forced choice, preferential looking test (PLT) became the basis for most studies of normal and abnormal development. In this version, the observer is masked to the positions of the striped and homogeneous stimuli. Instead of judging the infant's duration of fixation, the observer is forced to make a choice based on fixation direction only: Is the striped pattern on the infant's right or left? (Note: It is the observer who is forced to make the choice, not the infant! See Figure 5.) In diverse studies and clinical applications, features vary, but the typical test apparatus consists of a large gray screen with a small, central peephole (Fig 6). Stimulus apertures are located at a given distance to the left and right of the peephole. The grating targets can be positioned behind either aperture by rotating a wheel or changing

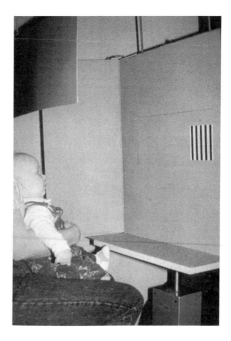

Figure 6 *Preferential looking test apparatus. (Reprinted with permission from Dobson et al [18].)*

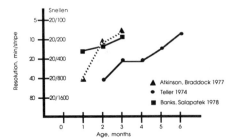

Figure 7 *Preferential looking test acuities in healthy infants.*

large cards behind the screen. Full descriptions of the testing procedures and statistical analysis can be found elsewhere [14].

The forced-choice technique has statistical features that yield precise, reproducible data, but the problem with the procedure is that it is time-consuming and laborious (numerous trials are required to obtain stable acuity thresholds). Success rates fall off rapidly for children older than 1 year, and monocular testing can lengthen testing time to undesirable levels, as well as increase the subject's fussiness. It also requires 3 adults to participate. Still, it has been used with success to determine age-related norms for binocular PLT acuity in infants (Fig 7) [15–17]. It is important to note that almost all PLT studies document variations of approximately 1 octave within and between age-matched infants. An *octave* is defined as "a doubling or halving of the angular subtense of the image" (e.g., 20/20 to 20/40 is lowering acuity by 1 octave). A stripe of 10 arcmin (3 cpd, 20/200) is 1 octave lower in frequency than a stripe of 5 arcmin (12 cpd, 20/100). Thus, all PLT results should be interpreted with this variability in mind.

Modifications in the Forced-Choice Paradigm

PLT as a Screening Test   Various investigators have attempted to refine the PLT technique to make it more practical for daily clinical use. The first such effort attempted to survey a large number of healthy infants to determine diagnostic stripe widths [18, 19] to be used as a vision test for well-baby screening. The test is rapid (less than 10 minutes) and widely applicable (90% of infants tested successfully completed binocular testing by inexperienced testers).

"Fast" PLT   In a parallel refinement of forced-choice paradigms, Gwiazda and co-workers [20] used slide projectors in an otherwise dark room. A unique stimulus presentation method started with frequencies 0.5 octave lower than accepted norms for the infant's age (with no certainty of bracketing threshold). In their "fast" method, the slides are arranged in order of increasing spatial frequency (staircase fashion). Their hypothesis held that this stimulus presentation provided the infant with more distinct alter-

natives (bright screens in a dark room), which would make the observer's job easier. These investigators also claimed that their method of progression through the various frequencies made the determination of threshold frequency more efficient. The method yielded another, rather surprising result: Infants seemed preferentially to fixate the *homogeneous* field as the grating stimulus approached threshold [21]. If this were the case for earlier PLT studies, threshold acuity might have been systematically underestimated. Banks and colleagues [22] repeated PLT under identical testing conditions and failed to reproduce this preference for homogeneous fields near threshold acuity.

Extending PLT to Older Children   The next refinement in forced-choice PLT borrowed operant techniques from audiometry studies to broaden the applicability of PLT to age groups for which traditional preferential looking had been most difficult (12 to 24 months old). Operant techniques utilize positive visual and auditory reinforcement of behavior (animated toys) conducive to completing PLT. Mayer and Dobson [23, 24] have used operant techniques to establish norms in age groups typically difficult to test. Their results in infants show good agreement with previously published, nonoperant studies.

Combining Staircase Presentation with Operant Techniques to Test Monocular Acuity   Wedding typical forced-choice and operant techniques with a transformed up-down staircase method of stimulus presentation, Mayer and associates [25] were able successfully to complete PLT, *including monocular testing*, on 85% of children from 11 days to 5 years of age. Acuity values in children with normal eyes agreed well with data from studies using the more traditional method of binocular testing with constant stimuli (see previous discussion). These investigators could detect acuity differences due solely to refractive error (normalization of PLT acuity with refractive correction) as well as those due to secondary amblyopia. In children with strabismic amblyopia, PLT acuities did not always agree with fixation behavior. The authors hypothesized that fixation preference may precede PLT acuity asymmetry in some cases but that PLT may act as a useful adjunct in occlusion therapy for strabismic amblyopia. In children with structural ocular disorders, PLT acuities were consistent with the severity of the disorder. In one of the earliest applications, the authors used PLT to guide occlusion therapy, with predictable results (abolition of interocular acuity difference, freely alternating fixation).

Acuity Card Techniques   Even with the modifications described earlier, the primary limitation of PLT persisted: The time and effort involved in performing reliable, complete, monocular testing was great enough to preclude use in a busy clinic setting, as well as to reduce significantly the number of children able to complete testing successfully. These problems prompted the development of the acuity card technique, which is essentially a simplified version of forced-choice PLT [26]. The cards are large rectangles with grating stimuli at each end. One grating is of spatial frequency within the normal resolution range for the infant being tested. The other is a high-frequency grating well above the resolution limit, thus appearing as a blank gray target with space-average luminance identical to its counterpart. The cards may be presented behind a screen to block out distracting stimuli in the environment (Fig 6). Unlike forced-choice paradigms, the examiner is not masked to stimulus frequency and is allowed to use *any* aspect of the child's behavior to make a determination regarding fixation preference. The examiner is given free reign in selecting the appropriate testing frequencies, as well as deciding when the child is no longer able to resolve the targets. As performed by the test's creators, acuity card testing is significantly faster than traditional PLT—2 to 6 minutes for a single acuity card test and 37 minutes for the complete battery. Testability runs in the 90 to 100% range for both monocular and binocular testing, except for newborns (too sleepy) and 24-month-olds (too fussy to patch, completing 100% of binocular testing but 75% of monocular testing). Interobserver acuity correlation is good. The acuity values obtained by the investigators compare favorably with established traditional PLT values (Fig 8) [26]. The authors make several cautionary points regarding the inherent variability and possible examiner bias in acuity card testing. They also emphasize the importance of high-quality gratings. Finally, and perhaps most importantly, they note that this is a resolution, not a recognition, task. It is well recognized that amblyopic children characteristically have recognition acuities considerably lower than resolution acuities. Thus, acuity card acuity will overestimate eventual Snellen performance.

Applications of PLT

Binocular Vision Birch [27] assessed monocular and binocular acuities as well as PLT responses to stereo targets in children 0 to 11 months old. She found interocular acuity differences of 1 octave in the first 5 months of life, which decreased to 0.5 octave by 9 to 11 months. The author found that, at this point in development, interocular acuity differences are in greatest decline as binocular vision is beginning to develop into a functionally superior state to monocular acuity. She concluded that the third and fifth months of life may mark a period of binocular competition culminating in small interocular acuity differences and the development of stereopsis.

Color Vision Hamer and co-workers [28] used preferential-looking paradigms to evaluate color discrimination in infants 1 to 3 months old. They found that by age 3 months, all infants could discriminate wavelengths of 550 or 633 nm from a surround of 589 nm. Fewer than 50%

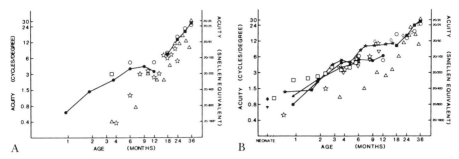

Figure 8   *Acuity card acuities in healthy infants: (A) monocular and (B) binocular. (Reprinted with permission from Teller et al [26].)*

of infants 1 month old could make such a discrimination. Packer and colleagues [29] found that by increasing test field size, discrimination performance increased at all ages and confirmed Hamer's conclusion that color discrimination failures in infants did not reflect receptor-level immaturity. Rather, post-receptor processing lags in development, causing loss of wavelength-specific visual information. Packer's group [29] also noted the correlation of bichromatic acuity (as determined in their study) with grating acuity, contrast sensitivity, and large spatial summation areas seen in infants and concluded that a common spatial resolution deficit may limit all three functions.

Meridional Variations in Acuity   PLT has been used extensively to investigate the oblique effect (preference for main-axis gratings over obliques) and meridional amblyopia. In Teller's original description of forced-choice PLT on infants less than 6 months old [14], no acuity differences were found for vertical versus diagonal gratings. The authors noted that the lack of orientation preference might reflect insensitivity of the PLT to infants' responses to higher spatial frequencies (where the oblique effect is demonstrated in adults) or a true indifference to orientation secondary to immature visual processing.

Gwiazda and associates [30] used PLT on 104 infants ranging from 17 to 45 weeks old. They found that for every age group, infants demonstrated an oblique effect for frequencies near threshold. This anisotropy was significantly greater in 1-year-olds than in older children and adults. The investigators ascribed their ability to detect an orientation preference to a more sensitive PLT technique and hypothesized that the oblique effect must diminish later in childhood.

To investigate the oblique effect in older children, Gwiazda and colleagues [31] measured grating acuity for four orientations in 111 children aged 3 to 8 years, including 9 with a history of significant astigmatism (1.75 to 3.5 D) that had disappeared at the time of the study. They verified their earlier hypothesis that anisotropy systematically diminished with age. Myopic children showed a preference for their less myopic meridian, either horizontal or vertical, over the more myopic one when tested at age 6 months. *This meridional preference was eradicated by optical correction.* These same children, when tested at age 6 years, had astigmatism of less than 0.5 D. The meridional effect persisted, however, implying uncorrectable acuity loss for their previously more myopic meridian (meridional amblyopia). This result implies that although an oblique effect and meridional preferences paralleling refractive error may be measurable within the first 4 to 6 months of life, true meridional amblyopia must not develop until later, since refractive correction eradicates the meridional preferences during the first year of life.

In parallel studies, Gwiazda and co-workers [32, 33] evaluated 70 infants aged 7 to 53 weeks with significant astigmatism (greater than 1 D). In several series of controlled experiments, they were able to support their earlier work by failing to demonstrate meridional amblyopia in children younger than 1 year.

PLT in Premature and Impaired Children   As early as 1970 [34], investigators were putting preferential looking to use in premature infants. Dubowitz and co-workers [35] used tracking techniques and PLT (Fantz technique) to detect visual function in preterm infants by the postconceptual age of 31 to 32 weeks. Visual development in premature infants followed that of full-term infants of a comparable post-conceptual age. This led the investigators to hypothesize that inherent maturational factors are more important in early visual development than is experience.

Manning and co-workers [36] used classical forced-choice PLT in 59 prematurely born infants. Their results indicated that before 2 months postterm, these infants were unable to complete PLT reliably, even with normal findings on ophthalmological examinations. Patients with developmental delays often had poorer PLT acuities than the ophthalmic examination would have predicted. In some children with strabismus, PLT did detect abnormal interocular acuity differences and served as a guide to occlusion therapy.

Brown and Yamamoto [37] applied the more streamlined acuity card procedure in an attempt to facilitate early visual assessment of high-risk infants seen in high-risk settings (intensive care units). Their technique was performed at the bedside with typical acuity cards. The test was repeated for infants who failed to complete the first trial. With additional trials, the completion rate approached 98%. Testing time was short. The acuity values obtained compare favorably with previous forced-choice and acuity card data on full-term infants. The acuity improvement seen with increasing age in these preterm infants is statistically significant and blends smoothly with data extrapolated from full-term infants.

PLT as a Guide to Occlusion Therapy   Several investigators have used PLT to guide decisions regarding occlusion therapy schedules. In studies of children with monocular congenital cataracts, PLT has been used to guide occlusion therapy with predictable results and better outcome than is historically associated with this condition [38–40]. It is in this setting, perhaps, where PLT holds its greatest promise.

Advantages and Disadvantages of PLT   There can be no doubt that PLT has dramatically increased the amount of information regarding preverbal visual function for both the clinician and the psychologist-investigator. The low cost of the equipment, along with its accessibility to minimally trained users, makes the test appealing and applicable in a broad range of settings. Refinements in the forced-choice technique have shortened the time required to collect, successfully and reliably, accurate data from normal and abnormal children across a wide age range. Certain caveats must be kept in mind. First, the test has an inherent variability of approximately 1 octave within and between children. Any acuity result must be understood as the potential spatial sensitivity ranging from one-half to two times the frequency so determined. This variability is not a disabling disadvantage but is a critical feature in interpreting results. Second, to a greater degree than OKN, PLT requires an alert, relatively cooperative child. Unfortunately, these qualities are often missing at the time of a medical or ophthalmic examination. Thus, PLT must often be rescheduled at a time when the child is in optimal testing condition. Third, as with OKN, the activity being monitored is a motor response. Failure to fixate a grating preferentially does not automatically imply the child cannot see the target. The other developmental capabilities involved in fixation behavior may be lagging behind resolution acuity. A good example is congenital oculomotor apraxia, a condition that makes obtaining a reliable PLT very difficult.

Finally, and perhaps most important, grating stimuli are inherently different from the standard recognition stimuli to which PLT acuity values are routinely compared (Snellen equivalents). To equate a PLT acuity value to a Snellen acuity is very misleading. As discussed on page 2, recognition tasks are more complex than resolution tasks. Thus, a child's PLT acuity is directly analogous only to other PLT acuities: age-matched norms for the same PLT technique, previous PLT results on the same child, or interocular comparisons. When these comparisons are made, PLT becomes a powerful tool for screening, diagnostic, and therapeutic decisions. *To use PLT results to predict future Snellen acuity is not valid.*

The danger in using PLT acuities as predictors for future recognition capability is adequately borne out by the literature. Mayer and colleagues [41] performed PLT and standard recognition acuity tests (Allen cards, Snellen single letters and rows) in a group of pediatric patients. All children, even those ophthalmologically normal, showed better grating acuities than recognition acuities. The discrepancy was significantly larger for children with amblyopia and foveal abnormalities, whereas for children with other ocular abnormalities, the resolution-recognition disparity matched that of children with normal eyes. In the amblyopes, the discrepancy was greater for strabismic amblyopia than for refractive or structural amblyopia. In fact, grating acuities in strabismic amblyopia did not correlate with recognition acuities! The authors mentioned possible explanations, including the heterogeneity of eye disorders, single versus linear acuity, and stimulus size and relative complexity. These findings were recently confirmed in a group of anisometropic amblyopes [42]. Teller grating card acuities were better than letter recognition acuities and did not worsen proportionately.

The critical point is that grating acuity provides information about visual processing that is complementary to standard recognition testing. Direct comparison of acuities is not appropriate.

Visual Evoked Potentials

Background and Literature Review The third method used to estimate visual acuity in preverbal children is the VEP. Full description of the nature and source of the waveform, as well as technical details concerning its generation and recording, is beyond the scope of this discussion, but excellent reviews are available [43, 44]. In brief, the VEP is a summed cortical response to a temporal change in some characteristic of a visual stimulus. It is actually a transient electroencephalogram (EEG) from which background cerebral "noise" must be subtracted. Monitoring electrodes are placed on the scalp over the occipital pole with grounding electrodes on the forehead, earlobe, or mastoid. The visual stimulus may be a simple flash or a more complex pattern. The pattern (checkerboard, sinusoidal gratings) may be presented transiently or continuously via pattern reversal. The waveform is generated by computer amplification and averaging to maximize signal-to-noise ratio. The salient features of the waveform are the amplitude of the first positive (upward) wave and the implicit time (the

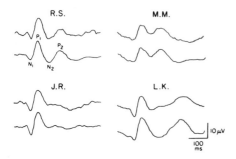

Figure 9 *Transient-pattern visual evoked potential waveform. Initials represent patients. (Reprinted with permission from Sokol et al [64].)*

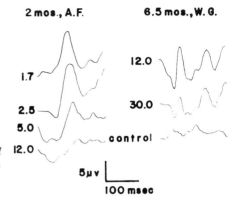

Figure 10 *Transient visual evoked potential with various spatial frequency stimuli.* Initials *represent patients. (Reprinted with permission from Marg et al [47].)*

interval elapsed between the stimulus presentation and peaking of the first positive wave). Figure 9 is a good example of a normal transient VEP, with P_1 representing the first positive wave.

A number of studies on normal adults have shown that pattern (not flash) VEPs may be used to estimate psychophysical recognition acuity, with good reproducibility and accuracy [45, 46]. Amplitude of the first positive wave diminishes and the implicit time increases as stripe width or check size decreases (increasing spatial frequency, acuity). Calculating acuity values traditionally utilizes the amplitude value rather than the implicit time. There are several ways of arriving at a threshold spatial frequency. The first is to select the highest spatial frequency that elicits a waveform detectably different from that of a blank stimulus of identical space-averaged luminance [47]. The second, shown to correlate well with adult Snellen acuity, involves extrapolation of a regression line fitting VEP amplitude to stimulus frequency through zero microvolt amplitude (i.e., the highest spatial frequency that, if tested, would render any positive wave) [46]. The latter method has gained wider acceptance. Figures 10 and 11 show the typical loss of amplitude and complexity with increasing spatial frequency in the immature visual system of the infant.

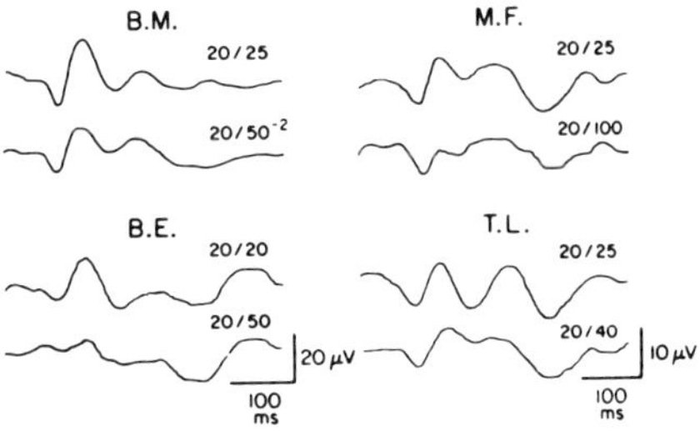

Figure 11 *Pattern-reversal visual evoked potentials with various spatial frequency stimuli.* Initials *represent patients. (Reprinted with permission from Sokol et al [64].)*

Marg and colleagues [47] used transient square-wave gratings to document VEP acuity of 20/400 at 1 month of age, improving to 20/20 by 4 to 6 months. Sokol [48] used pattern reversal checkerboards to document VEP acuity of 20/150 at 2 months, improving to 20/20 by 6 months. He explained the rapid improvement in acuity as reflecting the macular and foveal development that is concluded by the sixth month in term infants. Marg's estimates were somewhat higher, possibly because of difference in stimulus presentation; the transient stimulus method undoubtedly contributes luminance variations that are independent of spatial frequency and confound threshold determination. The results of these investigations are seen in Figure 12.

Norcia and Tyler [49] introduced the "sweep" VEP to infant acuity threshold measurements. In this technique, pattern reversal gratings spanning the expected acuity limits are rapidly presented in sequence within 10 seconds. This dramatically shortens the time required to collect the data. The method produced acuity values that differed somewhat from those of Marg [47] and Sokol [48]. At 1 month, infant VEP acuity was calculated at 20/80. The authors ascribed this higher acuity to the short duration of testing; quicker testing reduces state variation in the infants' responses, making the test more sensitive (akin to shortening PLT time, improving testability). Adult thresholds were not reached until 8 months of age, later than in previously published studies. The authors point out shortcomings in earlier studies that might have led to overestimation of threshold in the older infants (in Sokol's data [48], the frequencies sampled were well below the extrapolated threshold, ignoring important portions of the amplitude-frequency function).

Sokol and Jones [50] used pattern reversal checkerboards to investigate the variation in implicit time (or latency) of the VEP with infant age. Implicit times were consistently less variable than amplitudes and were consistently longer for smaller checks (as in adults). The implicit times also decreased with age for every check size. The implications of these findings are considerable. First, the failure of smaller checks to elicit any response until 12 to 16 weeks parallels the time course of foveal and macular devel-

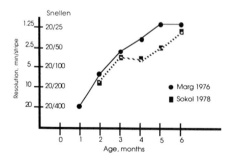

Figure 12 *Visual evoked potential acuities in healthy infants.*

opment (as discussed earlier). This confirms the hypothesis that, in adults, response to smaller checks is a function of the central 3 degrees of the visual field (fovea). Second, the implicit time progression for large checks is similar to that of amplitude in other infant studies (i.e., adult levels reached within the first 6 to 8 months of life). According to the authors, this reflects the early myelination of the optic nerve. The implicit times for small checks reach adult levels much more gradually, reflecting the ongoing but diminishing plasticity of the child's nervous system. This developmental profile is reflected in the sensitivity of the child's vision to deprivation (organic or therapeutic), which is greatest in the first 6 to 12 months and declines thereafter over 6 to 8 years. Thus, implicit time for small check size more accurately parallels clinical observations on visual development than does implicit time for either large checks or amplitude. The other advantage to implicit times is their lower variability, seen in adults as well as children.

Applications of VEP Acuity

VEP as Guide to Occlusion Therapy VEP acuity measurements have been used successfully to guide patching therapy in 8 neonates with monocular congenital cataracts who underwent early surgical and refractive correction [51]. VEP has also been used in children aged 5 months to 8 years to determine the absolute responses to patching in four different disorders of monocular visual deprivation [52].

Contrast Sensitivity VEP has been used to measure the contrast sensitivity function in infants [53–55]. Contrast sensitivity is determined by measuring the lowest detectable contrast for sine wave gratings of various frequencies. Adults show peak contrast sensitivity at spatial frequencies well below acuity threshold (at gratings of spatial frequencies equivalent to 20/100 to 20/200). VEP data, using the extrapolation techniques, show contrast sensitivity increasing over the first 3 months of age but remaining well below adult levels. The loss of contrast sensitivity at low frequencies seen in adults is not seen in infants younger than 2 months. Intraretinal lateral inhibitory processing, believed to be responsible for this effect [56], may be developing during this time.

Binocular Vision and the Sensitive Period VEP binocular summation refers to the larger amplitude of the VEP under binocular conditions. It is the subject of many studies, with seemingly contradictory or confusing results. Recently, Leguire and co-workers [57] reviewed the topic and present new data suggesting that a summation function they have configured may reflect the early portion of the human sensitive period during which binocular vision is developing (peaking at 3 months of age). In esotropes, the function is similar but incompletely expressed and is triggered by surgical alignment. These authors propose that optimal timing for surgical realignment would be at approximately 3 months of age.

Advantages and Disadvantages of VEP Acuity Perhaps the greatest advantage of VEP methods is that they are purely sensory. Unlike OKN and PLT, no motor response is required. VEP testing can be accomplished for children who would not be able to complete OKN or PLT testing. On the other hand, functional visual behavior requires considerable postcortical processing, which the VEP does not reflect. Thus, VEP acuity may represent acuity *potential*. Another disadvantage rests with our incomplete understanding about its generation and nature. VEP waveforms have been recorded in children with severe brain damage and behavioral blindness [58], as well as from an infant with complete absence of the occipital cortex [59]. VEP results must be interpreted with great caution in neurologically impaired patients. Another important disadvantage is the cost and complexity of the VEP equipment. Considerable experience is needed before VEP waveforms can be generated and interpreted with reliability and accuracy.

Comparison of OKN, PLT, and VEP Acuities

Comparison of the different modalities of acuity testing in preverbal children involves several considerations [42]. First, all three tests show increasing resolution acuity through the first year of life (see the Table). Second, within techniques and across laboratories, each test has an inherent uncertainty in acuity thresholds of approximately 1 octave. Individual infants, when tested with any one of the modalities, will also vary 1 octave. Third, the limited acuity in infants is probably secondary to neural rather than optical factors. Accommodation is well established by the eighth week postterm. Furthermore, optical blur has little effect on the low-frequency range in which infants respond, and testing distances have made no difference in threshold values. On the other hand, neural development is progressing rapidly over the first 6 to 12 months postpartum and more slowly over the next 6 years. Several testing parameters show developmental time courses remarkably parallel to known neurological development.

When comparing acuity values across techniques, OKN and PLT data tend to cluster, whereas VEP acuities are several orders of magnitude

Comparison of Visual Acuity Values for Various Techniques

Modality	Acuity at Various Ages			
	1 mo.	6 mo.	1 yr.	Age for 20/20 (months)
Optokinetic nystagmus	20/400	20/100	20/60	24–30
Preferential looking test	20/400	20/100	20/50	18–24
Visual evoked potentials	20/200	20/25	20/20	6–8

higher (see the Table). There are several possible reasons for this. The most obvious explanation lies in the marked differences between the nature of the stimuli used in the different tests. PLT gratings are classically stationary, whereas VEP pattern presentation generally involves both temporal and spatial modulation. Is it not possible that the temporal characteristics of VEP stimuli account for the higher acuity values [60]? Two studies comparing stationary with temporally modulated PLT stimuli, as well as temporal PLT with temporal VEP, showed that the stationary-temporal factor accounts for only a fraction of the PLT-VEP disparity [61, 62].

PLT acuity values are directly dependent on the statistical selection of a percentage value for the rate at which the observer must correctly choose stimulus location. Thus, some of the PLT-VEP discrepancy may reflect PLT criteria that are too strict. Indeed, lowering PLT criteria does narrow the gap by 1 to 1.5 octaves but does not eradicate it. Sokol and Moskowitz [63] found that clearly recognizable VEP waveforms could be generated by spatial frequencies that elicited no recognizable behavioral change on a PLT. By dropping the percentage-correct criterion to 55%, VEP and PLT acuities became statistically indistinguishable. However, significant correlation of VEP and PLT acuity values seen at higher criteria (70%) disappeared. Interestingly, implicit time of the VEP was significantly correlated with PLT acuity with both criteria.

Critical differences in data gathering may contribute to the difference between PLT and VEP acuities. To maximize the signal-to-noise ratio, VEP waveforms are summed and amplified by high-speed computer. The interpretation of PLT responses requires careful observation of global behavior; even the most experienced examiner may not be able to detect all the meaningful signal amidst the noise (e.g., involuntary or poorly controlled movements, partial gaze changes). Computer waveform analysis may always prove more efficient and provide greater sensitivity.

Finally, it is possible, if not likely, that a certain discrepancy exists between behavioral and electrophysiological tests regardless of methodological differences. The two tests tap fundamentally different capabilities of the nervous system. Relatively high-frequency information is apparently available to visual cortex early in development. Behavioral responses must require considerable postcortical processing, which lags behind the afferent visual processing in the VEP.

Sokol and co-workers [64] compared PLT and VEP testing with standard recognition tests in a pediatric population, attempting to determine relative testability as well as sensitivity to abnormal interocular acuity differences. Monocular PLT and VEP were completed in similar percentages of children older than 2 years (75 to 90%). In younger children, monocular VEP was more frequently completed than PLT. VEP acuities agreed with recognition tasks more often (66%) than PLT (50%). Both tests were found to be more sensitive to abnormal interocular acuity differences in children younger than 3 years than are Allen cards.

■ Conclusion

It is fair to state that all three techniques described in this chapter—OKN, PLT, VEP—can be used in a complementary fashion to evaluate visual function in children (as well as adults) who are unable to complete recognition acuity tests. However, it is not advisable to compare directly an acuity value from one test with that derived using a different technique. Each method provides a unique set of data on different levels of visual (and motor) processing. Thus, it is best to specify the type of test used to determine the acuity being cited (e.g., "20/200 PLT acuity," "20/80 VEP acuity"). OKN serves primarily in a screening role. PLT may soon serve as a more reliable screening test. Both VEP and PLT can currently serve as useful adjuncts in the diagnosis and treatment of children with monocular and binocular visual disorders, particularly in assessing progression or response to therapy. The Snellen equivalents are helpful for the examiner only on a conceptual basis. The modalities described here, being resolution tasks, differ fundamentally from the recognition acuities with which the clinician is so familiar. Although the two may parallel each other in healthy eyes, the resolution-recognition disparity becomes greater as visual acuity diminishes. Therefore, predicting Snellen acuity from any of these modalities is inappropriate and misleading.

■ References

1. DeLaey JJ. Assessment of visual acuity in childhood. Bull Soc Belge Ophtalmol 1982;202:21–40
2. Hubel DH, Wiesel TN. The period of susceptibility to the physiologic effects of unilateral eye closure in kittens. J Physiol (Lond) 1970;206:419–436
3. Miranda SB, Hack M, Fantz RL, et al. Neonatal pattern vision: a predictor of future mental performance. J Pediatr 1977;91:642–647
4. Westheimer G. Visual acuity. In: Moses RA, Hart WM, eds. Adler's physiology of the eye: clinical applications. St Louis: Mosby, 1987
5. Ohm J. Die klinische Bedeutung des optischen Drenystagmus. Klin Monatsbl Augenheilkd 1922;68:232
6. Gorman JJ, Cogan DG, Gellis SS. An apparatus for grading the visual acuity of infants on the basis of opticokinetic nystagmus. Pediatrics 1957;19:1088–1092
7. Dayton GO, Jones MH, Aiu P, et al. Developmental study of coordinated eye movements in the human infant: I. Visual acuity in the newborn human: a study based on induced optokinetic nystagmus recorded by electrooculography. Arch Ophthalmol 1964;71:865–870
8. Catford GV, Oliver A. Development of visual acuity. Arch Dis Child 1973;48:47
9. Fulton AB, Hansen RM, Manning KA. Measuring visual acuity in infants. Surv Ophthalmol 1981;25:325–332
10. Smith JL. Pediatric neuro-ophthalmology. In: Smith JL, ed. Neuro-ophthalmology. Springfield: Thomas, 1964:344–384
11. Enoch JM, Rabinowicz IM. Early surgery and visual correction of an infant born with unilateral eye lens opacity. Doc Ophthalmol 1976;41:371–377

12. Berlyne DE. The influence of the albedo and complexity of stimuli on visual fixation in the human infant. Br J Psychol 1958;49:315–318
13. Fantz RL. Pattern vision in young infants. Psychol Rec 1958;8:43–47
14. Teller DY, Morse R, Borton R, Regal D. Visual acuity for vertical and diagonal gratings in human infants. Vision Res 1974;14:1433–1439
15. Hoyt CS, Nickel BL, Billson FA. Ophthalmologic examination of the infant: developmental aspects. Surv Ophthalmol 1982;26:177–189
16. Fantz RL, Ordy JM, Udelf MS. Maturation of pattern vision in infants during the first six months. J Comp Physiol Psychol 1962;55:907–917
17. Enoch JM, Rabinowicz IM. Early surgery and visual correction of an infant born with unilateral eye lens opacity. Doc Ophthalmol 1976;41:371–382
18. Dobson V, Teller DY, Lee CP, Wade B. A behavioral method for efficient screening of visual acuity in young infants: I. Preliminary laboratory development. Invest Ophthalmol Vis Sci 1978;17:1142–1150
19. Fulton AB, Manning KA, Dobson V. A behavioral method for efficient screening of visual acuity in young infants: II. Clinical application. Invest Ophthalmol Vis Sci 1978;17:1151–1157
20. Gwiazda J, Brill S, Mohindra I, Held R. Preferential looking acuity in infants from two to fifty-eight weeks of age. Am J Optom Physiol Opt 1980;57:420–427
21. Held R, Gwiazda J, Brill S, et al. Infant visual acuity is underestimated because near threshold gratings are not preferentially fixated. Vision Res 1979;19:1377–1379
22. Banks MS, Stephens BR, Dannemiller JL. A failure to observe negative preference in infant acuity testing. Vision Res 1982;22:1025–1031
23. Mayer DL, Dobson V. Assessment of vision in younger children: a new operant approach yields estimates of acuity. Invest Ophthalmol Vis Sci 1980;19:566–570
24. Mayer DL, Dobson V. Visual acuity development in infants and young children as assessed by operant preferential looking. Vision Res 1982;22:1141–1151
25. Mayer DL, Fulton AB, Hansen RM. Preferential looking acuity obtained with a staircase procedure in pediatric patients. Invest Ophthalmol Vis Sci 1982;21:538–543
26. Teller DY, McDonald MA, Preston K, et al. Assessment of visual acuity in infants and children: the acuity card procedure. Dev Med Child Neurol 1986;28:779–789
27. Birch EE. Infant interocular acuity differences and binocular vision. Vision Res 1985;25:571–576
28. Hamer RD, Alexander K, Teller DY. Rayleigh discriminations in young human infants. Vision Res 1982;22:575–587
29. Packer O, Hartmann EE, Teller DY. Infant color vision: the effect of test field size on Rayleigh discriminations. Vision Res 1984;24:1247–1260
30. Gwiazda J, Brill S, Mohindra I, Held R. Infant visual acuity and its meridional variation. Vision Res 1978;18:1557–1564
31. Gwiazda J, Scheiman M, Held R. Anisotropic resolution in children's vision. Vision Res 1984;24:527–531
32. Gwiazda J, Mohindra I, Brill S, Held R. Infant astigmatism and meridional amblyopia. Vision Res 1985;25:1269–1276
33. Gwiazda J, Mohindra I, Brill S, Held R. The development of visual acuity in infant astigmats. Invest Ophthalmol Vis Sci 1985;23:1717–1723
34. Miranda SB. Visual abilities and pattern preferences of premature infants and full-term neonates. J Exp Child Psychol 1970;10:189
35. Dubowitz LM, Dubowitz V, Morante A. Visual function in the newborn: a study of preterm and full-term infants. Brain Dev 1980;2:15–29
36. Manning KA, Fulton AB, Hansen RM, et al. Preferential looking vision testing: application to evaluation of high-risk, prematurely born infants and children. J Pediatr Ophthalmol Strabismus 1982;19:286–293

37. Brown AM, Yamamoto M. Visual acuity in newborn and preterm infants measured with grating acuity cards. Am J Ophthalmol 1986;102:245–253
38. Jacobson JG, Mohindra I, Held R. Development of visual acuity in infants with congenital cataracts. Br J Ophthalmol 1981;91:559–565
39. Catalano RA, Simon JW, Jenkins PL, Kandel GL. Preferential looking as a guide for amblyopia therapy in monocular infantile cataracts. J Pediatr Ophthalmol Strabismus 1987;24:56–63
40. Robb RM, Mayer DL, Moore BD. Results of early treatment of unilateral congenital cataracts. J Pediatr Ophthalmol Strabismus 1987;24:178–181
41. Mayer DL, Fulton AB, Rodier D. Grating and recognition acuities of pediatric patients. Ophthalmology 1984;91:947–953
42. Friendly DS, Jaafar MS, Morillo DL. A comparative study of grating and recognition visual acuity testing in children with anisometropic amblyopia without strabismus. Am J Ophthalmol 1990;110:293–299
43. Sokol S. Visually evoked potentials: theory, techniques and clinical applications. Surv Ophthalmol 1976;21:18–44
44. Dobson V, Teller DY. Visual acuity in human infants: a review and comparison of behavioral and electrophysiologic studies. Vision Res 1978;18:1469–1483
45. Spekreijse H, Van der Twell LH, Zuidema T. Contrast evoked potentials in man. Vision Res 1973;13:1577–1601
46. Campbell FW, Maffei L. Electrophysiologic evidence for the existence of orientation and size detectors in the human visual system. J Physiol (Lond) 1970;207:635–652
47. Marg E, Freeman DN, Peltzman P, Goldstein PJ. Visual acuity development in human infants: evoked potential measurements. Invest Ophthalmol 1976;15:150
48. Sokol S. Measurement of infant visual acuity from pattern reversal evoked potentials. Vision Res 1978;18:33–39
49. Norcia AM, Tyler CW. Spatial frequency sweep VEP: visual acuity during the first year of life. Vision Res 1985;25:1399–1408
50. Sokol S, Jones K. Implicit time of pattern evoked potentials in infants: an index of maturation of spatial vision. Vision Res 1979;19:747–755
51. Beller R, Hoyt CS, Marg E, Odom JV. Good visual function after neonatal surgery for congenital monocular cataracts. Am J Ophthalmol 1981;91:559–565
52. Odom JV, Hoyt CS, Marg E. Effect of natural deprivation and unilateral eye patching on visual acuity of infants and children. Arch Ophthalmol 1981;99:1412–1416
53. Atkinson J, Braddick O, Braddick F. Acuity and contrast sensitivity of infant vision. Nature 1974;247:403
54. Banks MS, Salapatek P. Contrast sensitivity function of the infant visual system. Vision Res 1976;16:867–869
55. Banks MS, Salapatek P. Acuity and contrast sensitivity in 1, 2, and 3-month old infants. Invest Ophthalmol Vis Sci 1978;17:361–365
56. Estevez O, Cavonius CR. Low frequency attenuation in the detection of gratings: sorting out the artifacts. Vision Res 1976;16:481
57. Leguire LE, Rogers GL, Bremer DL. Visual-evoked response binocular summation in normal and strabismic infants: defining the critical period. Invest Ophthalmol Vis Sci 1991;32:126–133
58. Bodis-Wollner I, Atkin A, Raab E, Wolkstein M. Visual association cortex and vision in man: pattern-evoked occipital potentials in a blind boy. Science 1977;198:629
59. Dubowitz LMS, Mushin J, DeVries L, Arden GB. Visual function in the newborn infant: is is cortically mediated? Lancet 1986;1:1139–1141
60. Regan D. Assessment of visual acuity by evoked potential recording: ambiguity caused by temporal dependence of spatial frequency selectivity. Vision Res 1978; 18:439–443
61. Dobson V, Teller DY, Belgum J. Visual acuity in human infants assessed with

stationary stripes and phase-alternated checkerboards. Vision Res 1978;18:1233–1238

62. Sokol S, Moskowitz A, McCormack G, Augliere R. Infant grating acuity is temporally tuned. Vision Res 1988;28:1357–1366
63. Sokol S, Moskowitz A. Comparison of pattern VEPs and preferential looking behavior in 3-month-old infants. Invest Ophthalmol Vis Sci 1985;26:359–365
64. Sokol S, Hansen VC, Moskowitz A, et al. Evoked potential and preferential looking estimates of visual acuity in pediatric patients. Ophthalmology 1983;90:552–562

Postnatal Ocular Growth and Its Regulation

■■■■■■■ Donald S. Fong, M.D.

The prevalence of myopia in the United States in children 12 to 17 years of age is 25.7% among whites and 11.7% among blacks [1]. Myopia is at least the seventh cause of blindness in the United States and accounts for 15,000 legally blind persons. The most common form of myopia is low myopia, which develops in the postnatal period. An understanding of ocular growth is essential in our quest for a cure for myopia.

■ Postnatal Changes

Cornea and Lens

Although all the structures of the eye are formed at birth, they undergo some change and maturation. In the cornea, all the postnatal changes occur deep to the epithelium. The stroma shows decreasing cellularity. The anterior, banded portion of Descemet's membrane is formed in utero and shows little postnatal change. The posterior, nonbanded portion increases in thickness and is deposited by the endothelium throughout life [2]. The endothelium shows a 36% decrease in cell count during the first 2 years of life [3].

The lens grows throughout life. The birth weight of the lens (65 mg) doubles by 1 year of age and doubles again by the ninth decade [4].

Retina

The size of the retinal fovea and foveola decreases from the neonatal period to adulthood [5]. The rod-free zone is 1,000 μm in the neonate and 650 to 700 μm in the adult. The cone density increases from 18 cones per 100 μm in the neonate to 42 cones per 100 μm in adults. The inner segment of the neonatal cone is 7.5 μm wide and 10 μm long; in the adult, it is 2.0 μm wide and 25 μm long. Corresponding to the increase in inner segment length, the outer segment of the cone is 3 μm in the neonate and 60 μm long in the adult. Through these changes, the eyes develop increased resolution and better color vision.

The surface area of the retina and retinal pigment epithelium (RPE) increases two and a half times from the sixth week of gestation to the end of the first postnatal year [6]. The RPE layer shows increasing cell density in the macular area until 6 months of age and decreasing cell density in the other parts of the posterior segment. This differential change probably is due to centripetal migration of the cells rather than to mitosis [7].

Choroid and Sclera

There is little published data on postnatal choroidal or scleral changes. Postnatally, both structures increase in mass, but neither shows much differentiation. During fetal development, the sclera matures from the limbus to the posterior pole and from the inner to the outer portions. There is cytological maturation at the seventh week of gestation, shown by the loss of free ribosomes and the increase of rough endoplasmic reticulum and the Golgi apparatus [8]. Most of the postnatal scleral growth appears to occur in the area between the equator and the ora serrata [9].

■ Postnatal Biometry

Cycloplegic refraction, keratometry, and axial length measurements performed on eyes from the thirtieth week of gestation to the thirty-sixth year of age show the following measurements [10]: In the premature neonate, the cornea measures 53.6 ± 2.5 D; the lens, 43.5 ± 3.6 D; and the axial length, 15.1 ± 0.9 mm. In the term neonate, the cornea measures 51.2 ± 1.1 D; the lens, 34.4 ± 2.3 D; and the axial length, 16.8 ± 0.6 mm. The notable differences between the term and the preterm neonate are the reduced powers of the cornea and lens in term neonates.

Postnatally, the corneal curvature decreases from 51 D to 44 D during the first 6 months and then stabilizes. The lens decreases in power and reaches the adult average of 18 D in a linear fashion. Axial length increases during two postnatal periods. The first period, the infantile period, encompasses most of the growth (5 mm) and ends at approximately the third year of age. The second period, the juvenile period, results in only 1 mm of growth and ends at approximately the fourteenth year of age. Although the growth during the juvenile period is small, it is important for the determination of the final refraction. The magnitude and duration of these growth phases are, however, not related to any other known variable [11].

The mean refraction is 1.0 D for the premature neonate (30 to 35 weeks) and +0.4 D for the term neonate (39 to 41 weeks). This difference is due to the maturation of the cornea and lens. There is little change in the overall refraction of the eye during the first 6 to 7 years of age; from that time to 20 to 36 years, there is almost 1.5 D of myopic change. The onset of this refractive change appears to correspond to the beginning of formal schooling.

The magnitude of postnatal growth of the eye is impressive. The diameter increases by 40% and the volume by 300%. Yet, during this entire process, the visual image remains focused on the retina! In addition, in 200 emmetropic eyes examined by Sorsby and colleagues [12], the powers of each component of refraction (cornea, anterior chamber depth, lens, and vitreous chamber depth) varied by 20%. This precision in coordinating growth among components of various powers, so that a focused image is constantly maintained, cannot be random and suggests a regulatory system.

■ Coordination of Postnatal Growth

Evidence

Evidence for a regulatory system of ocular growth has accumulated in several animal models, including the chick [13], monkey [14], tree shrew [15], and cat [16]. However, several caveats must be considered before interpreting and applying the results from the different animal models. Although the chick regulatory system can be readily manipulated, the chick eye is different from that of humans [17]. Both the chick cornea and lens can accommodate, and lenticular accommodation is mediated by striated muscle. The chick retina is afoveal, cone dominated, and contains no retinal vessels. Furthermore, the chick eye possesses a *pecten,* which is an erectile membrane extending from the disc into the vitreous body, and cartilage in the inner sclera. Nonhuman primates are the closest animal model for human diseases, but conditions that affect and produce ocular growth changes in these animals cannot be assumed to have the same effect in humans. With these cautions in mind, there is good evidence that eyes tend to grow in a regulated fashion toward emmetropia.

The first piece of evidence is the observation that chicks raised with lenses of different powers in front of their eyes tend to develop eyes that have a shift in their noncycloplegic refractive state [18]. The ability of eyes to down-regulate and up-regulate ocular growth is further evidence of this regulatory system. For example, chick eyes that are exposed to constant darkness become hyperopic. Upon return to a light environment, the eyes increase their ocular growth [19].

Characteristics of the Regulatory System

One requirement for such a regulatory system is the quality of visual stimuli. Chicks raised with translucent occluders over their eyes develop eyes with increased axial lengths [20]. Raviola and Wiesel [14] reported that prolonged retinal exposure to formless images can lead to ocular growth in monkeys. These investigators monocularly sutured the eyes of neonatal monkeys so that only formless images could project through the eyelid onto the retina. After a period of time, the sutured eye measured a greater axial length than the unoccluded eye and showed the choroidal attenuation and peripapillary scleral crescents typical of human myopia. Because only lid-sutured monkeys raised in the light developed myopia, and those monkeys raised in the dark did not, Raviola and Wiesel suggested that deprivation of visual stimuli, and not the lid-suturing alone, was the critical factor.

One mechanism for growth induction is accommodation, although other mechanisms may also be important. For example, in stump-tail monkeys, cycloplegia with topical atropine arrests the development of axial elongation [14], but in rhesus macaque monkeys, neither cycloplegia nor optic nerve section arrests the ocular growth. In chicks, optic nerve section fails to arrest ocular growth [19]. Furthermore, chicks with occluders over half the retina developed myopia only in the occluded half [21]. These observations suggest that the regulation of ocular growth in certain species is locally controlled by the retina and does not involve brain-derived responses such as accommodation.

This regulatory system also appears to function only during a certain period of development. Adult monkeys cannot be made myopic and older chicks can only be made less myopic. Interestingly, small periods (2 hours) of continuous normal vision can prevent the development of axial elongation in chicks [22].

Finally, the myopic axial elongation in chick eyes appears to be due to actual growth and not just stretching. More DNA, protein, and proteoglycan synthesis occurs in myopic than in nonmyopic chick scleras [23].

■ Postnatal Ocular Growth Factors

Intraocular Pressure

Several possible mediators involved in ocular growth have been identified. One such mediator is intraocular pressure (IOP). IOP was shown to be the growth force of the embryonic eye when cannulation of the vitreous cavity, during development, arrests the growth of chick eyes [24]. Evidence supporting the role of IOP are the observations that some infant humans and monkeys have higher IOP [25] than adult humans and monkeys and that eyes with infantile glaucoma tend to be large. On the other hand, however, none of the monkeys in Raviola and Wiesel's animal model [15] demonstrated elevated IOP when measured under anesthesia. The IOP in these monkeys, though, has not been measured in the unanesthetized state.

Insulinlike Growth Factors

Insulinlike growth factors (IGF) are another possible mediator of ocular growth. These peptides are homologous to insulin and have major effects on cell growth and differentiation in cell culture. Human corneal endothelial cells exposed to IGF-I synthesize DNA, and Northern blot analysis has detected IGF-I in the cornea [26]. IGF-II expression and type 2 IGF receptor expression in the rat follow the sequence of tissue growth and differentiation, both spatially and temporally [27]. Lentropin, a vitreous-derived factor that stimulates chick lens fiber differentiation, has been shown to be inhibited by monoclonal antibody specific to human IGF-I, suggesting that lentropin is related to the IGFs [28].

Vasoactive Intestinal Peptide

Vasoactive intestinal peptide (VIP) is a 28–amino acid peptide that has been shown to be elevated in myopic rhesus macaque [29, 30] and myopic Green monkey eyes [31]. The hypothesis is that the blurred visual images are detected by the retinal cells that are sensitive to contrast. These cells then secrete VIP, which may in turn cause ocular growth.

VIP is similar in structure to secretin and glucagon. Although initially described in the gastrointestinal tract, VIP is found throughout the body. VIPergic nerves innervate the superficial limbal blood vessels, aqueous humor outflow apparatus, iris nerve fibers, large blood vessels, and ciliary bodies of many species [32]. Third ventricular injection of VIP causes a rise in IOP [33].

Dopamine

Dopamine and its metabolite 3,4-dihydroxyphenylacetic acid (DOPAC), have been found to be reduced in myopic eyes of white leghorn chicks [34]. Administration of apomorphine, a dopamine agonist, has been shown to cause a dose-dependent reduction in axial but not equatorial elongation. In addition, the apomorphic effect can be nullified by the administration of haloperidol, a dopamine antagonist. In a seemingly contradictory fashion, however, haloperidol acting alone also causes a reduction in axial elongation.

Lens-Derived Growth Factor

There may also be a lens-derived growth factor [35, 36]. Unilateral lensectomies in neonatal monkeys produce eyes that are shorter than the unmanipulated eyes of control monkeys. From Raviola and Wiesel's lid-sutured myopia model [15], blurred images (such as from aphakia) should produce elongated eyes, not short eyes. This reduction in ocular length caused by aphakia was shown to persist even after some of the eyes were fitted with extended-wear soft contact lenses. These observations suggest that the lens may be an important factor for eye growth.

■ Abnormal Ocular Growth

Disturbances in either the regulatory system or its mediators may result in myopia. Myopia from infantile glaucoma is one example in which an excess of one mediator—increased IOP—results in enlarged eyes [37]. Myopia with orbital hemangiomas is an example of a disturbance in the regulatory system leading to ocular growth. Unilateral hemangiomas of the eyelid and orbit have been shown to indent the cornea and cause unilateral astigmatism. This astigmatism forms aberrant images that act like the formless images in the lid-sutured chick and monkey models and lead to myopia [38]. Other forms of visual deprivation and distortion during infancy can also lead to axial myopia. This is seen in eyes with breaks in Descemet's membrane, congenital cataracts, corneal opacities, ptosis, and vitreous hemorrhage [39–41].

Near-work may also disturb the regulatory system. Evidence for this hypothesis includes the following observations: (1) Occupations involving increased near-work tend to have a higher prevalence of myopia. (2) Myopia tends to develop at the age of 6 years when reading and schooling begins. (3) Younger Eskimos, with a higher rate of literacy, have a higher prevalence of myopia than do older Eskimos. (4) Caged cats and monkeys that live in a small environment with more near visual stimuli have more myopia than do their wild counterparts.

It has been suggested that printed text may appear as blurred images to the majority of the retina (the nonfoveal retinal neurons) and lead to ocular growth. Printed text may appear blurry because the nonfoveal neurons have large receptive fields and can not resolve the individual letters in printed material. These neurons are able to detect and respond only to the small contrast difference between the letters and the white page. The contrast between text and page is approximately ten, whereas the contrast outside on a sunny day is one hundred to one thousand times greater. Finally, printed text is a chromatic, and most natural scenes have color.

■ Treatment of Myopia

There is currently no consensus on methods either to prevent the development of myopia or to retard its progression. The basis for certain treatments may be drawn from the experimental models.

Since reading is believed to disturb the local regulatory system by the mechanism of blurred visual images and decreased contrast, a well-lit environment to maximize contrast is theoretically beneficial. The chick data, showing that a period of 2 hours per day of normal vision prevents myopia, suggest that daily periods of natural scenery exposure is also theoretically important.

The role of cycloplegics in preventing the progression of myopia has been demonstrated in several studies involving atropine. One study composed of 62 patients compared the refraction of atropinized eyes and the control fellow eyes in the same patients [42]. After 2 years, the treated eye measured +0.17 D and the untreated eye −0.99 D. Another study looked at 253 patients binocularly treated with atropine and 146 similar control children. At 4 years, the final myopia in the treated children measured one-half the amount in the control children [43].

Although these cycloplegic trials show encouraging results, several problems limit the usefulness of the results. Noncompliance is one problem; one-third of the treated patients left the trial in one study [44]. In addition, the chronically dilated pupil may predispose the treated eye to increased cumulative photic damage. As much as twenty-five times the amount of solar radiation may reach the retina in dilated eyes. Finally, the appearance of a child wearing bifocals may discourage both the parents and the child from continuing with therapy.

Intraocular pressure–lowering drops have also been examined as therapy for myopia [44]. One study randomized 51 children to treatment with timolol 0.25% and 51 children to control drops. At 2 years, no difference in refraction was noted, even though there was a 2– to 3–mm Hg IOP decrease in the treated eyes.

Surgical procedures for the correction of myopia aim mainly to change the refraction of the eyes rather than prevent or retard the progression of myopia. The surgical options include clear lens extraction and kerato-refractive surgery (keratomileusis, epikeratophakia, radial keratotomy, excimer laser keratoplasty), but there are few indications for them in the pediatric age group. Scleral reinforcement aims to limit eye growth and entails strengthening the posterior sclera in pathological myopia with a band of fascia lata or other suitable material. Although this procedure is widely practiced in Eastern Europe, it is rarely used in the United States and almost never on children.

■ Comments

Starting from birth, the eye changes in both size and refraction. The maintenance of emmetropia throughout this growth phase depends on the coordinated growth of each of the refractive components of the eye. Regulatory mechanisms have been demonstrated and characterized in several animal models. Several mediators have also been identified that may regulate the ultimate size of the globe. Disturbance of either the regulatory system or its mediators may result in myopia.

The author would like to thank Elio Raviola, MD, PhD, for review of the manuscript.

■ References

1. Sperduto RD, Seigel D, Roberts J, Rowland M. Prevalence of myopia in the United States. Arch Ophthalmol 1983;101:405–407
2. Murphy C, Alvarado J, Juster R. Prenatal and postnatal growth of the human Descemet's membrane. Invest Ophthalmol Vis Sci 1984;25:1402–1415
3. Murphy C, Alvarado J, Juster R, Maglio M. Prenatal and postnatal cellularity of the human corneal endothelium. Invest Ophthalmol Vis Sci 1984;25:312–322
4. Weale RA. A biography of the eye: development, growth and age. London: HK Lewis, 1982:92
5. Yuodelis C, Hendrickson A. A qualitative and quantitative analysis of the human fovea during development. Vision Res 1986;26:847–855
6. Robb RM. Increase in retinal surface area during infancy and childhood. J Pediatr Ophthalmol Strabismus 1982;19(4):16–20
7. Robb RM. Regional changes in retinal pigment epithelial cell density during ocular development. Invest Ophthalmol Vis Sci 1985;26:614–620
8. Sellheyer K, Spitznas M. Development of the human sclera—a morphological study. Graefes Arch Clin Exp Ophthalmol 1988;226:89–100
9. Streeten BW. Development of the human retinal pigment epithelium and the posterior segment. Arch Ophthalmol 1969;81:383–394
10. Gordon RA, Donzis PB. Refractive development of the human eye. Arch Ophthalmol 1985;103:785–789
11. Curtin BJ. The myopias: basic science and clinical management. Philadelphia: Harper & Row, 1985:29–37
12. Sorsby A, Benjamin B, Sheridan M. Refraction and its components during the growth of the eye. Medical Research Council special report series No. 301. London: Her Majesty's Stationery Office, 1961
13. Wallman J, Adams JI. Developmental aspects of experimental myopia in chicks: susceptibility, recovery and relation to emmetropization. Vision Res 1987;27: 1139–1163
14. Raviola E, Weisel TN. An animal model of myopia. N. Engl J Med 1985;312: 1609–1615
15. Sherman SM, Norton TT, Casagrande VA. Myopia in the lid-sutured tree shrew (*Tupaia glis*). Brain Res 1977;124:154–157
16. Ni J, Smith EL. Effect of chronic optical defocus on the kitten's refractive status. Vision Res 1989;29:929–938
17. Sturkie P. Avian physiology. New York: Springer-Verlag, 1986:37–48
18. Schaeffel F, Glasser A, Howland HC. Accommodation, refractive error and eye growth in chickens. Vision Res 1988;28:639–657
19. Troilo D, Gottlieb MD, Wallman J. Visual deprivation causes myopia in chicks with optic nerve section. Curr Eye Res 1987;6:993–999
20. Wallman J, Turkel J, Trachtman J. Extreme myopia produced by modest change in early visual experience. Science 1978;201:1249–1251
21. Wallman J, Gottlieb MD, Rajaram V, Fugate-Wentzek LA. Local retinal regions control local eye growth and myopia. Science 1987;237:73–77

22. Judge SJ. Does the eye grow into focus? Nature 1990;345:477–478
23. Christensen AM, Wallman J. Increased DNA and protein synthesis in scleras of eyes with visual-deprivation myopia. Invest Ophthalmol Vis Sci 1989;30 (ARVO suppl):402
24. Coulombre AJ. The role of intraocular pressure in the development of the chick eye: I. Control of eye size. J Exp Zool 1956;133:211–225
25. Rousseau CJ, Bito LZ. Intraocular pressure of rhesus monkeys (*Macaca mulatta*): II. Juvenile ocular hypertension and its apparent relationship to ocular growth. Exp Eye Res 1981;32:407–417
26. Hyldahl L, Engstrom W, Schofield PN. Stimulatory effects of insulin-like growth factors on DNA synthesis in the human embryonic cornea. J Embryol Exp Morphol 1986;98:71–83
27. Cuthbertson RA, Beck F, Senior PV, et al. Insulin-like growth factor II may play a local role in the regulation of ocular size. Development 1989;107:123–130
28. Beebe DC, Silver MH, Belcher KS, et al. Lentropin, a protein that controls lens fiber formation, is related functionally and immunologically to the insulin-like growth factors. Proc Natl Acad Sci USA 1987;84:2327–2330
29. Stone RA, Laties AM, Raviola E, Weisel TN. Increase in retinal vasoactive intestinal polypeptide after eyelid fusion in primates. Proc Natl Acad Sci USA 1988;85: 257–260
30. Raviola E, Wiesel TN, Reichlin S, et al. Increase of retinal vasoactive intestinal polypeptide (VIP) after neonatal lid fusion in the rhesus macaque. Invest Ophthalmol Vis Sci 1991;32 (ARVO suppl):1203
31. Fong DS, Wiesel TN, Raviola E, Reichlin S. Is lid-fusion myopia caused by an increase in retinal vasoactive intestinal polypeptide (VIP)? Invest Ophthalmol Vis Sci 1991;32 (ARVO suppl):1203
32. Stone RA. Vasoactive intestinal polypeptide and the ocular innervation. Invest Ophthalmol Vis Sci 1986;27:951–957
33. Nilsson SFE, Sperber GO, Bill A. Effects of vasoactive intestinal polypeptide (VIP) on intraocular pressure, facility of outflow and formation of aqueous humor in the monkey. Exp Eye Res 1986;43:849–857
34. Stone RA, Lin T, Laties AM, Iuvone PM. Retinal dopamine and form-deprivation myopia. Proc Natl Acad Sci USA 1989;86:704–706
35. Wilson JR, Fernandes A, Chandler CV, et al. Abnormal development of the axial length of aphakic monkey eyes. Invest Ophthalmol Vis Sci 1987;28:2096–2099
36. Tigges M, Tigges J, Fernandes A, et al. Postnatal axial eye elongation in normal and visually deprived rhesus monkeys. Invest Ophthalmol Vis Sci 1990;31:1035–1046
37. Costenbader FD, Kwitko ML. Congenital glaucoma: an analysis of seventy-seven consecutive eyes. J Pediatr Ophthalmol 1967;9(2):9–15
38. Robb RM. Refractive errors associated with hemangiomas of the eyelids and orbit in infancy. Am J Ophthalmol 1977;83:52–58
39. Rabin J, Van Sluyter RC, Malach R. Emmetropization: a vision-dependent phenomenon. Invest Ophthalmol Vis Sci 1981;20:561–564
40. Angell LK, Robb RM, Berson FG. Visual prognosis in patients with ruptures in Descemet's membrane due to forceps injuries. Arch Ophthalmol 1981;99:2137–2139
41. Miller-Meeks MJ, Bennett SR, Keech RV, Blodi CF. Myopia induced by vitreous hemorrhage. Am J Ophthalmol 1990;109:199–203
42. Bedrossian RH. The effect of atropine on myopia. Ophthalmology 1979;86:713–717
43. Brodstein RS, Brodstein DE, Olson RJ, et al. The treatment of myopia with atropine and bifocals: a long term prospective study. Ophthalmology 1984;91:1373–1379
44. Jensen H. Timolol maleate in the control of myopia. Acta Ophthalmol [Suppl] (Copenh) 1988;185:128–129

Amblyopia

Samuel E. Navon, M.D., Ph.D.
Craig A. McKeown, M.D.

The term *amblyopia* (Gk., *amblyios:* dull, *-ops:* vision) literally means "a dullness of vision." Its use, however, is much more specific, referring to "a unilateral or bilateral decrease in visual acuity caused by form vision deprivation or abnormal binocular interaction for which no organic causes can be detected by the physical examination of the eye and which, in appropriate cases, is reversible by therapeutic measures" [1]. By this definition, amblyopia affects 1.0 to 4.0% of the general population [2]. In fact, it is estimated that amblyopia is responsible for loss of vision in more people younger than 45 years than all other ocular diseases and trauma combined. The toll of this disorder is even greater because the risk of the amblyope sustaining blinding trauma to the normal eye is significantly higher than that of the general population [3].

In this chapter, we will provide an understanding of the clinically relevant abnormalities that characterize amblyopia, describe the major physiological and histological changes found in the amblyopic visual system, and review important aspects of the therapy of amblyopia.

■ Clinical Features of Amblyopic Vision

Visual perception is formed by several distinct components, only one of which is the acuity measured in the standard letter chart (Snellen acuity). In addition to decreased Snellen acuity, the amblyopic visual system exhibits well-defined abnormalities in several other facets of visual perception. An understanding of these abnormalities is important for several reasons. First, when present, they can aid in the diagnosis of amblyopia. This is especially useful when amblyopia must be distinguished from other causes

Table 1 *Abnormalities Found in Amblyopia*

Decreased visual acuity
Abnormal contour interaction
Eccentric fixation
Decreased contrast sensitivity
Decreased brightness perception
Binocular suppression of amblyopic eye
Increased perception and reaction times

of decreased visual acuity. Second, if an abnormality can be quantified, its measurement could be used to follow the effectiveness of therapy. This might also aid in determining the end point of treatment. Finally, understanding the visual abnormalities in amblyopia gives insight into the pathophysiology of the disease. As we will see below, some of the most fundamental pathophysiological changes present in amblyopia were first inferred on the basis of careful clinical observations. Table 1 summarizes the major abnormalities found in amblyopia; we will review the most important ones here.

Decreased Visual Acuity

The hallmark of amblyopia is decreased foveal acuity. From a practical standpoint, a commonly used diagnostic criterion is a loss of visual acuity of two or more lines on the Snellen chart. As will be discussed later, the degree of amblyopia is dependent on many factors such as the age of the patient during amblyogenesis, the length and type of visual deprivation, and the presence of monocular versus binocular involvement.

One of the most interesting features of amblyopia is a normalization of visual acuity in dim light. At low levels of illumination, the visual acuity of the amblyopic eye is often found to be equal to, or occasionally even better than, that of the normal fellow eye [4, 5]. This phenomenon is demonstrated in Figure 1, which shows the visual acuity obtained at different levels of illumination for normal subjects, patients with macular edema or diabetic retinopathy, and those with amblyopia. In patients with organic macular disease, there is typically a dramatic and immediate loss of vision when neutral density filters are used to decrease background illumination. In sharp contrast, amblyopic subjects showed a negligible loss of vision under the same circumstances. Their vision paralleled that of normal subjects under progressively dimmer background illuminations. This phenomenon is highly specific for amblyopia and therefore has useful diagnostic potential, especially when examining an adult with vision loss of unknown origin.

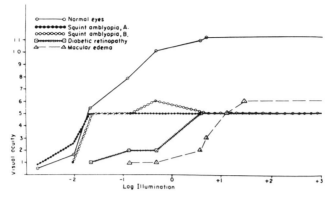

Figure 1 *Visual acuity as a function of background illumination. The curve for normal eyes represents the average of the measurements of 10 normal eyes. The curves for strabismic (squint) amblyopia and organic disease represent individual cases. (Reprinted from von Noorden and Burian [5]. Copyright © 1959, American Medical Association. Used with permission.)*

Abnormal Contour Interaction

It is not uncommon for amblyopes to demonstrate a significant decrease in acuity for objects placed in a row compared with acuity for the same objects viewed separately. This is referred to as the *crowding phenomenon* and represents an abnormality of contour interaction between the point of fixation and adjacent objects. Abnormal contour interaction is a hallmark of amblyopic vision, although crowding is probably present to a smaller degree in normal subjects as well [6, 7]. This phenomenon is not present with organic vision loss. Therefore, its presence is particularly noteworthy during the initial evaluation of a patient. The crowding phenomenon becomes more pronounced during the course of treatment (i.e., single-object acuity improves more rapidly than does line acuity). Therefore, during this period it is important for both single-letter and line acuities to be recorded. It is highly desirable that as the end point of therapy is reached, these two types of acuity approach each other. If normal line acuity cannot be achieved, there may be a greater risk that the vision of the amblyopic eye will regress when therapy is discontinued. Thus, at least at the completion of treatment, the presence or absence of the crowding phenomenon may have significant prognostic value.

Normal Light Perception

Although many aspects of visual function are abnormal in amblyopic vision (see Table 1), the ability to perceive a simple light signal is normal

[8]. This function is referred to as the *visual threshold* and is defined as "the dimmest amount of light perceptible." Amblyopes appear to have normal visual thresholds both foveally and peripherally.

Conclusions

The clinical characteristics just described have been investigated in detail and used to gain insight into the nature of the defect in amblyopia. A review of the many studies is beyond the scope of this chapter, but their results can be used to arrive at several important conclusions:

1. *Amblyopic visual perception simulates that of the peripheral retina under reduced illumination.* The normalization of visual acuity under reduced illumination demonstrates that the amblyopic eye is at its worst under bright (ambient) illumination, which is needed for optimal form vision. This behavior plainly sets amblyopia apart from vision loss due to organic lesions, in which the opposite behavior is generally exhibited.
2. *The amblyopic visual system contains abnormally large receptive fields.* A receptive field is a discrete area of the visual field that is processed by the visual system as a single unit. Thus, a group of photoreceptors act together to transmit a receptive field to the visual cortex. The presence of abnormally large receptive fields in amblyopia has been inferred from the existence of the crowding phenomenon. In other words, visual signals from adjacent contours interfere with one another because the summation of visual information takes place over an abnormally large area. The prediction of enlarged retinal receptive fields in amblyopic eyes has been confirmed by quantitative measurements [9].
3. *The simple function of light perception is normal in amblyopia.* The amblyopic process appears to include a dissociation between light sense (normal) and the acuity function (impaired).

■ Pathophysiological Features

The animal model has proved invaluable for studying the electrophysiological and histological changes caused by stimulus deprivation in the immature visual system. In these experiments, animals are raised with varying types of visual deprivation (i.e., monocular versus binocular, strabismic versus form [or total] deprivation) during different periods of their visual maturation. The visual system lends itself particularly well to such studies because of the elegant and discrete organization of visual pathways from each eye to the visual cortex.

Retina

Visual information travels from the retina to cortical areas along at least two parallel pathways [10, 11]. Each pathway appears to be supplied by a discrete type of retinal ganglion cell. X-type ganglion cells have a relatively high density in the fovea. These cells have small receptive fields, respond best to high spatial frequencies (i.e., small dots, fine lines), and are relatively poor at discriminating quickly flickering images. Y-type ganglion cells are more evenly distributed across the retina. These cells have large receptive fields, respond best to low spatial frequencies, and can detect high flicker frequencies. Ikeda and Tremain [12, 13] have reported a significant reduction in the spatial resolving powers of retinal X cells in kittens with strabismic amblyopia and in those treated with unilateral or bilateral instillation of atropine, which induced an ametropic amblyopia.

Additional evidence supporting retinal involvement in amblyopia came from measuring visual thresholds as a function of the wavelength of light. Using this technique, increased lateral inhibition between retinal cone cells was demonstrated in the amblyopic eye [14]. This finding suggests a possible retinal contribution to two abnormalities of amblyopic vision: decreased acuity under bright illumination and increased spatial summation.

Afferent pupillary defects have been noted in amblyopic eyes with varying incidence (10 to 93%) [15, 16]. The more sensitive the examining technique, the higher the detection rate of an abnormality. The presence of an afferent pupillary defect suggests that an abnormality exists at the retinal level because fibers that mediate the pupillary reaction to light branch from the visual pathway prior to the lateral geniculate nucleus. There is no apparent relationship between the magnitude of the pupillary defect and the degree of amblyopia [15]. Therefore, this abnormality is probably not an integral component of the defect causing the reduced acuity in amblyopia.

Lateral Geniculate Nucleus

The lateral geniculate nucleus serves as the relay station between retinal ganglion fibers and those that project to the visual cortex. When viewed in cross section, the lateral geniculate nucleus is divided into six layers (Fig 2). Fibers originating from ipsilateral ganglion cells go to layers 2, 3, and 5. Fibers from contralateral ganglion cells go to layers 1, 4, and 6. This segregated organization is ideal for studying the effects of visual deprivation. In kittens and infant monkeys raised with the eyelid of one eye sutured from birth for 3 months, the activity of geniculate cells receiving input from the deprived eye was diminished and significant histological changes were present [17, 18]. In layers supplied by the sutured eye, cells were decreased by approximately 30% in size and contained shrunken nuclei

Ipsilateral retinal ganglion cells

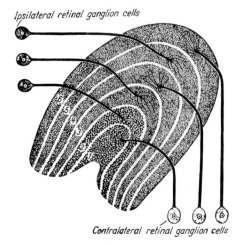

Contralateral retinal ganglion cells

Figure 2 *Diagram of a transverse section through the right lateral geniculate body. The layers are numbered from ventral to dorsal. Contralateral fibers project onto layers 1, 4, and 6. Ipsilateral fibers project onto layers 2, 3, and 5. (Reprinted from P Glees, Verh Anat Ges 1959;55:60. Used with permission.)*

and nucleoli (Fig 3). Eyelid closure for shorter periods of time (2 months versus 3) produced similar but less severe changes, and no changes were seen when visual deprivation was carried out in adult cats. As with humans, it appears that a period of visual immaturity exists during which the normal development of the visual system is highly dependent on adequate exposure to formed images. Histological changes similar to those described earlier have recently been observed in an amblyopic human [19].

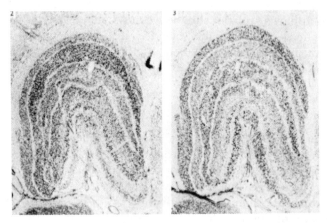

Figure 3 *The lateral geniculate nucleus of the contralateral (left) and ipsilateral (right) sides of an infant monkey after 3 months of eyelid suture. The cells in laminae 1, 4, and 6 of the contralateral side and laminae 2, 3, and 5 of the ipsilateral side are smaller and paler-staining than those in the adjacent laminae of the same side and than those in the corresponding laminae of the other side (× 25). (Reprinted from Headon and Powell [18] with permission.)*

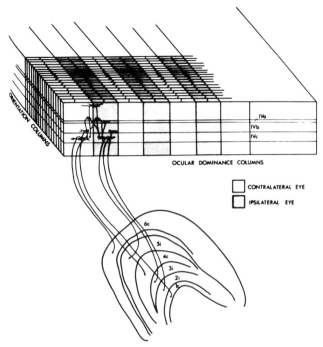

Figure 4 *Organization of the visual cortex. Fibers from the lateral geniculate body are schematically shown projecting to ocular dominance columns of the visual cortex. These columns are further organized into orientation slabs. A complex cell in an upper layer is shown receiving input from two neighboring ocular dominance columns but from the same orientation column. (Reprinted from Hubel and Wiesel [20] with permission.)*

Visual Cortex

The lateral geniculate nucleus transmits visual information via the optic radiation to reach the visual cortex. The organization of the visual cortex can be studied by using intracellular microelectrodes to record electrical activity from single cells during visual stimulation. Using this technique, Hubel and Wiesel [20] showed that the incoming information continues to be highly ordered. Figure 4 schematically illustrates the visual cortex. Six layers can be distinguished, all but one receiving binocular input at the cellular level. In addition, ocular orientation columns can be distinguished, which are highly sensitive to the linear orientation of the visual stimulus.

Microelectrode recordings from the visual cortex of a normal adult cat are shown in Figure 5. As can be seen, there is normally a small but significant dominance of input from the eye that is contralateral to the side of

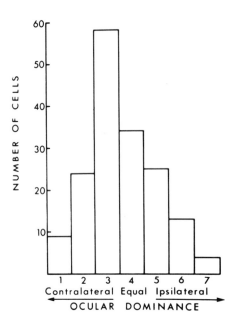

Figure 5 *Ocular dominance distribution of 223 cells recorded from striate cortex of adult cats in a series of 45 penetrations. Intracellular recordings of the electrical activity of cells of the visual cortex were made using a microelectrode. Responses were categorized according to the degree of influence by the ipsilateral or contralateral as follows: Cells of group 1 were driven only by the contralateral eye. For cells of group 2, there was marked dominance of the contralateral eye; for group 3, slight dominance. Cells in group 4 showed no obvious difference between the 2 eyes. For cells in group 5, the ipsilateral eye dominated slightly; in group 6, markedly. In group 7, the cells were driven only by the ipsilateral eye. (Reprinted from Hubel and Wiesel [24] with permission.)*

cortex that is being studied. Hubel and Wiesel [21, 22] further used this elegant technique to demonstrate that abnormal visual experience during early life can dramatically alter the functional domains of the 2 eyes in the visual cortex. When single-cell recordings were made from the visual cortex of kittens in which one eye had been deprived of vision, the following changes were observed:

1. *A reduction in the number of cortical cells receiving input from the deprived eye.* As shown in Figure 6, when visual cortex contralateral to the deprived eye was studied, there was a striking shift in ocular dominance to the side of the nondeprived eye. Similarly, when recordings were made from the other side of the same cortex, input was obtained only from the contralateral (nondeprived) side (data not shown). The number of cortical cells responding to the amblyopic eye can be increased if that eye is used and the previously normal eye is deprived [23]. This probably represents the physiological basis of occlusion therapy.
2. *A reduction in the number of binocularly driven visual cortical cells.* Depending on the degree of visual deprivation, a reduction from the norm of 80% (see Fig 5) down to no binocular input at all (see Fig 6) was observed. This reduction in binocular input also occurs in alternating strabismus *without* induced amblyopia (Fig 7) [24]. The last finding may explain the loss of stereopsis in strabismic patients without amblyopia.

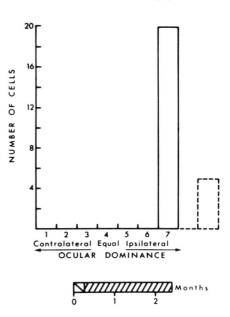

Figure 6 *Ocular dominance distribution of 25 cells recorded in the visual cortex of a 2¹/₂-month-old kitten. During the first week, the eyes were not yet open; on the eighth day, the lids of the right eye were sutured, and they remained closed until the time of the experiment. The left eye opened normally on the ninth day. Recordings were made from the left visual cortex, contralateral to the eye that had been closed. Five of the cells, represented by the interrupted column on the right, could not be driven from either eye. The remaining 20 were driven only from the normally exposed (left, or ipsilateral) eye and were therefore classed as group 7 (see Figure 5 for classification scheme). (Reprinted from Wiesel and Hubel [22] with permission.)*

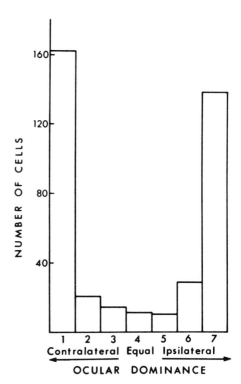

Figure 7 *Loss of binocular input in strabismus without amblyopia. A large squint was created in 4 kittens by dividing the right medial rectus muscle 8 to 10 days after birth, just at the time the eyes were beginning to open. Visual cortex intracellular recordings were then performed as described in Figure 5. (Reprinted from Hubel and Wiesel [24] with permission.)*

3. *A relative increase in the number of cortical cells responding to a contour orientation that was the only one present during the period of visual development.* This is believed to be the basis of meridional amblyopia [25].

More recently, positron emission tomography has been used to investigate, noninvasively, changes in the metabolic activity of the visual cortex in amblyopic human subjects [26]. This technique demonstrates a striking reduction in the ability of visual stimulation of an amblyopic eye to induce glucose metabolism in the amblyopic visual cortex. These results provide a satisfying correlation to the findings of Hubel and Wiesel described previously.

■ Types of Amblyopia

Amblyopia is caused by either form vision deprivation or abnormal binocular interaction, or both. Although many clinical situations can produce amblyopia, they can all be explained on the basis of strabismus, ametropia, stimulus deprivation, or a combination of these etiologies.

Strabismic Amblyopia

Characteristics   Amblyopia is often seen in conjunction with strabismus at the time the strabismus is documented by a visit to an ophthalmologist [27]. In this situation, it often cannot be known with certainty whether the amblyopia is the consequence or the cause of the strabismus. Amblyopia is most likely to develop in patients with constant tropia who favor one eye for fixation and is, therefore, uncommon in intermittent exotropes. In addition, this type of amblyopia is always unilateral. Figure 8 schematically illustrates the factors that produce amblyopia in strabismus. The image received by the fovea of the deviated eye is not only different from that

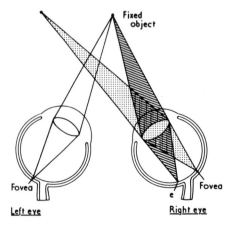

Figure 8   *Strabismic amblyopia. The image of the visual object fixed by the left eye falls on nasal retinal elements (e) of the right eye (diplopia). The image of a second object, located to the left of the object fixed by the left eye, falls on the fovea of the right eye (confusion). (Reprinted from GK von Noorden, Factors involved in the production of amblyopia. Br J Ophthalmol 1974;58:158–164. Used with permission.)*

of the fixating, sound eye but is also out of focus (unless the object happens to lie at the same distance from the object of interest). The severity of the amblyopia cannot be consistently correlated with the angle of strabismic deviation [28].

Therapy The upper age limit for amblyopia therapy is generally accepted from clinical experience to be 8 to 9 years [29, 30]. Occlusion of the fixating eye is the treatment of choice, and there is considerable difference of opinion on whether full-time or part-time occlusion should be used in selected cases. Efforts to improve vision are best made prior to surgical correction of strabismus for several reasons. First, fixation behavior will be much harder to determine once the eyes are surgically aligned. Second, optimal acuity may maximize the chances of restoring binocular vision. Finally, parent motivation toward patching might be increased by the visual reminder of strabismus.

Ametropic Amblyopia

Characteristics With sufficient hyperopia, the accommodative effort may inadequately focus images onto the retina near and at distance. The affected eyes are deprived of sharp retinal images, and this loss of high spatial frequencies can produce a type of bilateral amblyopia known as *isoametropic amblyopia*. In contrast, in high myopia objects close to the patient's face will be in focus and amblyopia is considerably less likely to be induced.

When significant anisometropia (unequal refractive error between the 2 eyes) is present, the binocular interaction is abnormal due to the superimposition of a focused and a defocused image originating from a single fixation point (Fig 9). This greatly reduces the amount of refractive error needed to produce amblyopia.

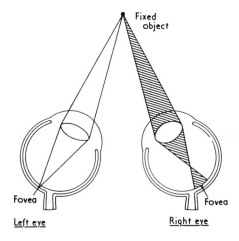

Figure 9 *Ametropic amblyopia. The fovea of the right myopic eye receives a blurred image of the object fixed by the left emmetropic eye. (Reprinted from GK von Noorden, Factors involved in the production of amblyopia. Br J Ophthalmol 1974;58:158–164. Used with permission.)*

In anisohyperopia, amblyopia is much more likely to occur because only that amount of accommodation necessary to focus the image in the less hyperopic eye is utilized. The more hyperopic eye probably never enjoys clear images. For this reason, when the excess of hyperopia in one eye is 2 D or even less, amblyopia may be present. In anisomyopia, the more myopic eye can be used for near work and the less myopic eye for distance. Thus, sharply focused images will be available to both eyes at distances up to their respective near points. When one or both eyes are myopic, amblyopia in either eye is unusual unless the difference between the eyes is considerable (greater than 5 or 6 D) [31]. Therefore, when amblyopia is present in patients with only mild to moderate degrees of myopia, further examination to rule out organic causes for the decreased acuity should be considered [32]. The severity of amblyopia cannot be consistently correlated with the degree of anisometropia [33].

Similar to these situations, uncorrected astigmatism present early in life results in the deprivation of sharp contours of a specific orientation. From the preceding discussion, it can be seen how this could result in meridional amblyopia [24]. This might explain the inability of some adult astigmatics to achieve normal acuity even after full correction of their refractive error.

Therapy A significant number of children with ametropic amblyopia are more than 5 years old when diagnosed because refractive errors are frequently not detected until routine school screening examinations [29, 30]. Any course of therapy begins with correcting the underlying refractive error. If the amblyopia is mild, spontaneous improvement may occur over several weeks to months. Part-time occlusion may be preferable if binocular interaction is present, the amblyopia is mild, and the child is in school. With pronounced anisometropia, contact lenses may be preferable to reduce the amount of aniseikonia. However, disadvantages inherent to contact lenses, such as noncompliance, infection, and other problems, must be considered. With isoametropic amblyopia due to significant bilateral hyperopia, therapy consists of constant wear of spectacles or contact lenses. In this situation, improvement is usually gradual (over months to several years), and 20/20 acuity is often not obtainable.

Stimulus Deprivation Amblyopia

Characteristics Stimulus deprivation, shown schematically in Figure 10, has the most potential to cause severe amblyopia. Except for transient forms, the loss of vision often does not respond well to therapy and is more severe than in patients with strabismus or anisometropia. If present in the first 3 months of life, stimulus deprivation can lead to profound and permanent reduction in visual acuity as well as nystagmus. Table 2 categorizes the major causes of stimulus deprivation. For any given cause

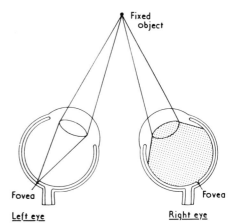

Figure 10 *Stimulus deprivation amblyopia. The media opacity in the right eye prevents image formation on the fovea; only diffuse light can enter the eye. (Reprinted from GK von Noorden, Factors involved in the production of amblyopia. Br J Ophthalmol 1974; 58:158–164. Used with permission.)*

and severity, unilateral cases are considerably more amblyogenic than are bilateral cases [34]. This may be due to a preservation of binocular interaction with the latter.

Therapy   Of critical importance in the treatment of stimulus deprivation amblyopia is the removal of barriers to well-focused retinal images as soon as possible, preferably within the first 6 weeks of life in cases of congenital stimulus deprivation. Total occlusion at a high percentage (75 to 90%) of the time may be necessary to reverse the severe visual loss in some children. The occluded eye must be carefully checked at each follow-up visit for the development of occlusion amblyopia in the sound eye [35].

Mimickers of Amblyopia   Clinically, one may suspect a diagnosis other than, or in addition to, amblyopia if adequate amblyopia treatment improves the vision up to a certain level but is unable to restore the expected level of acuity to the eye. In general, amblyopia may be mimicked by any irreversible defect in the afferent visual system caused by subophthalmoscopic morphological changes. This underscores the importance of maintaining a high index of suspicion toward entities such as optic nerve glioma.

It is also not uncommon for amblyopia to coexist with organic ocular disease. For example, amblyopia has been described as a major cause of

Table 2   *Causes of Stimulus Deprivation*

Ptosis (complete)
Corneal opacities
Congenital cataracts
Other media opacities
Iatrogenic origin (occlusion amblyopia)

vision loss in juvenile glaucoma, with estimates of its incidence as high as 78% [36]. Standard amblyopia management (discussed next) for these patients can restore a significant amount of vision that would otherwise have been irreversibly lost [37].

■ Treatment of Amblyopia

Treatment Modalities

The most important step in the treatment of amblyopia is removing obstacles to clear vision. There is no hope of reversing an amblyopic defect as long as the inciting factors are still present. Not only must media opacities such as congenital cataracts and eyelid lesions be removed, but refractive errors must also be corrected.

The most common method to treat amblyopia is occlusion of the better eye. There are no rigid rules for the amount of occlusion time per day or how long therapy should be carried out. In high-percentage occlusion, the better eye is covered 75 to 90% of the time. Low-percentage occlusion may be sufficient if the amblyopia is not severe.

Cycloplegia of the better eye may result in enough blurring to cause the patient to use the amblyopic eye. Atropine is most commonly used. The emmetropic child will then generally respond by using the amblyopic eye for near fixation but may continue to use the better eye for distance. With hyperopia, however, the atropinized eye may be penalized at distance and at near.

Other methods of treatment, such as pleoptics and the CAM visual stimulator are expensive, inconvenient, and either no better or less effective than occlusion therapy [38, 39]. These methods are not generally used in the United States.

Principles of Treatment

In considering methods for reducing the morbidity due to amblyopia, prevention cannot be overemphasized. This is underscored by the fact that the reversibility of amblyopic vision loss decreases significantly with age. Education and awareness by the primary care physician is essential, because he or she is often the first person to detect an abnormality. The red reflex of every baby should be checked at birth. Vision screening programs are essential, and newer techniques such as photorefraction are promising.

The daily amount of occlusion and overall length of therapy must be determined individually for each patient and should be open to modification during the course of treatment. Setting a goal for optimal visual acuity will depend on the severity of the amblyopia, the risk of inducing occlusion amblyopia in the dominant eye, and the psychological costs to the patient and family.

Table 3 *Causes of Suboptimal Results of Amblyopia Therapy*

Noncompliance
Uncorrected refractive error
Irreversibility of the amblyopia
Failure to prescribe sufficient treatment

Follow-up evaluations should be spaced at intervals of 1 week for each year of life when high-percentage occlusion is employed. These evaluations should always include assessment of vision in the better eye to allow for early detection of occlusion amblyopia. Ideally, treatment is discontinued when the target acuity is reached and subsequent office visits show no further improvement. Not surprisingly, 20/20 vision is frequently not achieved. Table 3 lists the possible causes of suboptimal results.

Until the visual system is fully mature, routine follow-up is necessary to detect recurrence of amblyopia after cessation of treatment. There is a significant risk that amblyopia will recur, even following successful primary treatment. For these patients, additional part-time occlusion may be needed to maintain a good outcome.

■ References

1. von Noorden GK. Mechanisms of amblyopia. Adv Ophthalmol 1977;34:93–115
2. von Noorden GK. Binocular vision and ocular motility: theory and management of strabismus, ed 4. St Louis: Mosby, 1990:208–245
3. Tommila V, Tarkkanen A. Incidence of loss of vision in the healthy eye in amblyopia. Br J Ophthalmol 1981;65:575–577
4. von Noorden GK, Burian HM. Visual acuity in normal and amblyopic patients under reduced illumination: I. Behavior of visual acuity with and without neutral density filter. Arch Ophthalmol 1959;61:533–535
5. von Noorden GK, Burian HM. Visual acuity in normal and amblyopic patients under reduced illumination: II. The visual acuity at various levels of illumination. Arch Ophthalmol 1959;62:396–399
6. Cibis L, Hurtt J, Rasicovich A. A clinical study of separation difficulty in organic and in functional amblyopia. Am Orthopt J 1968;18:66–72
7. Stuart JA, Burian HM. A study of separation difficulty: its relationship to visual acuity in normal and amblyopic eyes. Am J Ophthalmol 1962;53:471–477
8. Wald G, Burian HM. The dissociation of form vision and light perception in strabismic amblyopia. Am J Ophthalmol 1944;27:950–963
9. Hommer K, Schubert G. Die absolute Grosse der fovealen receptorischen Feldzentren und der Panum-Areale. Graefes Arch Ophthalmol 1963;166:205–210
10. Enroth-Cugell C, Robson JG. The contrast sensitivity of retinal ganglion cells of the cat. J Physiol (Lond) 1966;187:517–552
11. Cleland BG, Dubin MW, Levick WR. Sustained and transient neurones in the cat's retina and lateral geniculate nucleus. J Physiol (Lond) 1971;217:473–496
12. Ikeda H, Tremain KE. Amblyopia resulting from penalisation: neurophysiological studies of kittens reared with atropinisation of one or both eyes. Br J Ophthalmol 1978;62:21–28
13. Ikeda H, Tremain KE. Amblyopia occurs in retinal ganglion cells in cats reared with convergent squint without alternating fixation. Exp Brain Res 1979;35:559–582

14. Harwerth RS, Levi DM. Increment threshold spectral sensitivity in anisometropic amblyopia. Vision Res 1977;17:585–590

15. Greenwald MJ, Folk ER. Afferent pupillary defects in amblyopia. J Pediatr Ophthalmol Strabismus 1983;20:63–67

16. Krueger KE. Pupillenstorungen und amblyopie. Ber Dtsch Ophthalmol Ges 1961; 63:275–278

17. Wiesel TN, Hubel DH. Effects of visual deprivation on morphology and physiology of cells in the cat's lateral geniculate body. J Neurophysiol 1963;26:978–993

18. Headon MP, Powell TPS. Cellular changes in the lateral geniculate nucleus of infant monkeys after suture of the eyelids. J Anat 1973;116:135–145

19. von Noorden GK, Crawford MLJ, Levacy RA. The lateral geniculate nucleus in human anisometropic amblyopia. Invest Ophthalmol Vis Sci 1983;24:788–790

20. Hubel DH, Wiesel TN. Laminar and columnar distribution of geniculo-cortical fibers in the macaque monkey. J Comp Neurol 1972;146:421–450

21. Hubel DH, Wiesel TN. Receptive fields of cells in striate cortex of very young, visually inexperienced kittens. J Neurophysiol 1963;26:994–1002

22. Wiesel TN, Hubel DH. Single-cell responses in striate cortex of kittens deprived of vision in one eye. J Neurophysiol 1963;26:1003–1017

23. von Noorden GK, Crawford MLJ. Morphological and physiological changes in the monkey visual system after short-term lid suture. Invest Ophthalmol Vis Sci 1978; 17:762–767

24. Hubel DH, Wiesel TN. Binocular interaction in striate cortex of kittens reared with artificial squint. J Neurophysiol 1965;28:1041–1059

25. Mitchell DE, Freeman RD, Millodot M, Haegerstrom G. Meridional amblyopia: evidence for modification of the human visual system by early visual experience. Vision Res 1973;13:535–558

26. Demer JL, von Noorden GK, Volkow ND, Gould KL. Imaging of cerebral blood flow and metabolism in amblyopia by positron emission tomography. Am J Ophthalmol 1988;105:337–347

27. Costenbader FD. Infantile esotropia. Trans Am Ophthalmol Soc 1961;59:397–429

28. von Noorden GK, Frank JW. Relationship between amblyopia and the angle of strabismus. Am Orthopt J 1976;26:31–33

29. Mein J, Harcourt B. Diagnosis and management of ocular motility disorders. St Louis: Blackwell, 1986:181–193

30. Greenwald MJ, Parks MM. Treatment of amblyopia. In: Tasman W, Jaeger EA, eds. Duane's clinical ophthalmology, vol 1. Philadelphia: Lippincott, 1990: chap 11, 1–9

31. Jampolsky A, Flom BC, Weymouth FW, Moses LE. Unequal corrected visual acuity as related to anisometropia. Arch Ophthalmol 1955;54:893–905

32. Horwich H. Anisometropia amblyopia. Am Orthopt J 1964;14:99–104

33. Helveston EM. Relationship between degree of anisometropia and depth of amblyopia. Am J Ophthalmol 1966;62:757–759

34. von Noorden GK. Classification of amblyopia. Am J Ophthalmol 1967;63:238–244

35. Burian HM. Occlusion amblyopia and the development of eccentric fixation in occluded eyes. Am J Ophthalmol 1966;62:853–856

36. Barsoum-Homsy M, Chevrette L. Incidence and prognosis of childhood glaucoma: a study of 63 cases. Ophthalmology 1986;93:1323–1327

37. Burton BJ. Successful treatment of functional amblyopia associated with juvenile glaucoma. Graefes Arch Clin Exp Ophthalmol 1988;226:150–153

38. Keith CG, Howell ER, Mitchell DE, Smith S. Clinical trial of the use of rotating grating patterns in the treatment of amblyopia. Br J Ophthalmol 1980;64:597–606

39. Veronneau-Troutman S, Dayanoff SS, Stohler T, Clahane AC. Conventional occlusion vs. pleoptics in the treatment of amblyopia. Am J Ophthalmol 1974;78: 117–120

Duane's Syndrome

Vera O. Kowal, M.D.
Craig A. McKeown, M.D.

■ Classification

Duane's syndrome is a congenital eye movement disorder character-ized by retraction of the globe and narrowing of the palpebral fissure on attempted adduction and includes variable limitations of abduction, adduction, or both. Vertical eye movements on attempted adduction are also frequently noted. During the late nineteenth century, this syndrome was described in some detail by Heuck [1], Stilling [2], Türk [3], Bahr [4], Sinclair [5], and Wolff [6]. In 1905, Alexander Duane [7] published a series of 54 cases of this retraction syndrome. He summarized the literature and offered theories on pathogenesis and treatment. Since then, his name has become attached to the syndrome, though in Europe it is still referred to as the Stilling-Türk-Duane syndrome. Duane's syndrome is by no means rare, and it has intrigued ophthalmologists for decades. Of particular inter-est are the pathophysiology of this anomaly as well as its electromyographic characteristics and associated developmental malformations.

Although Duane's syndrome has typically been subdivided into three clinical types (Table 1), as described by Huber [8], many cases of congenital retraction syndromes cannot be classified into a single type. In fact, an entire spectrum of retraction syndromes exists, with a high level of variabil-ity among individual patients. Huber's classification scheme, based on clini-cal presentation and electromyography (EMG), may be useful because it includes the most common variations.

Subsequently, Huber analyzed the EMG findings of the extraocular muscles in Duane's syndrome patients and noted that all had one common feature: paradoxical, anomalous innervation of the lateral rectus muscle of the affected eye. He classified three EMG discharge patterns, generally corresponding to the three clinical types (Table 2). Huber also noted that anomalous vertical movements frequently occurred in all three types. In

Table 1 *Huber's Clinical Classification of Duane's Syndrome*

Type I
Marked limitation or complete absence of abduction
Normal or slightly defective adduction
Widening of the palpebral fissure on attempted abduction
Narrowing of the palpebral fissure and retraction of the globe on attempted
  adduction
Type II
Limitation or complete defect of adduction with exotropia of the affected eye
Abduction normal or slightly limited
Narrowing of the palpebral fissure and retraction of the globe on attempted
  adduction
Type III
Limitation or absence of both abduction and adduction
Narrowing of the palpebral fissure and retraction of the globe on attempted
  adduction

Source: Adapted from Huber [8].

Table 2 *Huber's Classification of Electromyographic Discharge Patterns in Duane's Syndrome*

Type I
Lateral rectus muscle with minimum activity on attempted abduction and peak
  activity on adduction
Normal medial rectus muscle
Type II
Lateral rectus muscle with peak activity on both abduction and attempted adduction
Normal medial rectus muscle
Type III
Simultaneous activity of medial and lateral rectus muscles on both attempted
  abduction and adduction
Complete absence of normal agonist-antagonist relationship

Source: Adapted from Huber [8].

some instances, horizontal deviations that change in magnitude during upgaze and downgaze can produce A-, V-, or X-pattern strabismus.

Maruo and colleagues [9] confirmed Huber's clinical and EMG classifications when they observed 266 cases of Duane's syndrome and performed EMG studies in 126 of them. Ahluwalia and co-workers [10] have proposed a subclassification of Huber's system known as *Khurana's modification*, but it has not come into general use.

■ Epidemiological Features

Prevalence

Of all congenital oculomotor anomalies, Duane's syndrome is the most common. Its prevalence is difficult to determine because not all cases come to the attention of the ophthalmologist. In a review of a series of 500 patients with a broad range of ocular motility disturbances, Ahluwalia [10]

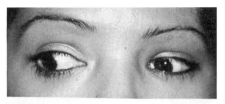
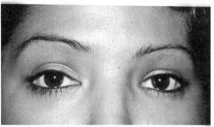
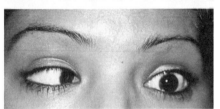

Figure 1 *Duane's syndrome type I. (Top) Right gaze with retraction of the left globe and narrowing of the left palpebral fissure. (Middle) Primary gaze. (Bottom) Left gaze with limited abduction of the left eye.*

could elicit a clinical picture of Duane's syndrome in 20 (4%). In all reports, Duane's type I (Fig 1) is by far the most common, followed by types III and II. In the study of 266 patients by Maruo and co-workers [9], 198 (74.4%) exhibited type I, 45 (16.9%) type III, and 22 (8.3%) type II. In 1 patient the type could not be identified. The majority of the patients with bilateral involvement (40 of 53) in this series had Duane's type III. One of the bilateral cases was mixed, with one eye demonstrating type I and the other type III.

Sex Distribution

For unknown reasons, Duane's syndrome appears to be more common in women. In the study of 266 patients by Maruo and associates [9], 145 (54.5%) were female. Other authors have reported similar sex distributions: Pfaffenbach and colleagues [11], 106 (57.0%) female patients of 186 total; Isenberg and Urist [12], 58 (57.4%) female patients of 101 total; Raab [13], 45 (64.3%) female patients among 70 cases; and Ahluwalia [10], 11 (55.0%) female patients among 20 cases. Kaufmann and co-workers [14] reported no difference in the sex ratio, whereas Tredici and von Noorden [15] noted a preponderance of male patients (42 [60.0%] of 70 cases). No reasonable explanation has been offered for this apparent sex distribution.

Laterality

Duane's syndrome involves the left eye more frequently than the right and is usually unilateral. Maruo and colleagues [9] reported bilateral involvement in 53 of 266 cases (19.9%) and unilateral involvement in 213 cases (80.1%). Among the unilateral cases, the left eye was affected in 156 cases (73.2%). These results are similar to those reported by Pfaffenbach and co-workers [11], with 34 (18.3%) bilateral and 144 (77.4%) unilateral cases. In 8 (4.3%), the laterality was not indicated. Of the unilateral cases, the left eye was affected in 107 (74.3%) cases. Isenberg and Urist [12] had similar results, noting bilateral involvement in 16 of 101 cases (15.8%) and unilateral involvement in 85 cases (84.2%). Among the unilateral cases, the left eye was affected in 56 cases (65.9%). Kirkham [16] reported bilateral involvement in 20 patients (18.2%) and unilateral involvement in 90 (81.8%). Of the 90 patients with unilateral involvement, the left eye was affected in 66 cases (73.3%). Raab [13] reported that 7 of 70 cases (10%) were bilateral and 63 (90%) unilateral. Among the unilateral cases, 47 (74.6%) involved the left eye. Combining these five clinical studies yields 725 patients with Duane's syndrome, excluding the 8 patients in which laterality was not indicated. Bilateral involvement was seen in 130 cases (17.9%) and unilateral in 595 (82.1%). Among the patients with unilateral involvement, the right eye was affected in 163 cases (27.4%) and the left eye in 432 cases (72.6%). The reason for the left eye being affected more frequently than the right eye is unknown.

■ Clinical Presentation

Age at Presentation

The age at which patients initially present may differ from the age at which the anomaly was first noticed. Maruo and co-workers [9] noted that 59.0% (157) of their patients were younger than 10 years at their first visit. Pfaffenbach and colleagues [11] reported 36.0% (67) presenting in early infancy and 35.5% (66) in childhood or youth, whereas 28.5% (53) did not notice the anomaly until adulthood.

Heredity

Most cases of Duane's syndrome occur sporadically, but it is estimated that an autosomal dominant pattern is seen in approximately 5.0% of cases [11]. One study showed a positive family history of Duane's syndrome in 4 of 70 patients (5.7%), although a specific inheritance pattern was not discussed [13].

Amblyopia and Anisometropia

Early evidence by Kirkham [16] suggested that amblyopia and aniso-metropia were far more common in patients with Duane's syndrome than in the general population. Defining amblyopia as a visual acuity of less than or equal to 20/40, Kirkham found amblyopia in 25.0% of his 110 patients. Recent studies have shown that amblyopia is not more common in patients with Duane's syndrome than in the general population. Maruo and associates [9] found a 3.6% prevalence of amblyopia in 220 patients with Duane's syndrome, and Tredici and von Noorden [15] noted a 3.0% prevalence in 70 patients. By most estimates, these figures agree with the prevalence of amblyopia in the general population [17]. It has been observed that most patients with Duane's syndrome and strabismus in the primary position adopt a head turn to achieve single binocular vision, thereby avoiding the development of amblyopia.

Kirkham [16] also reported that 40.0% of his 110 cases had anisometropia exceeding 1 D, but more recent reports do not support this finding. Raab [13] found anisometropia in 17.0% of 70 patients, and Tredici and von Noorden [15] found the same percentage in 72 patients. Again, these reports are in concordance with the frequency of anisometropia in the general population.

Eye Position and Head Position

Horizontal alignment was evaluated in 54 patients with unilateral Duane's syndrome [13], and orthotropia was seen in 40.7%. Of those patients with heterotropia, esodeviation was present in the majority of patients with Duane's type I, whereas exodeviation was more common in Duane's type III.

Variable head positions (face turns) in Duane's syndrome are usually attributed to maintenance of fusion. Raab [13] found that many patients who were orthotropic in primary gaze (14 of 62 [22.6%]), nevertheless had face turns. The face turn compensates for the underacting muscle. Another possibility is that a face turn is used to avoid the visual annoyance of an anomalous vertical movement.

Vertical Deviations

Anomalous vertical movements are a prominent feature of Duane's syndrome. Raab [13] reported a frequency of 25.0% (18 of 72 eyes), and Isenberg and Urist [12] found a frequency of 44.6% (45 of 101 patients). The vertical movements consist of an upshoot or downshoot of the affected eye during attempted adduction. Occasionally, the cornea may disappear from view (Fig 2). The mechanism does not appear to be overaction of the

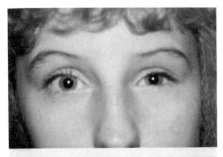

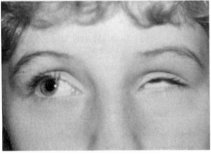

Figure 2 *Vertical upshoot. (Top) Primary gaze. (Bottom) Right gaze with vertical upshoot of the left eye.*

oblique muscles, since surgical correction of the obliques is not effective [11]. It appears that cocontraction of the horizontal rectus muscles allows them to slide over the globe resulting in a vertical deviation [18], sometimes referred to as the *leashing effect.*

■ Associated Malformations

Another feature of Duane's syndrome that deserves attention is its frequent association with other ocular lesions and systemic congenital malformations. The true frequency of associated anomalies is difficult to evaluate, since minor abnormalities may escape detection unless specifically investigated. Patients with Duane's syndrome appear to have a significant increase in the number of associated congenital malformations [9, 11, 19], with estimates of incidence ranging from 10 to 20 times greater than in the general population. In the study by Pfaffenbach's group [11] of 186 patients with Duane's syndrome, 62 (33.3%) had 1 or more additional malformations, 32 (17.2%) had 2 or more congenital anomalies, and 15 (8.1%) had 3 or more congenital malformations. Most of these frequencies represent minimal estimates because not all the patients had additional studies to detect unsuspected malformations. It is likely that Duane's syndrome is a heterogeneous disorder, and it is doubtful that a single mechanism is responsible for all varieties.

Ocular Malformations

Of 186 patients with Duane's syndrome, Pfaffenbach and colleagues [11] found 15 (8.1%) with ocular abnormalities. Maruo and co-workers [9] found 37 (13.9%) of 266 patients with ocular abnormalities. Many associated ocular abnormalities have been reported, primarily in the form of case reports. However, no clear pattern has emerged. The ocular abnormalities described include dysplasia of the iris stroma, nystagmus, pupillary anomalies, cataracts, microphthalmos, persistent hyaloid arteries, choroidal colobomas, distichiasis, crocodile tears (gustolacrimal reflex), heterochromia, ptosis, and epibulbar dermoid [9–11, 19, 20].

Systemic Malformations

Among the systemic complications, some are isolated anomalies and others are grouped together in "malformation syndromes." The most commonly reported systemic anomalies in 186 patients [11] included skeletal abnormalities involving the spinal column, facies, extremities and digits, or trunk in 34 (18.3%); congenital ear malformations and hearing abnormalities in 14 (7.5%); and central nervous system disorders in 10 (5.4%). Malformation syndromes seen in association with Duane's syndrome include Goldenhar's syndrome, or oculoauriculovertebral dysplasia (consisting of epibulbar dermoids, auricular malformations with appendages, pretragal blind-ended fistulas, and vertebral anomalies); and Klippel-Feil anomaly (consisting of cervical fusion, short neck, low posterior hairline, and pseudopterygia) [19]. Duane's syndrome in association with perceptive deafness and the Klippel-Feil anomaly has been called *cervicooculoacousticus* or the *Wildervanck syndrome.*

Cross and Pfaffenbach [19] hypothesized that Duane's retraction syndrome is a result of dysgenesis sometime during the fourth to tenth week of gestation. This hypothesis is based on the fact that most of the associated anomalies occurring with Duane's syndrome involve structures that are developing during this time. Perhaps a common teratogenic stimulus at an early stage of embryogenesis is responsible [19].

Because of the wide variety of systemic malformations associated with Duane's syndrome, a thorough physical examination may be appropriate in all patients presenting with this syndrome. Likewise, a screening examination for strabismus in patients with skeletal, vertebral, and auricular abnormalities might reveal more frequent association with Duane's syndrome.

■ Pathophysiological Features

Duane's syndrome has been well described clinically; however, the etiology and pathophysiology have intrigued ophthalmologists since early clinical descriptions. Early observations revealed abnormalities of the medial or lateral rectus muscle, or both, which led investigators to conclude that Duane's syndrome was due to a local, myogenic phenomenon [3, 7, 21]. It was believed that the cause of the abduction deficiency was fibrosis of the lateral rectus muscle and that limitation of adduction was due to a posterior insertion of the medial rectus muscle.

With the introduction of EMG, paradoxical innervation of the medial and lateral rectus muscles was described [18, 22]. This evidence suggested a neurogenic cause of Duane's syndrome, involving either a supranuclear lesion or a cranial nerve anomaly. Also on the basis of EMG findings, the phenomenon of globe retraction, once believed to have a mechanical cause, could be explained by cocontraction of the horizontal rectus muscles [18].

Subsequently, Huber [8] distinguished three types of Duane's syndrome based on EMG recordings and clinical findings, and speculated on the pathophysiological features of each type. According to Huber, Duane's type III, consisting of limited or absent abduction and adduction, could be caused by an absent abducens nerve with oculomotor innervation to the lateral rectus muscle. Duane's type II, with limited or absent adduction and relatively normal abduction, could be explained by dual innervation of the lateral rectus muscle by both the abducens and oculomotor nerves. Duane's type I, with limited or absent abduction and relatively normal adduction, could be caused by a partial double innervation of the lateral rectus muscle.

Case reports by Hotchkiss [23] and Miller [24] and their co-workers describe the intracranial and orbital abnormality in 2 patients with bilateral Duane's type III and unilateral type I, respectively. Both patients exhibited the typical clinical features of Duane's syndrome. In both, postmortem studies revealed absence of the abducens nucleus and abducens nerve on the affected side(s) (Fig 3). The oculomotor nuclei and nerves were normal in both patients. The lateral rectus muscles were innervated by a branch from the inferior division of the oculomotor nerve. In addition, fibrosis of the lateral rectus muscles was limited to those areas of the muscle with the poorest innervation. This anatomical evidence strongly supports EMG evidence that Duane's syndrome is caused by a developmental neurological anomaly.

Further evidence was described previously by Cross and Pfaffenbach [19], who showed that most associated malformations involve structures that differentiate during the fourth to tenth week of gestation, coincidental with the development of the third, fourth, and sixth cranial nerves. They postulated that a teratogenic stimulus early in embryogenesis could result in Duane's syndrome.

Unfortunately, the origin of this disturbance of development of the central nervous system is still unclear. Variations in pathogenicity and timing of teratogenic events, whether genetic or environmental, could account for the wide spectrum of malformations and the differences in ocular motility abnormalities seen in the different types of Duane's syndrome.

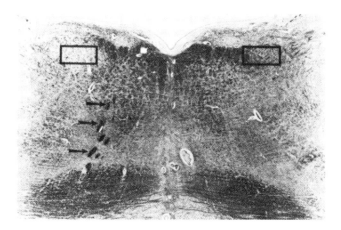

Figure 3 *Unilateral Duane's syndrome; section through pons at level of caudal portion of abducens nucleus. Right abducens nucleus is present* (box, left side of section) *and portions of fascicle of abducens nerve can be identified* (arrows). *In region normally occupied by left abducens nucleus* (box, right side of section), *no consistent cellular structures are seen (myelin-Nissl, × 11.5). (Reprinted by permission from Miller et al. [24].)*

Duane's syndrome is thus a combination of neurological and mechanical abnormalities. It involves a congenital neurological anomaly, with subsequent development of fibrosis and contractures over time.

Although Duane's syndrome is a well-recognized congenital ocular motility abnormality, several cases of acquired retraction syndromes have been reported that are clinically similar to Duane's [25–27]. One case involved a patient who had a left trigeminal rhizotomy for tic douloureux [25]. Postoperatively, he had a left sixth nerve palsy and developed the typical findings of Duane's syndrome on the same side. Another case of acquired retraction syndrome occurred following a lateral orbitotomy (Krönlein's approach) for a cavernous hemangioma [26]. A third case of acquired retraction syndrome was seen in a patient with rheumatoid arthritis [27]. The pathogenesis was unclear but was believed to be secondary to myopathy or vasculitis associated with collagen vascular disease. The term *Duane's syndrome* should be reserved for the congenital form. Acquired forms should be called *acquired retraction syndromes* or *pseudo-Duane's syndrome* [28].

■ Evaluation

A thorough ocular examination is required in patients with Duane's syndrome, with special attention to the presence of other ocular or systemic malformations. Measurements of ocular misalignment, ocular range of motion, head turn, globe retraction, palpebral fissure size, and upshoots or downshoots are indicated. In cooperative patients, traction testing can be used to evaluate force generation and restriction of motion. Photographic documentation may be considered. In addition, a complete systemic evaluation by a pediatrician, family practitioner, or internist may be appropriate to rule out associated malformations.

On occasion, it can be difficult to distinguish acquired from congenital retraction syndromes. In acquired cases, history and early normal photographs or ocular examinations are useful. Ocular EMG can confirm that the retraction syndrome is due to innervational, not structural, anomalies. However, ocular EMG is technically difficult and is not readily available. Evidence that may support an acquired retraction syndrome is the presence of diplopia, as diplopia in the preferred gaze direction is usually absent in the adult with congenital Duane's syndrome [28].

■ Treatment

Over the years, there has been considerable controversy regarding the appropriate surgical management of Duane's syndrome. If fusion can be maintained with a mild to moderate head turn, surgery is not usually performed. The goal of surgery in Duane's syndrome is the elimination or improvement of an unacceptable head turn, the elimination or reduction of significant misalignment of the eyes, the reduction of severe retraction, and the improvement of upshoots and downshoots. Surgery does not eliminate the fundamental abnormality of innervation, and no surgical technique has been successful in completely eliminating the abnormal eye movements. In general, surgery should be undertaken cautiously and expectations clearly defined to the patient.

Many different surgical procedures have been advocated. Since Duane [7] first suggested using simple horizontal muscle recession procedures to manage Duane's syndrome surgically, they have been used with success [9, 29]. As the pathophysiology of Duane's syndrome has become more clear, the appropriateness of simple recession procedures has been confirmed. The muscle to be recessed is selected by evaluating the direction of gaze with the greatest limitation of motion and by the presence or absence of an esotropia or exotropia. For instance, if limitation of abduction with an esotropia is present, the medial rectus muscle of the affected eye is usually recessed. Conversely, with limitation of adduction and an exotropia, recession of the lateral rectus muscle may be considered. Occasionally, recessions are performed on both horizontal rectus muscles of an affected eye, particularly when globe retraction is severe. The amount of recession is determined by preoperative measurements of deviation in primary position as well as the limitation of motion on duction, version, and traction testing. The restriction present with passive stretching is usually due to the development of contractures. In a study by Pressman and Scott [29] of 19 patients with Duane's syndrome who underwent horizontal muscle recession, abnormal head position was eliminated in 79.0%, and all had a significant reduction of this problem. The recessions were done by the adjustable suture technique when possible. Upshoots and downshoots are sometimes improved by recession alone but may require other approaches, such as posterior fixation sutures or splitting of the horizontal rectus muscles.

Gobin [21] and others have advocated vertical rectus muscle transposition procedures in combination with recession of the medial rectus muscle. Molarte and Rosenbaum [30] recently reported a series of 13 patients with type I Duane's syndrome who underwent vertical rectus transposition surgery. The procedure involved transposition of the entire superior and inferior rectus muscle insertions to the region of the lateral rectus muscle insertion. Several months later, 6 of the patients underwent a second operation, a medial rectus recession, for residual esotropia or face turn. The abnormal face turn was improved in all of the patients and eliminated in 73%. In addition, abduction ability was increased, and the binocular diplopia-free field size was enlarged in all patients. Although abduction is increased, adduction is usually sacrificed to some degree [21, 30]. The increase in abduction is often not utilized, since the patient has learned to turn his head to the side and continues to do so postoperatively. Transposition procedures may increase the tendency for upshoots and downshoots [18, 30] and may also induce vertical deviations. Simultaneous surgery on multiple rectus muscles, as advocated by Gobin [21], may result in anterior segment ischemia, especially in adults. Molarte and Rosenbaum [30] staged the surgery by performing primary transposition procedures followed by, if necessary, medial rectus recession as a secondary procedure at a later date.

Resection procedures of either the lateral or medial rectus muscles have generally not been successful [9, 21, 29]. The globe retraction is often increased and range of motion worsened, presumably because of the anomalous innervation with cocontraction in the presence of contractures. Resection procedures are generally contraindicated in Duane's syndrome.

In summary, simple horizontal muscle recession procedures, vertical rectus muscle transposition procedures, or combinations of the two may be successful in improving or eliminating head turns and misalignment of the eyes. The choice of procedure must be individualized.

■ **References**

1. Heuck G. Über angeborenen vererbten Beweglichkeitsdefect der Augen. Klin Monatsbl Augenheilkd 1879;17:253–279
2. Stilling J. Untersuchungen Über die Entstehung der Kurzsichtigkeit. Wiesbaden, Germany: JF Bergmar, 1887:13
3. Türk S. Bemerkungen zu einem Falle von Retractionsbewegung des Auges. Zentralbl Prakt Augenheilkd 1899;23:14–18
4. Bahr K. Vorstellurg eines Falles von Eigenartiger Muskelanomalie eines Auges. Ber Dtsch Ophthalmol Ges 1896;25:334–336

5. Sinclair WW. Abnormal associated movements of the eyelids. Ophthal Rev 1895; 14:307–319

6. Wolff J. The occurrence of retraction movements of the eyeball together with congenital defects in the external ocular muscles. Arch Ophthalmol 1900;29:297–309

7. Duane A. Congenital deficiency of abduction, associated with impairment of adduction, retraction movements, contraction of the palpebral fissure and oblique movements of the eye. Arch Ophthalmol 1905;34:133–159

8. Huber A. Electrophysiology of the retraction syndromes. Br J Ophthalmol 1974; 58:293–300

9. Maruo T, Kubota N, Arimoto H, Kikuchi R. Duane's syndrome. Jpn J Ophthalmol 1979;23:453–468

10. Ahluwalia BK, Gupta NC, Goel SR, Khurana AK. Study of Duane's retraction syndrome. Acta Ophthalmol (Copenh) 1988;66:728–730

11. Pfaffenbach DD, Cross HE, Kearns TP. Congenital anomalies in Duane's retraction syndrome. Arch Ophthalmol 1972;88:635–639

12. Isenberg S, Urist MJ. Clinical observations in 101 consecutive patients with Duane's retraction syndrome. Am J Ophthalmol 1977;84:419–425

13. Raab EL. Clinical features of Duane's syndrome. J Pediatr Ophthalmol Strabismus 1986;23:64–68

14. Kaufmann H, Kolling G, Hartwig H. Das Retraktionssyndrom von Stilling-Türk-Duane. Klin Monatsbl Augenheilkd 1980;178:110–115

15. Tredici TD, von Noorden GK. Are anisometropia and amblyopia common in Duane's syndrome? J Pediatr Ophthalmol Strabismus 1985;22:23–25

16. Kirkham TH. Anisometropia and amblyopia in Duane's syndrome. Am J Ophthalmol 1970;69:774–777

17. von Noorden GK. Binocular vision and ocular motility: theory and management of strabismus, ed 3. St Louis: Mosby, 1985:371–377

18. Scott AB, Wong GY. Duane's syndrome: an electromyographic study. Arch Ophthalmol 1972;87:140–147

19. Cross HE, Pfaffenbach DD. Duane's retraction syndrome and associated congenital malformations. Am J Ophthalmol 1972;73:442–450

20. Terashima M, Hayasaka S. Multiple congenital anomalies associated with Duane's syndrome. Ophthalmic Paediatr Genet 1990;11:133–137

21. Gobin MH. Surgical management of Duane's syndrome. Br J Ophthalmol 1974; 58:301–306

22. Strachan IM, Brown BH. Electromyography of extraocular muscles in Duane's syndrome. Br J Ophthalmol 1972;56:594–599

23. Hotchkiss MG, Miller NR, Clark AW, Green WR. Bilateral Duane's retraction syndrome: a clinical-pathologic case report. Arch Ophthalmol 1980;98:870–874

24. Miller NR, Kiel SM, Green WR, Clark AW. Unilateral Duane's retraction syndrome (type 1). Arch Ophthalmol 1982;100:1468–1472

25. Smith JL, Damast M. Acquired retraction syndrome after sixth nerve palsy. Br J Ophthalmol 1973;57:110–114

26. Sood GC, Srinath BS, Krishnamurthy G. Acquired Duane's retraction syndrome following Kronlein's operation. Eye Ear Nose Throat Mon 1975;54:308–310

27. Baker RS, Robertson WC Jr. Acquired Duane's retraction syndrome in a patient with rheumatoid arthritis. Ann Ophthalmol 1980;12:269–272

28. Bixenman WW [and replies by Baker RS, Smith JL]. Letters to the editor. Ann Ophthalmol 1980;12:906–913

29. Pressman SH, Scott WE. Surgical treatment of Duane's syndrome. Ophthalmology 1986;93:29–38

30. Molarte AB, Rosenbaum AL. Vertical rectus muscle transposition surgery for Duane's syndrome. J Pediatr Ophthalmol Strabismus 1990;27:171–177

Brown's Syndrome

Eddy Anglade, M.D.
Craig A. McKeown, M.D.
Richard M. Robb, M.D.

Brown's syndrome is an ocular motility disorder featuring a limitation of passive as well as active elevation in adduction. The disorder may be congenital or acquired and constant or intermittent in nature. Although the exact etiology remains uncertain, current research indicates that all forms of the syndrome share an abnormality in the tendon-trochlear assembly.

■ Historical Perspective

The superior oblique tendon sheath syndrome, as described by Harold Whaley Brown in 1950 [1], was characterized as an inability to elevate the affected eye in adduction. This was presumed to be the result of a congenital palsy of the ipsilateral inferior oblique with secondary shortening of the anterior sheath of the superior oblique tendon during development. Brown later conceded that this theory did not adequately explain the etiology of the disorder bearing his name [2]. Indeed, the precise etiology of Brown's syndrome remains elusive.

■ Clinical Features

Physical Findings

Several findings on physical examination are considered essential to the diagnosis of Brown's syndrome [1–5]. Most evident is the inability to elevate the affected eye in adduction (Fig 1). Elevation improves in the primary position and in abduction. There is little or no overaction of the

63

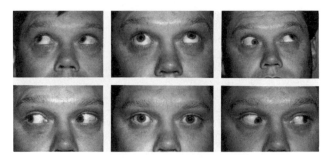

Figure 1 *Brown's syndrome involving the right eye.*

ipsilateral superior oblique muscle. Typically, exotropia occurs in upgaze. Discomfort may be felt in the region of the trochlea on attempted elevation in adduction. Head position abnormalities are common, with chin-up posture as well as face turn to place the affected eye in abduction. Variable head tilts may also be seen, as well as widening of the palpebral fissure on adduction. A positive traction test with retroplacement of the globe with the forceps during passive elevation places the superior oblique tendon on stretch and accentuates the restriction to elevation in adduction in Brown's syndrome [6]. There is also significant limitation of extortion with the globe retroplaced.

Grading System

Based on these clinical features, Eustis and colleagues [7] designed a grading system for describing the severity of Brown's syndrome. The mild form exhibits restricted elevation in adduction with no hypotropia or downshoot in adduction. In the moderate form, elevation is restricted in adduction, and there is an associated hypotropia or downshoot in adduction but no hypotropia in primary position. Severe Brown's syndrome is noted for restricted elevation and marked downshoot in adduction, with hypotropia present in primary position.

Congenital and Acquired Brown's Syndrome

In the congenital form of Brown's syndrome, the motility disturbance is constant and is unlikely to resolve spontaneously [8]. Conversely, the acquired form may be constant or intermittent, and spontaneous improvement occurs in some cases [8]. Acquired forms of Brown's syndrome may be seen in association with such conditions as trauma, inflammation, and metastatic disease. Some cases of acquired Brown's syndrome may respond to medical management.

Amblyopia

Brown [2] did not believe that amblyopia was a significant feature of the syndrome in his series of 126 patients. However, fusion was demonstrated in only 98 of the patients. Subsequently, several authors [9, 10] have reported that amblyopia may be seen in Brown's syndrome, especially when the eyes are not aligned in the preferred head position. Clark and Noel [9] found amblyopia in 7 of 28 consecutive cases.

■ Differential Diagnosis

The differential diagnosis of Brown's syndrome includes other possible causes of limited elevation of the globe such as double-elevator palsy, blow-out fractures, inferior oblique palsy, superior oblique overaction, and Duane's retraction syndrome. Double-elevator palsy may be distinguished by limitation of elevation in primary position and in abduction as well as in adduction. Ptosis may also be seen.

Trauma resulting in orbital floor blow-out fractures, with entrapment or scarring of inferior orbital tissues, is usually distinguished by restriction of elevation in abduction as well as in adduction [11]. Positive traction test in both abduction and adduction is also seen. Occasional cases, however, may show elevation deficiencies that are greater in adduction and are difficult to distinguish from Brown's syndrome.

Superior oblique overaction can result in hypotropia on adduction and may resemble Brown's syndrome. Inferior oblique palsy may also resemble Brown's syndrome by causing a hypotropia in adduction and elevation. The two conditions can be generally differentiated from Brown's syndrome by traction testing, which demonstrates free elevation in adduction. In addition, version testing in superior oblique overaction reveals an A-pattern, unlike the typical V-pattern seen in Brown's syndrome.

Duane's retraction syndrome, with an associated downshoot in adduction, can resemble Brown's syndrome but is distinguished by its characteristic globe retraction and narrowing of the palpebral fissure on attempted adduction.

■ Pathophysiological Features

Congenital Brown's Syndrome

Tendon or Trochlear Anomalies The majority of patients with congenital, constant Brown's syndrome are believed to have anomalies of the superior oblique tendon or the tendon-trochlear complex, or both. Parks [12] has proposed that a reduction in the normal elasticity of the superior oblique muscle and tendon could result in an inability to elevate the eye in adduction. This idea gained support when it was found that tendon sheath stripping failed as a therapy for Brown's syndrome. Moreover, there is no true anterior sheath of the superior oblique tendon.

It has been suggested that Brown's syndrome may parallel the orthopedic disorder digital tenosynovitis stenosans [10, 13, 14], in which thickening and stenosis occur at the pulley entrance of a digital tendon. At the point where the tendon is restricted, it becomes enlarged secondarily. It has been proposed that in similar fashion, the passage of an enlarged superior oblique tendon might have restricted movement through the trochlea. In a study of the trochlear region in the fetus and embryo, Sevel [15] noted the presence of thick trabeculae between the tendon and trochlea which, in the normal fetus, have almost completely disappeared by full term. He proposed that persistence of thickened trabecular remnants might result in Brown's syndrome. Helveston and co-workers [16] conducted studies of human cadaveric and exenterated tissue specimens and proposed a telescoping or sliding theory of superior oblique tendon movement through the trochlea, not unlike laminar flow in fluid dynamics. Only the central tendon fibers make the full excursion, whereas the peripheral fibers move relatively less (Fig 2). Thus, any process that interferes with the telescoping or sliding movement of the individual tendon fibers could result in Brown's syndrome.

Inferior Oblique and Inferior Orbital Abnormalities Prior to our current understanding of the limitation of movement of the superior oblique tendon in Brown's syndrome, structural abnormalities of the inferior oblique and adjacent structures were believed to play a role. Girard [17] described anomalous check ligaments at the insertion of the inferior oblique, resulting in its pseudoparalysis. Romaine [18] proposed that in cases of Brown's syndrome in which no abnormality of the superior oblique muscle or tendon was found at surgery, exploration of the area surrounding the inferior oblique, Lockwood's ligament, and the inferior rectus should be undertaken. This is particularly important following trauma.

Paradoxical Innervation Inadequate or paradoxical innervation to the inferior oblique has been offered as a possible etiological mechanism for Brown's syndrome. Breinin [19] demonstrated normal electromyographic patterns from the inferior oblique muscles in 2 patients with Brown's syndrome. Using simultaneous electromyography, Papst and Stein [20] demonstrated co-contraction of the superior oblique and inferior oblique on elevation and adduction in 2 patients with Brown's syndrome, thus drawing a parallel (i.e., co-contraction) between Brown's syndrome and Duane's retraction syndrome. In 1971, Ferig-Seiwerth and Celic [21] demonstrated paradoxical innervation in 1 of 3 patients with Brown's syndrome and proposed that congenital Brown's syndrome might be due to

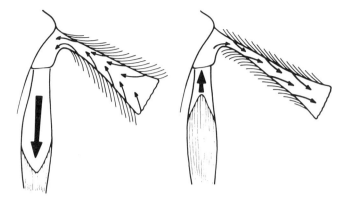

Figure 2 *Telescopic action of the superior oblique tendon while passing through the trochlea.*

a central innervational disorder. Subsequent studies [22], however, have demonstrated normal electromyographic findings of the inferior and superior oblique muscles in patients with Brown's syndrome.

Acquired Brown's Syndrome

Acquired Brown's syndrome may be seen following surgery and trauma or in association with inflammatory diseases. An iatrogenically induced Brown's syndrome is commonly seen after tucking the superior oblique tendon [8, 23]. Acquired Brown's syndrome has also been described following frontal and ethmoid sinus surgery, blepharoplasty, and scleral buckling procedures [5, 24, 25]. Brown's syndrome has been associated with rheumatoid arthritis (adult and juvenile), sinusitis, and metastasis in the region of the trochlea [26–29], suggesting an inflammatory etiology in these forms of acquired Brown's syndrome. Direct as well as indirect trauma can result in Brown's syndrome.

■ Therapy

Therapeutic interventions for Brown's syndrome vary, of course, with the etiology and severity of motility disturbance. Observation alone is used in mild congenital Brown's syndrome. Visual acuity and binocular status should be monitored closely in young children. Spontaneous resolution may occur in acquired and intermittent cases. Systemic and locally injected corticosteroids have been used in treating some cases of acquired Brown's syndrome.

Surgical indications include hypotropia in the primary position with significant diplopia in adults or concern over loss of binocularity in a child

[1, 30], anomalous head position [30], loss of a compensatory head position in a child with resultant hypotropia and, rarely, for cosmetically unacceptable downshoot in adduction [7, 31]. Surgery is directed at improving the patient's field of single binocular vision, head position, and versions [7, 32].

The techniques of correcting Brown's syndrome have evolved as understanding of its pathophysiology grew. Tendon sheath stripping advocated early by Brown [1] was based on the misconception that the syndrome was due to a contracted anterior sheath surrounding the superior oblique tendon. This procedure has been abandoned because it is ineffective. Tenectomy of the posterior tendon, Z-tenotomy, tendon recession, and split tendon lengthening were evaluated by Parks [12, 33] as a means of reducing the incidence of overcorrection or postoperative superior oblique palsy and were found to be unsatisfactory.

Currently, tenotomy and tenectomy are the preferred procedures for weakening the superior oblique tendon and relieving restriction of elevation in adduction in Brown's syndrome. Postoperatively, restriction of elevation is relieved, but varying degrees of superior oblique palsy supervene in up to 85% of patients [7] when either tenotomy or tenectomy is used alone. Repeat procedures for iatrogenic superior oblique palsy were reported in 82% of patients in one study [33]. In an effort to decrease the incidence of superior oblique palsy, Parks and Eustis [31] reported successful results in 94% of patients with the use of simultaneous superior oblique tenotomy and a 14-mm inferior oblique recession. Overcorrection was not a significant complication; however, some degree of inferior oblique muscle underaction was seen postoperatively in 75% of eyes, and it has been subsequently recommended that the inferior oblique recession be reduced to 10 mm. Consideration of the surgical anatomy during tenotomy may be of particular importance in preventing overcorrection. Wilson and co-workers [8] have stressed the importance of preserving the union of the sub–Tenon's capsular portion of the intermuscular septum that surrounds the superior oblique tendon in its position nasal to the superior rectus muscle. It is believed that the intact intermuscular septum may serve as an insertion for the proximal end of the cut tendon, with the force of the superior oblique being transmitted by the preserved septum. The use of a silicone expander for more quantitative weakening of the superior oblique, proposed recently by Wright and colleagues [34, 35], is currently being evaluated.

■ References

1. Brown HW. Congenital structural muscle anomalies. In: Allen JA, ed. Strabismus ophthalmic symposium I. St Louis: Mosby, 1950:205–236
2. Brown HW. True and simulated superior oblique tendon sheath syndromes. Doc Ophthalmol 1973;34:123–136

3. Mein J, Harcourt B. Diagnosis and management of ocular motility disorders. Oxford: Blackwell Scientific, 1986:301–304

4. Parks MM, Mitchell PR. Ophthalmoplegic syndromes and trauma. In: Tasman W, Jaeger EA, eds. Duane's clinical ophthalmology, vol 1. Philadelphia: Lippincott, 1990: chap 20, 5–7

5. Parks MM, Brown M. Superior oblique tendon sheath syndrome of Brown. Am J Ophthalmol 1975;79:82–86

6. Guyton DL. Exaggerated traction test for the oblique muscles. Ophthalmology 1981;88:1035–1040

7. Eustis HS, O'Reilly C, Crawford JS. Management of superior oblique palsy after surgery for true Brown's syndrome. J Pediatr Ophthalmol Strabismus 1987;24: 10–16

8. Wilson EM, Eustis HS, Parks MM. Brown's syndrome. Surv Ophthalmol 1989;34:153–172

9. Clarke WN, Noel LP. Brown's syndrome: fusion status and amblyopia. Can J Ophthalmol 1983;18:118–123

10. Sandford-Smith JH. Intermittent superior oblique tendon sheath syndrome. Br J Ophthalmol 1973;57:865–870

11. Jackson OB Jr, Nankin SJ, Scott WE. Traumatic simulated Brown's syndrome: a case report. J Pediatr Ophthalmol Strabismus 1979;16:160–162

12. Parks MM. The superior oblique tendon (lecture). Trans Ophthalmol Soc UK 1977;97:288–304

13. Sandford-Smith JH. Superior oblique tendon sheath syndrome and its relationship to stenosing tenosynovitis. Br J Ophthalmol 1973;57:859–865

14. Sandford-Smith JH. Superior oblique tendon sheath syndrome. Br J Ophthalmol 1975;59:385–386

15. Sevel D. Brown's syndrome—a possible etiology explained embryologically. J Pediatr Ophthalmol Strabismus 1981;18:26–31

16. Helveston EM, Merriam WW, Ellis FD, et al. The trochlea: a study of the anatomy and physiology. Ophthalmology 1982;89:124–133

17. Girard LJ. Pseudoparalysis of the inferior oblique muscle. South Med J 1956; 49:342–349

18. Romaine HH. Motility surgery. NY State J Med 1963;63:1511–1514

19. Breinin GM. New aspects of ophthalmoneurologic diagnosis. Arch Ophthalmol 1957;58:375–388

20. Papst W, Stein HJ. Zur Ätiologie des Musculus-obliquus-superior-Sehnenscheidensyndroms. Klin Monatsbl Augenhielkd 1969;154:506–518

21. Ferig-Seiwerth F, Celic M. A contribution to the knowledge of superior tendon sheath syndrome (Brown's syndrome). In: Orthoptics—proceedings of the Second International Orthoptic Congress, Amsterdam, May 11–13, 1971. Amsterdam: Excerpta Medica, 1972:354–359

22. Catford GV, Hart JCD. Superior oblique tendon sheath syndrome: an electromyographical study. Br J Ophthalmol 1971;55:155–160

23. Helveston EM, Ellis FD. Superior oblique tuck for superior oblique palsy. Aust J Ophthalmol 1983;11:215–220

24. Blanchard CL, Young LA. Acquired inflammatory superior oblique tendon sheath (Brown's) syndrome: report of a case following frontal sinus surgery. Arch Otolaryngol 1984;110:120–122

25. Lowe RF. Bilateral superior oblique tendon sheath syndrome: occurrence and spontaneous recovery in one of uniovular twins. Br J Ophthalmol 1969;53:466–471

26. Booth-Mason S, Kyle GM, Rossor M, Bradbury P. Acquired Brown's syndrome: an unusual cause. Br J Ophthalmol 1985;69:791–794

27. Clark E. A case of apparent intermittent overaction of the left superior oblique. Br Orthopt J 1966;23:116–117

28. Killian PJ, McClain B, Lawless OJ. Brown's syndrome: an unusual manifestation of rheumatoid arthritis. Arthritis Rheum 1977;20:1080–1084

29. Smith E. Aetiology of apparent superior oblique tendon sheath syndrome. Trans Ophthopt Assoc Aust 1965;7:32

30. Nutt AB, Mein J. The significance and management of abnormal head postures. Trans Ophthalmol Soc Aust 1963;23:57–71

31. Parks MM, Eustis HS. Simultaneous superior tenotomy and inferior oblique recession in Brown's syndrome. Ophthalmology 1987;94:1043–1048

32. Crawford JS, Orton RB, Labow-Daily L. Late results of superior oblique muscle tenotomy in true Brown's syndrome. Am J Ophthalmol 1980;89:824–829

33. Parks MM. Surgery for Brown's syndrome. In: Symposium on strabismus. Transactions of the New Orleans Academy of Ophthalmology. St Louis: Mosby, 1978: 157–177

34. Wright K. Superior oblique silicone expander for Brown's syndrome and for superior oblique overaction. American Association of Pediatric Ophthalmology and Strabismus Fifteenth Annual Meeting, 1989

35. Wright KW, Min B, Park C. Comparison of superior oblique tendon expander to tenotomy for the management of superior oblique overaction and Brown's syndrome. Bolton Landing, NY, American Association of Pediatric Ophthalmology and Strabismus, 1990

Neonatal Conjunctivitis

Cynthia Grosskreutz, M.D., Ph.D.
Lois B. H. Smith, M.D., Ph.D.

Neonatal conjunctivitis is defined as inflammation of the conjunctiva in an infant younger than 1 month old. It is characterized by redness and swelling of the eyelids and palpebral conjunctiva and purulent discharge with one or more polymorphonuclear cells per high-power field on a Gram-stained conjunctival smear [1].

The first prophylactic treatment for neonatal conjunctivitis was performed in 1881 by Credé [2], who used silver nitrate to prevent infection with *Neisseria gonorrhoeae*. Over the past century, this practice has been the mainstay for the prevention of neonatal conjunctivitis. The list of causes of neonatal conjunctivitis has continued to expand and now includes *Chlamydia, Staphylococcus, Streptococcus,* and *Neisseria* species and herpes virus as well as chemical conjunctivitis. The recognition of causes of neonatal conjunctivitis not affected by silver nitrate has prompted a search for new and broader prophylactic agents. Several recent studies have examined neonatal ocular prophylaxis with topical tetracycline ointment and erythromycin ointments as well as parenteral administration of ceftriaxone and kanamycin, but neonatal conjunctivitis remains a problem in the United States and in other parts of the world.

■ Bacterial Flora in the Conjunctiva at Birth

The bacteria found in the conjunctiva of the newborn reflect the mode of delivery. In infants delivered vaginally, the bacteria are characteristic of the flora of the female genital tract. In a study of 100 eyes, Isenberg and colleagues [3] examined the bacteria isolated from conjunctival cultures taken within 15 minutes of delivery. Both aerobic and anaerobic cultures were investigated. Anaerobic organisms accounted for 78.4% of the cultures and aerobic organisms for 21.6%. The anaerobic organisms most frequently isolated were *Lactobacillus* (40.5% of aerobic and anaerobic) and *Bifidobacterium* species (18.9%), diphtheroids (6.3%), *Propionibacterium acnes* (6.3%), and *Bacteroides* species (5.4%). Of the aerobic organisms isolated, *Staphylococcus epidermidis* was the most common (9.0% of aerobic and anaerobic), followed by *Corynebacterium* (6.3%) and *Streptococcus* species (2.7%) and *Escherichia coli* (1.8%).

The conjunctival flora following cesarean section is a function of the time elapsed between membrane rupture and actual delivery. Isenberg and co-workers [4] found that more than three-fourths of the infants delivered by cesarean section within 3 hours of membrane rupture had sterile conjunctival cultures. In neonates delivered by cesarean section more than 3 hours after membrane rupture, the bacterial populations were between those of infants delivered vaginally and those delivered by cesarean section less than 3 hours after membrane rupture.

■ Pathogenetic Role of Sexually Transmitted Diseases

It has been reported that 42% of neonates exposed to *N. gonorrhoeae* during delivery and 31% exposed to *Chlamydia trachomatis* develop conjunctivitis [5]. Neonatal infection caused by herpes simplex virus develops in 40 to 60% of newborns exposed to active genital herpes virus [6]. The prevalence of *Chlamydia* infection is on the rise both in the developing world and in industrialized nations. In one study carried out in Nairobi, Kenya, more than 50% of the infants with neonatal conjunctivitis demonstrated both *N. gonorrhoeae* and *C. trachomatis* as causative agents [7]. The incidence of gonococcal neonatal conjunctivitis is 0.3 per 1,000 live births in the United States [8] and 40 per 1,000 live births in Kenya [5]. The incidence of neonatal conjunctivitis caused by *C. trachomatis* is reported to be 5 to 60 per 1,000 live births in the United States and as high as 80 per 1,000 live births in Kenya [5].

■ Causes of Neonatal Conjunctivitis

Chemical Conjunctivitis

Chemical conjunctivitis is the most common form of neonatal conjunctivitis. It is related to the prophylactic use of 1% silver nitrate drops and develops rapidly in up to 90% of the infants so treated. Chemical conjunctivitis due to silver nitrate is usually self-limiting and resolves in 24 to 48 hours.

Bacterial Conjunctivitis

Microbial causes of neonatal conjunctivitis may be bacterial or viral. The relative frequencies with which various pathogens give rise to neonatal conjunctivitis is, not surprisingly, related to the particular maternal patient population. In a study in Kenya, Laga and colleagues [5] found the most common cause of neonatal conjunctivitis to be *C. trachomatis* (32%), followed by *N. gonorrhoeae* (12%), *Hemophilus* species (7%), *Streptococcus pneumoniae* (6%), *Staphylococcus aureus* (6%), *N. gonorrhoeae* with *C. trachomatis* (3%), and other bacteria (3%). More than half of the *N. gonorrhoeae* strains identified were penicillinase-producing. In a study at the Mount Sinai Hospital in New York City, Jarvis and co-workers [9] found a substantially different distribution of etiological pathogens. Staphylococcal species predominated (30.2%), followed by culture-negative (normal) flora (22.1%), chemical conjunctivitis (7.4%), and gonococcal and chlamydial conjunctivitis (3.1% each); results were unobtainable in 10%. These investigators also grouped together as "other pathogens" 25% of the cases of neonatal conjunctivitis, including: *E. coli* (9 cases), *Streptococcus viridans* (4), *Streptococcus faecalis* (2), *S. pneumoniae* (2), *S. aureus* with *E. coli* (2), *S. aureus* with *Pseudomonas aeruginosa* (1), *Serratia* species (1), *Klebsiella oxytoca* (1), *Enterococcus* species (1), and *Hemophilus parainfluenza* (1). In contrast to the report from Kenya [4], none of the 3 cases of gonococcal neonatal conjunctivitis in the New York study were caused by penicillin-resistant *N. gonorrhoeae* [9].

Viral Conjunctivitis

Neonatal herpes simplex virus infection may affect the eyes as well as the skin with oral and vaginal lesions. If the mother has a history of a genital herpetic infection, especially during pregnancy, neonatal herpes virus should be suspected. Infection can occur prior to birth (i.e., intrauterine infection) or during the birth process. The mortality is high for disseminated disease, and conjunctivitis may be the presenting symptom [10]. Nahmias and colleagues [11] reported a series of 297 neonates with herpes simplex virus infection and found ocular pathology in 17%. The incidence of the various ophthalmic findings was as follows: conjunctivitis, 10%; keratitis, 7%; chorioretinitis or chorioretinal scarring, 4%; cataracts, 1%; and optic atrophy, less than 1%.

Yanoff and co-workers [12], reported dizygotic twins born prematurely to a mother suspected of having a vaginal herpetic infection. Both infants developed herpes simplex encephalitis. The second twin died from disseminated herpes virus and was also diagnosed with a unilateral keratoconjunctivitis and bilateral endophthalmitis. At autopsy, the baby was shown to have a necrotizing retinitis and necrosis of the ciliary body and iris. Herpes simplex virus type II was cultured from the conjunctiva of both eyes and the cerebrospinal fluid.

Approximately 70% of neonatal herpes simplex virus infections are type II. Interestingly, in cases of herpes simplex infection with ocular involvement in which the virus was subtyped, 39% were type I. All cases of neonatal chorioretinitis, however, involved type II.

■ Diagnosis

Because of the potentially disastrous outcome of untreated neonatal conjunctivitis, diagnosis of the etiological agent must be made and appropriate treatment initiated as soon as possible. Neonatal conjunctivitis first presents as a diffuse, often hyperacute conjunctivitis with a papillary reaction [13]. Follicles are rarely seen prior to 6 to 8 weeks of life due to the immature nature of the infant's immune system, so that their absence is not a useful diagnostic sign (an intense follicular response in an adult is often helpful in making the diagnosis of chlamydial conjunctivitis). The clinical course may give a clue as to the etiological agent, although the disease patterns are not sufficiently different to be pathognomonic of any specific cause.

Conjunctivitis due to *N. gonorrhoeae* usually has its onset during the first 2 to 5 days of life [14]. The conjunctivitis begins with a serosanguineous discharge and inflammation of the eyelids. Within a day, the eyelids become markedly edematous, there is prominent chemosis, and the discharge becomes thick and purulent. Untreated, the infection may progress to involve the cornea and deeper layers of the conjunctiva.

Neonatal conjunctivitis caused by *C. trachomatis* typically has its onset during the first 3 weeks of life, with the average onset at 14 days of age [15]. The clinical presentation can be highly variable, ranging from mild inflammation to severe edema of the eyelids with copious purulent discharge. The cornea is rarely affected, and the disease involves primarily the tarsal conjunctiva.

Neonatal conjunctivitis due to herpes simplex infection characteristically occurs during the first 2 weeks of life. It may be unilateral or bilateral. The appearance of vesicular skin lesions may herald the onset of a more widespread infection, and the lesions can appear on the eyelid margins. The presence of microdendrites or geographical ulcers is the most common corneal involvement in neonates. The conjunctivitis is typically associated with nonspecific eyelid edema, injection of the bulbar conjunctiva, and a watery discharge.

Chandler and Rapoza [16] have suggested a comprehensive strategy for working up a neonate who develops conjunctivitis. In addition to an ocular evaluation, a complete physical examination is also necessary to determine the degree of systemic involvement. Initial laboratory workup should include conjunctival smears (Gram's stain and Giemsa stain), chlamydial assay, bacterial cultures (reduced blood agar, cooked meat or thioglycolate broth, chocolate agar in CO_2, or Thayer-Martin media), and viral cultures if clinically indicated. Serological titers of IgG and IgM have not been found useful in making the diagnosis of chlamydial conjunctivitis [15]. Preliminary diagnoses can be made on the basis of the appearance of the conjunctival smears [16]. A smear from an infant with a chemical conjunctivitis would be characterized by the presence of neutrophils and occasional lymphocytes, whereas a smear from an infant with bacterial conjunctivitis would contain bacteria and neutrophils. Intracellular gram-negative diplococci are present in up to 95% of culture-positive cases of gonococcal conjunctivitis. The smear from a conjunctiva infected with *Chlamydia* organisms would show neutrophils, lymphocytes, plasma cells, and basophilic intracytoplasmic inclusions in epithelial cells. Finally, the conjunctival smear from an infant with viral ophthalmia neonatorum would be expected to show lymphocytes, plasma cells, multinucleate giant cells, and eosinophilic intranuclear inclusions.

■ Treatment

Bacterial Conjunctivitis

Although prevention of neonatal conjunctivitis should be the primary goal, systematic prophylaxis of newborns is not possible in all parts of the world, and it is not always effective even when administered appropriately. Until recently, the standard therapy recommended for gonococcal neonatal conjunctivitis consisted of frequent topical aqueous penicillin G and, in addition, systemically administered penicillin G [14]. With the emergence of resistant strains of *N. gonorrhoeae*, this treatment has fallen out of favor.

Ceftriaxone, in a single intramuscular dose of 125 mg, is highly effective therapy against gonococcal neonatal conjunctivitis [17]. Intramuscular ceftriaxone has the added advantage of also treating extraocular gonococcal infections. This third-generation cephalosporin is effective against penicillinase-producing *N. gonorrhoeae* as well, an important consideration as the prevalence of penicillin resistance of *N. gonorrhoeae* has risen to as high as 53% in some parts of the world [5]. Another third-generation cephalosporin, cefotaxime, has also been shown to be effective against both penicillinase-producing and non-penicillinase-producing gonococcal conjunctivitis at a dose of 100 mg intramuscularly [18].

Kanamycin, 75 mg intramuscularly, followed by either gentamicin eye ointment for 3 days [19] or tetracycline ointment for 7 days [17], has also been shown to be highly effective against gonococcal ophthalmia neonatorum. The drawbacks to these regimens, however, are the need for continued topical application of ointment and the inferior efficacy of kanamycin in treating nonocular sites of gonococcal infections. Nonetheless, parenteral kanamycin and tetracycline ointment are readily available worldwide and are less expensive than ceftriaxone.

Several excellent choices exist for treating gonococcal ophthalmia neonatorum. Problems arise, however, when *N. gonorrhoeae* is not the sole infecting organism. Coinfection with *C. trachomatis* is common in infants diagnosed with gonococcal conjunctivitis, as is infection by *C. trachomatis* alone. Treatment of chlamydial conjunctivitis must be aimed not only at the ocular colonization, but also toward eradication of the nasopharyngeal carriage and the possible subsequent development of *C. trachomatis* pneumonia. Oral erythromycin estolate or ethylsuccinate suspension, 25 mg/kg twice daily for 14 to 21 days, is the systemic treatment of choice for chlamydial conjunctivitis [20].

Viral Conjunctivitis

Although the efficacy of treatment of herpes simplex conjunctivitis or vesicular blepharitis has not been fully established, the use of topical trifluorothymidine should be considered [21]. If, in addition, the neonate has herpetic keratitis, 1% trifluorothymidine drops should be given every 2 hours while the infant is awake. If the conjunctivitis does not respond to this therapy, another antiviral agent should be used. If systemic symptoms or ocular manifestations other than conjunctivitis or keratitis arise, the use of systemic acyclovir or vidarabine should be initiated [22].

■ Complications

Complications of untreated neonatal conjunctivitis caused by *N. gonorrhoeae* are common. Prior to the institution of neonatal ocular prophylaxis by Credé in the late nineteenth century, neonatal conjunctivitis was the leading cause of blindness in children. In one study, 16% of infants with gonococcal conjunctivitis had corneal lesions [7]. Additional complications include ulceration of the cornea with perforation, iridocyclitis, anterior synechiae and, rarely, panophthalmitis.

Long-term ocular sequelae from chlamydial conjunctivitis is extremely rare [23], but conjunctivitis often is the presenting sign of chlamydial infection in the newborn. Other complications of neonatal chlamydial infection include chlamydial pneumonia and rectal and vaginal infections. Schachter and associates [15] showed culture-positive evidence of chlamydial conjunctivitis in 18% of infants at risk (i.e., those born to mothers with positive cervical cultures) as well as a rate of 16% for chlamydial pneumonia and 14% for rectal and vaginal infections. Serological evidence of exposure was present in 60% of the infants at risk.

As with chlamydial conjunctivitis, the initial presentation of herpes simplex infection in a newborn may be conjunctivitis, which is the most frequent ocular symptom of the acute infection. The conjunctivitis may be the only manifestation of the infection, or it may proceed to involve the skin, mouth, and central nervous system and to disseminate to visceral organs. Even with the best antiviral therapy, the disseminated form of the disease has a mortality of 57%, and central nervous system involvement is associated with 10% mortality.

In a study of 32 children followed for up to 15 years after their neonatal herpetic infections, el Azazi and co-workers [24] found a surprisingly high rate of ocular sequelae: visual acuity of worse than 20/200 in 37%, exotropia in 34%, skew deviation in 31%, chorioretinal scars in 28%, tonic deviation in 22%, optic atrophy in 22%, corneal scars in 6%, cataracts in 3%, and esotropia in 3%. The rate of ocular abnormalities was particularly high (94%) in children with neurological deficits resulting from their neonatal herpetic infections.

One potential complication of prophylaxis for neonatal conjunctivitis that is not frequently addressed in the ophthalmic literature is the effect on bonding. The use of silver nitrate has been criticized because of the high incidence of chemical conjunctivitis, with its swelling of the eyelids and subsequent lack of visual contact of the infant with the caregivers. Similar arguments have been made with respect to the blurring of vision after topical application of ointment. Delaying of prophylactic instillation of medications has been suggested as one possible solution to this problem. Muhe and Tafari [25] have shown, however, that delaying prophylaxis for more than 4 hours after delivery results in a risk of ophthalmia neonatorum four and a half times greater than if the medications are administered immediately after birth.

■ Prophylaxis

As mentioned, the use of 1% silver nitrate instilled in the conjunctiva shortly after birth has been the mainstay of prophylaxis for neonatal conjunctivitis over the past century. Concerns about the chemical conjunctivitis ensuing from silver nitrate use and the spectrum of this agent's antimicrobial activity have caused its use as the primary prophylactic agent to be questioned in recent years. Several alternate protocols have been studied.

Topical application of a single dose of either 1% silver nitrate, 0.5% erythromycin ophthalmic ointment, or 1% tetracycline ophthalmic ointment was studied by Hammerschlag and colleagues [26], who concluded that these three therapies were equally effective in preventing gonococcal neonatal conjunctivitis but did not significantly reduce the incidence of chlamydial conjunctivitis. In another study, 1% silver nitrate and 1% tetracycline ointment were shown to reduce the incidence of chlamydial conjunctivitis but not to abolish it [27]. Despite the conflicting results of these two studies with respect to the treatment of chlamydial conjunctivitis, neither tetracycline nor silver nitrate drops eradicate the nasopharyngeal colonization nor do they prevent the *C. trachomatis* pneumonia.

Jarvis and co-workers [9] reported the use of an intramuscular injection of 50,000 units of aqueous penicillin along with the instillation of 1% tetracycline ointment. They found an incidence of 3.1 cases of neonatal conjunctivitis per 1,000 live births, of which only 3% were gonococcal. None of their cases of gonococcal neonatal conjunctivitis were caused by penicillin-resistant *N. gonorrhoeae*.

Because of the low incidence of neonatal conjunctivitis in several industrialized countries, routine prophylaxis has been abandoned. Sweden stopped requiring the use of prophylactic antibiotics in 1982, and they have not been used in the United Kingdom for more than 25 years. However, Sweden does require antibiotic prophylaxis if the mother has received no prenatal care.

Sexually transmitted diseases play a major role in the majority of cases of neonatal conjunctivitis. Several authors have suggested that the principal aim of ocular prophylaxis at birth should be to prevent gonococcal conjunctivitis since it has the highest potential for resulting in ocular morbidity [26, 27]. Chlamydial conjunctivitis, however, remains a problem. Because of the lack of a reliable topical agent for its prevention, along with the importance of eradicating the microorganism from the nasopharynx, the most effective method of control may be the screening and treatment of pregnant women. The patterns of health care delivery and prenatal care make this a challenging proposal in both the United States and other parts of the world.

■ References

1. Fransen L, Klauss V. Neonatal ophthalmia in the developing world: epidemiology, etiology, management and control. Int Ophthalmol 1988;11:189–196
2. Credé CSR. Die verhutuna der augenentzundung der neugeborenen. Arch Gynäkol 1881;18:367–370
3. Isenberg SJ, Apt L, Yoshimori R, Alvarez SR. Bacterial flora of the conjunctiva at birth. J Pediatr Ophthalmol Strabismus 1986;23:284–286
4. Isenberg SJ, Apt L, Yoshimori R, et al. Source of the conjunctival bacterial flora at birth and implications for ophthalmia neonatorum prophylaxis. Am J Ophthalmol 1988;106:458–462
5. Laga M, Plummer FA, Nzanze H, et al. Epidemiology of ophthalmia neonatorum in Kenya. Lancet 1986;2:1145–1149
6. Nahmias AJ, Josey WE, Naib ZM, et al. Perinatal risk associated with maternal genital herpes simplex virus infection. Am J Obstet Gynecol 1971;110:825–837
7. Fransen L, Nsanze H, Klauss V, et al. Ophthalmia neonatorum in Nairobi, Kenya: the roles of *Neisseria gonorrhoeae* and *Chlamydia trachomatis*. J Infect Dis 1986;153:862–869
8. Johnson D, McKenna H. Bacteria in ophthalmia neonatorum. Pathology 1975;7:199–201

9. Jarvis VN, Levine R, Asbell PA. Ophthalmia neonatorum: study of a decade of experience at the Mount Sinai Hospital. Br J Ophthalmol 1987;71:295–300

10. Nahmias AJ, Hagler WS. Ocular manifestations of herpes simplex in the newborn (neonatal ocular herpes). Int Ophthalmol Clin 1972;12:191–213

11. Nahmias AJ, Bisintine AM, Caldwell DR, Wilson L. Eye infections with herpes simplex viruses in neonates. Surv Ophthalmol 1976;21:100–105

12. Yanoff M, Allman MI, Fine BS. Congenital herpes simplex virus, type 2, bilateral endophthalmitis. Metab Pediatr Syst Ophthalmol 1982;6:287–295

13. Whitcher JP. Neonatal ophthalmia: have we advanced in the last 20 years? Int Ophthalmol Clin 1990;30:39–41

14. Glasgow LA, Overall JC Jr. Infections of the newborn. In: Behrman RE, Vaughan VC III, Nelson WE, eds. Textbook of pediatrics. Philadelphia: Saunders, 1983: 408–409

15. Schachter J, Grossman M, Sweet RL, et al. Prospective study of perinatal transmission of *Chlamydia trachomatis*. JAMA 1986;255:3374–3377

16. Chandler JW, Rapoza PA. Ophthalmia neonatorum. Int Ophthalmol Clin 1990; 30:36–38

17. Laga M, Naamara W, Brunham RC, et al. Single-dose therapy of gonococcal ophthalmia neonatorum with ceftriaxone. N Engl J Med 1986;315:1382–1385

18. Lepage P, Bogaerts J, Kestelyn P, Mehaus A. Single-dose cefotaxime intramuscularly cures gonococcal ophthalmia neonatorum. Br J Ophthalmol 1988;72:518–520

19. Fransen L, Nsanze H, D'Costa L, et al. Single-dose kanamycin therapy of gonococcal ophthalmia neonatorum. Lancet 1984;2:1234–1237

20. Rodriguez EM, Hammerschlag MR. Diagnostic methods for *Chlamydia trachomatis* disease in neonates. J Perinatol 1987;7:232–234

21. Rotkis WM, Chandler JW. Neonatal conjunctivitis. In: Tassman W, Jaeger E, eds. Duane's clinical ophthalmology, vol 4. Philadelphia: Lippincott, 1990: chap 6, 1–7

22. Whitley RJ. Herpes simplex virus infections of the central nervous system: a review. Am J Med 1988;85(suppl 2A):61–67

23. Chandler JW. Controversies in ocular prophylaxis of newborns. Arch Ophthalmol 1989;107:814–815

24. el Azazi M, Malm G, Forsgren M. Late ophthalmologic manifestations of neonatal herpes simplex virus infection. Am J Ophthalmol 1990;109:1–7

25. Muhe L, Tafari N. Is there a critical time for prophylaxis against neonatal gonococcal ophthalmia? Genitourin Med 1986;62:356–357

26. Hammerschlag MR, Cummings C, Roblin PM, et al. Efficacy of neonatal ocular prophylaxis for the prevention of chlamydial and gonococcal conjunctivitis. N Engl J Med 1989;320:769–772

27. Laga M, Plummer FA, Piot P, et al. Prophylaxis of gonococcal and chlamydial ophthalmia neonatorum: a comparison of silver nitrate and tetracycline. N Engl J Med 1988;318:653–657

Kawasaki Syndrome

Monte D. Mills, M.D.
Lois B. H. Smith, M.D., Ph.D.

Kawasaki syndrome is a clinical entity, also called *mucocutaneous lymph node syndrome*, first described by Tomisaka Kawasaki and colleagues in 1967 [1]. The primary features include fever, skin and mucous membrane changes, and lymphadenopathy. Conjunctivitis and iritis are a frequent and early finding, and the ophthalmology consultation can be an important factor in making an early diagnosis.

The syndrome frequently presents with abrupt onset of fever of 101° to 104°, lasting for 1 to 2 weeks despite antibiotics. Patients are typically infants or toddlers, although the disease has been reported in children as old as 5 years. Beginning by the third to fifth day of fever, skin changes develop that include a polymorphous exanthem of the trunk as well as erythema and edema of the palms and soles. The truncal rash starts as multiple discrete lesions, frequently targetlike with central clearing, which become confluent with time. The skin changes in the extremities are variable but frequently include prominent erythema of the palms and soles and edema early in the course, with subsequent desquamation of the periungual skin and nail changes.

Mucous membrane changes occur beginning in the first 10 days of illness, with erythema, edema, and cracking of the lips and oral mucosa. Changes in the tongue, similar to those seen in scarlet fever, have been called *strawberry tongue,* with hypertrophy of the lingual papillae. The lymphadenopathy is most prominent in the cervical region but may be present systemically and is nontender and nonsuppurative. Cardiac involvement, the most serious complication of Kawasaki syndrome, is usually not seen until the third week of illness or later. Findings may include myocarditis, coronary arteritis, thrombosis, and aneurysm.

Less frequent findings include diarrhea, arthralgia, arthritis, proteinuria, pyuria and nephrosis, cholangitis, cholecystitis, aseptic meningitis, urethritis and, in boys, meatitis. Laboratory abnormalities include anemia,

Table 1 *Diagnostic Criteria for Kawasaki Syndrome*

Fever of 5 days or longer plus at least four of the following:
1. Bilateral conjunctival injection
2. Oropharyngeal mucous membrane changes
   a. Injected pharynx
   b. Erythema and fissuring of lips
   c. Strawberry tongue, hypertrophy of lingual papillae
3. One or more changes of extremities
   a. Peripheral edema
   b. Erythema of palms and soles
   c. Desquamation of palms and soles
   d. Periungual desquamation
4. Rash
5. Cervical lymphadenopathy
Symptoms not explained by any known disease process

Source: Adapted from Morens et al. [26].

leukocytosis with leftward shift, thrombocytosis peaking at 750,000 to 1,500,000 platelets, an elevated erythrocyte sedimentation rate, and elevated acute-phase reactants including C-reactive protein, cryoprecipitate, and immune complexes.

Because of the protean manifestations, early clinical descriptions used many and conflicting definitions of the syndrome. Diagnostic criteria were therefore established by the Kawasaki Disease Research Committee in Japan in 1984 and were endorsed by the U.S. Centers for Disease Control (CDC) (Table 1).

■ Ocular Manifestations

Because of the prominence and early appearance of the eye findings, the consulting ophthalmologist is in a unique position to diagnose Kawasaki syndrome. Conjunctivitis, one of the primary diagnostic criteria, is frequently an early sign. Within the first 5 to 7 days of fever, bilateral bulbar conjunctival erythema that spares the limbus and palpebral conjunctiva is noted. The erythema may resemble episcleritis and is occasionally associated with subconjunctival hemorrhage. There is usually no exudate, although this has been reported [2–4]. The conjunctivitis usually persists for 2 to 3 weeks untreated [5]. Rarely, a superficial punctate keratitis has been reported; usually the cornea is uninvolved [6].

Anterior uveitis originally was believed to be unusual, but several prospective series with careful slit-lamp examination have shown 78 to 100% of patients have anterior chamber cells and flare or keratic precipitates [3, 5, 7–12]. The iritis is nongranulomatous, with no synechiae, recurrence, or glaucoma. Less common anterior segment pathological findings include subepithelial scarring of the conjunctiva in a single case following exudative conjunctivitis [12].

Posterior segment abnormalities were not reported in the original papers defining the syndrome. However, papilledema, vitreous opacities, exudative retinitis, cotton-wool spots, and preretinal membrane formation have all been noted [9, 11, 13]. Although the incidence of posterior segment pathological processes is not known, it appears low. Variable criteria for the diagnosis of Kawasaki syndrome also may have led to inclusion of several similar syndromes in the literature.

The ocular differential diagnosis is extensive, and the lack of pathognomonic signs or specific laboratory confirmation makes the role of the clinician crucial in the diagnosis. Therefore, it is essential that all children suspected of having Kawasaki syndrome have thorough ophthalmic evaluation as well as appropriate medical and laboratory workup.

■ Ocular Differential Diagnosis

Stevens-Johnson Syndrome and Bacterial Toxin Mediated Syndromes

Stevens-Johnson syndrome, or erythema multiforme major, is a clinical syndrome of fever, rash, and mucositis that frequently follows an upper respiratory viral syndrome or occurs as a systemic drug reaction. This syndrome is distinguished by severe corneal and conjunctival bullae, vesicles, and desquamation with pseudomembrane formation and, later, symblepharon formation. The differential diagnosis of Kawasaki syndrome is summarized in Table 2. The rash of Stevens-Johnson syndrome frequently includes target-shaped lesions that may become confluent with time, very much like Kawasaki syndrome. However, the Stevens-Johnson lesions progress to bullae and desquamation on skin as well as conjunctiva and mucous membranes. In contrast, Kawasaki syndrome should have no blistering, vesicle formation, or pseudomembrane on conjunctiva or skin. Stevens-Johnson syndrome itself also lacks adenopathy, but this is frequently not a reliable distinguishing feature as the syndrome often is associated with other conditions that stimulate adenopathy.

Streptococcal or staphylococcal toxin-mediated syndromes, including scarlet fever, staphylococcal scalded skin, and toxic shock syndrome, may exhibit prominent erythematous rash, strawberry tongue, and fever. However, these diseases usually lack conjunctivitis; if present, the conjunctivitis is usually exudative except in the toxic shock syndrome. The characteristic rashes of each are different. The rash of scarlet fever consists of diffuse, finely papillary lesions beginning on the neck and spreading downward. The rash of toxic shock is desquamative or bullous, with positive Nikolsky's sign (bullae formation with gentle traction). These syndromes are also distinguished by their association with infection with toxin-producing or-

Table 2 *Differential Diagnosis of Kawasaki Syndrome*

Bacterial infection
Streptococcal toxin-mediated syndromes (scarlet fever)
Staphylococcal toxin-mediated syndromes (toxic shock syndrome, scalded skin syndrome)
Leptospirosis
Yersinia pseudotuberculosis sepsis
Rickettsial infection
Rocky Mountain spotted fever
Tick typhus
Viral infection
Measles
Adenovirus
Enterovirus
Autoimmune disorder
Stevens-Johnson syndrome
Juvenile rheumatoid arthritis
Reiter's syndrome
Behçet's syndrome
Systemic lupus erythematosus
Inflammatory bowel disease
Sarcoidosis

ganisms, as well as the clinical setting. Exudative pharyngitis and tonsillitis with group A streptococci are found in scarlet fever; staphylococcal skin or cutaneous infection is found in scalded skin syndrome; and vaginitis or foreign-body infection with *Staphylococcus aureus* is found in toxic shock. A conjunctival source has been reported in scalded skin syndrome [14]. Aside from conjunctivitis, eye findings are unusual in these diseases. Rarely, focal posterior uveitis has been reported [3]. The presence of iritis should therefore suggest Kawasaki syndrome.

Juvenile Rheumatoid Arthritis

Juvenile rheumatoid arthritis may occasionally present with a red eye and may cause fever, arthralgia, and rash. However, the anterior uveitis is usually insidious in onset and severe, with synechiae formation, cataract, glaucoma, and recurrence, which are not usual features of Kawasaki syndrome [11]. In addition, there usually are no oral mucosal or extremity cutaneous changes in juvenile rheumatoid arthritis.

Viral Infections

Acute viral exanthems—adenovirus, measles, and enterovirus—frequently present with acute fever, rash, and conjunctivitis. Adenovirus conjunctivitis is distinguished by conjunctival follicles and involvement of palpebral conjunctiva, pseudomembranes, and exudation; superficial punctate keratitis and subepithelial infiltrates may also occur. These are not features commonly seen in Kawasaki syndrome. Measles occasionally includes mild anterior uveitis with red eye and distinctive rash. The limbal flush helps distinguish this cause of red eye from Kawasaki syndrome, which typically spares the limbal conjunctiva from the erythema. Also, there usually are no extremity changes or strawberry tongue in measles.

Rickettsial and Spirochetal Infections

Rickettsial infections, such as Rocky Mountain spotted fever and tick typhus, are another unusual infectious cause of acute fever, rash, and red eye. However, the petechial nature of the rash as well as the history of tick bite are often clues in these diseases. Frequently, there is no conjunctivitis or ocular findings; occasional nonexudative conjunctivitis without iritis has been reported. Laboratory serological testing is available.

Leptospirosis is caused by a zoonotic spirochete. The uncommon but widespread syndrome includes acute fever, rash, conjunctivitis, iritis, adenopathy, and oral mucosal changes [15]. Patients usually are older children and adults exposed to animals that harbor the causative organism. Although the disease is unusual, it should be ruled out by serological workup, culture, or dark-field examination of serum because it can present in a fashion identical to Kawasaki syndrome.

Miscellaneous Autoimmune Disorders

Reiter's syndrome includes iritis, urethritis, and arthritis; occasionally, it is associated with low-grade fever or rash. The differential diagnosis generally is not confusing, as Reiter's syndrome typically occurs in adults or children older than age 10. The red eye is typically unilateral, with ciliary flush and anterior uveitis.

Although rare in young children, Behçet's syndrome may cause an acute conjunctivitis in association with oral and genital ulcers. Other autoimmune disorders, including systemic lupus erythematosus, inflammatory bowel disease, and sarcoidosis (extremely rare in this age group), may cause similar syndromes. These diseases do not usually present with a bilateral conjunctivitis and do not generally make the differential diagnosis difficult, although an atypical case may be confusing. Serological evaluation can be helpful.

■ Epidemiological Features

The annual incidence of Kawasaki syndrome in the United States varies by location and year and has been reported to be from 4.5 to 9.1 cases per 100,000 children younger than 5 years. Although this incidence may seem low, local epidemics or clusters may show increased rates over brief periods. During epidemics in Boston, Houston, Rochester, Hawaii, North Carolina, Maryland, and Denver, the annual incidence was as high as 66 per 100,000 children younger than 5 years [16].

The incidence has been reported to be greater in Japan, with pandemics occurring every 3 years [17]. In the United States, a higher incidence is found among Oriental children (41.4 per 100,000 children younger than 5 years) than among whites (6.5 per 100,000) and blacks (8.9 per 100,000) of similar age [16]. A preponderance of male patients has been reported in several studies, in a ratio of approximately 1.4:1 [18]. Peak onset is approximately 1 year of age, and the syndrome is rare in children older than 5.

Socioeconomic level has been shown to correlate with Kawasaki syndrome, with an increase in higher socioeconomic groups in the United States in some controlled studies [19]. Other statistical risk factors include proximity of the patient's home to standing water [16] and recent use of rug shampoo [19, 20]. Despite the epidemiological evidence suggesting infectious transmission, multiple cases are rarely reported in families [21, 22].

The mortality of Kawasaki syndrome is almost entirely due to cardiac involvement. The rate of myocardial and coronary artery involvement varies depending on the methods of evaluation. Angiography is probably the most sensitive method of evaluating coronary arteries and reveals a rate of abnormalities varying from 10 to 60%. The larger studies in the United States have shown a rate of approximately 20% [23, 24]. Modern two-dimensional echocardiography has been reported to be 95% sensitive to coronary artery aneurysm, although data from studies using echocardiography are not strictly comparable to those using angiography.

Many patients with coronary aneurysm or even occlusion have no symptoms of heart failure or angina [25]. Electrocardiographic abnormalities have been reported in up to 50% of Kawasaki syndrome patients, most of whom will be asymptomatic. Sudden death may be the first sign of cardiac involvement. In the United States, 0.9 to 2.8% of affected children will die from sudden cardiac death (coronary thrombosis, ruptured aneurysm, myocardial infarction) or, less often, from congestive heart failure [26].

■ Pathological Features

Because of the self-limited nature of the ocular involvement with Kawasaki syndrome, relatively few cases involving histopathology are available. Conjunctival biopsies have shown mild inflammation of the subconjunctival connective tissue with polymorphonuclear and plasma cells. These conjunctival findings are nonspecific but can rule out Stevens-

Johnson syndrome when special immunohistochemical staining is performed [3].

Autopsies of fatal cases have revealed abnormalities of the retinal vasculature, uvea, and sclera. Vasculitis of the ophthalmic artery with central retinal artery occlusion and ischemia of inner retina has been reported in 1 fatal case [27]. Diffuse polymorphous inflammatory infiltrate throughout the uvea, including the iris and ciliary body, has been reported in other cases. The inflammation consisted of lymphocytes, plasma cells, and occasional polymorphonuclear cells. Focal inflammation of sclera with vasculitis of the episclera has also been reported [28].

Reports of systemic pathological abnormalities have been more numerous. Frequent findings have included focal arteritis of primary branches of the aorta, including the coronary, splenic, renal, pulmonary, mesenteric, and hepatic arteries. Inflammation is typically confined to the arterial media, with focal necrosis and aneurysm formation. Granulomas and giant cells are not seen. Some cases of sudden death have shown thrombosis within vessel lumina [29]. Other cardiac lesions include pericarditis, myocarditis, and valvulitis. Despite angiographic evidence of resolution of aneurysms, mural lesions may remain for life and may play a role in coronary atherosclerosis [23, 24, 30]. The lifelong consequences of these lesions are not known.

Other systemic findings include smaller thymus, with depletion of the thymus lymphocytes during acute illness [31].

Kawasaki syndrome may be identical to a pathological syndrome, infantile periarteritis nodosa, that was described in 1958 [29]. This syndrome was characterized as a polyarteritis with fatal coronary artery lesions identical to those seen in Kawasaki syndrome.

Immunological abnormalities in Kawasaki syndrome include lymphocytosis with polyclonal increase in B cells [32], polyclonal increase in IgG and IgA production [33, 34], and normal or reduced total T cells with an increase in the T4/T8 (helper-suppressor) ratio [35]. An increase in the expression of the Ia-DR antigen, interpreted as activation of the T4 cell line, has been measured [34].

Serum acute-phase reactants and lymphokines, including tumor necrosis factor, interleukin 1A, cryoprecipitate, and C-reactive protein have also been detected.

Studies of the HLA typing of patients in Japan and Israel have revealed evidence of HLA-Bw22 association [36]. However, this has not been confirmed in the U.S. population.

■ Etiological Features

Much of the epidemiological evidence suggests an infectious etiology for Kawasaki syndrome. Communitywide epidemics, the acute course of the illness, and the young age of patients all imply an infectious etiology. Proposed mechanisms have included bacteria-mediated or bacterial toxin–mediated causes. However, there has been no serological or cultural evidence of known streptococcal or staphylococcal toxin or toxin-producing infection reproducibly associated with the syndrome [16, 37]. *Propionibacterium acnes,* a ubiquitous organism normally considered non-pathogenic, has been isolated from the lymph nodes of affected patients. The organism has been proposed to produce a toxin, although none has been identified. A coronary vasculitis similar to Kawasaki syndrome is produced by inoculating mice with *Lactobacillus casei* cell wall extract [38].

Soon after the syndrome was first reported, a rickettsialike organism was observed by electron microscopy of tissues from infected patients. However, serological tests to known rickettsiae are negative, no organism has been isolated, and Kawasaki syndrome is unresponsive to antibiotics [18].

Search for a viral etiology has been less fruitful. All serological and culture studies of viruses, including adenovirus, parainfluenza, coronavirus, rotavirus, herpesvirus, and retrovirus, have shown no consistent association [26, 38–41].

An arthropod vector has been proposed by some investigators, and the association with recent carpet shampoo in the patient's home has been used as epidemiological supporting evidence [19]. Antibodies to house-dust mite have been reported in a small series [20]. The association with nearby surface water in one epidemic may implicate a mosquito or other waterborne vector [41].

In contrast to the evidence for an infectious cause of Kawasaki syndrome, an autoimmune mechanism is supported mostly by laboratory findings. An increased T4/T8 (helper-suppressor) ratio with increased T-cell activation suggests a regulatory abnormality of the T-cell line [42]. The increase in circulating B cells and antibodies as well as lymphokines may be secondary to abnormal regulatory effects of the T cells. The experimental effect of circulating lymphokines in inducing HLA expression on endothelial cells has been proposed as a cause of the vasculitis [43]. Kawasaki syndrome serum has been found to be experimentally cytotoxic against stimulated endothelial cells, probably via an antibody pathway [44]. Circulating immune complexes may also damage endothelial cells, either directly or via platelet activation [45]. Abnormal antineutrophil cytoplasm antibodies (ANCA) have been reported [46], but usually antinuclear antibody and rheumatoid factor serological findings are negative. ANCA are also seen in Wegener's granulomatosis, a vasculitis syndrome of presumed autoimmune etiology involving the conjunctiva, mucosa of paranasal sinuses, and kidneys.

The association with HLA-Bw22 also suggests an autoimmune role in the disease.

■ Treatment

After many unsuccessful trials of steroids and antibiotics, high-dose intravenous gamma globulin was found to be effective in reducing dramatically the rate of coronary artery involvement. First reported anecdotally, this therapy has been studied in a well-controlled U.S. study and confirmed to reduce the rate of coronary lesions from 23 to 8%. Japanese studies have shown a reduction of the lesions from 42 to 15% in an Oriental population [47]. The dose used, 400 mg/kg/day for 4 consecutive days starting within 10 days of onset of fever, was arrived at empirically and is currently under investigation. Single-dose immunoglobulin therapy was effective in an uncontrolled trial [48]. Immunoglobulin therapy dramatically reduces fever, conjunctivitis, leukocytosis, and leftward shift as well as other signs of Kawasaki syndrome, often after the first dose [49].

The mechanism of activity of gamma globulin therapy is not completely understood. Because the causative agent of Kawasaki syndrome is not known, a direct antietiological agent effect of the infused antibodies is one possibility. If the agent is common and induces humoral immunity, pooled gamma globulin may impart immunity (e.g., as in hepatitis A). The antibodies may also block nonspecific Fc receptors on lymphocytes and macrophages, inhibiting immune activation and function. Direct inhibition of lymphokine production and inhibition of the stimulated expression of endothelial antigens may also play a role. Experimental studies have shown no effect of the therapy on IgG production, in vitro coagulation parameters, and circulating immune complexes [50].

Aspirin has been used with gamma globulin to reduce platelet aggregation, but aspirin alone is not effective in reducing the incidence of coronary artery aneurysm formation [51]. Typically, high doses of aspirin (30 to 100 mg/kg/day) are required to affect platelet function. In addition, Kawasaki syndrome may cause poor gastrointestinal absorption of the aspirin, reducing serum levels of the drug [52].

■ Conclusion

Much remains to be learned about the enigmatic Kawasaki syndrome. Investigation into the etiological agent is still in the early stages. There are as yet no specific diagnostic tests, and the condition remains a clinical syndrome. For this reason, consulting ophthalmologists are in a unique position to assist in prompt diagnosis of this potentially treatable condition. The prominent and early findings, including anterior uveitis and bilateral conjunctival injection sparing the limbus, should suggest this syndrome in acutely ill children and initiate prompt ophthalmological evaluation. Unexplained high fever, rash, peripheral edema, oral mucosal changes, and adenopathy are other important signs. Morbidity is due primarily to coronary arteritis, which is found in up to 20% of patients in the United States. Treatment with gamma globulin is effective in reducing coronary artery abnormalities if therapy is begun promptly.

■ References

1. Kawasaki T, Kosaki F, Okawa S, et al. A new infantile acute febrile mucocutaneous lymph node syndrome (MLNS) prevailing in Japan. Pediatrics 1974;54:271–276
2. Ammerman SD, Rao MS, Shope TC, Ragsdale CG. Diagnostic uncertainty in atypical Kawasaki disease, and a new finding: exudative conjunctivitis. Pediatr Infect Dis 1985;4:210–211
3. Puglise JV, Rao NA, Weiss RA, et al. Ocular features of Kawasaki's disease. Arch Ophthalmol 1982;100:1101–1103
4. Smith LBH, Newburger JW, Burns JC. Kawasaki disease and the eye. Med Times 1989;117:39–42
5. Rennebohm RM, Burke MJ, Crowe W, Levinson JE. Anterior uveitis in Kawasaki's disease. Am J Ophthalmol 1981;91:535–537
6. Smith LBH, Newburger JW, Burns JC. Kawasaki syndrome and the eye. Pediatr Infect Dis J 1989;8:116–118
7. Burns JC, Joffe L, Sargent RA, Glode MP. Anterior uveitis associated with Kawasaki syndrome. Pediatr Infect Dis J 1985;4:258–261
8. Germain BF, Moroney JD, Guggino GS, et al. Anterior uveitis in Kawasaki disease. J Pediatr 1980;97:780–781
9. Jacob JL, Polomeno RC, Chad Z, Lapointe N. Ocular manifestations of Kawasaki disease (mucocutaneous lymph node syndrome). Can J Ophthalmol 1982;17:199–202
10. Lapointe N, Chad Z, Lacroix J, et al. Kawasaki disease: association with uveitis in seven patients. Pediatrics 1982;69:376–379
11. Ohno S, Miyajima T, Higuchi M, et al. Ocular manifestations of Kawasaki disease (mucocutaneous lymph node syndrome). Am J Ophthalmol 1982;93:713–717
12. Ryan EH, Walton DS. Conjunctival scarring in Kawasaki disease: a new finding? J Pediatr Ophthalmol Strabismus 1983;20:106–108
13. Verghote M, Rousseau E, Jacob JL, Lapointe N. An uncommon clinical sign in mucocutaneous lymph node syndrome. Acta Paediatr Scand 1981;70:591–593
14. Sheagren JN. Staphylococcal infections. In: Wyngaarden JB, Smith LH Jr, eds. Cecil textbook of medicine, ed 17. Philadelphia: Saunders, 1985:1543–1551
15. Wong ML, Kaplan S, Dunkle LM, et al. Leptospirosis: a childhood disease. J Pediatr 1977;90:532–537
16. Bell DM, Brink EW, Nitzkin JL, et al. Kawasaki syndrome: description of two outbreaks in the United States. N Engl J Med 1981;304:1568–1575
17. Yanagawa H, Kawasaki T, Shigematsu I. Nationwide survey on Kawasaki disease in Japan. Pediatrics 1987;80:58–62
18. Wortmann DW, Nelson AM. Kawasaki syndrome. Rheum Dis Clin North Am 1990;16:363–375
19. Ichida F, Fatica NS, O'Loughlin JE, et al. Epidemiologic aspects of Kawasaki disease in a Manhattan hospital. Pediatrics 1989;84:235–241
20. Fatica NS, Ichida F, Engle MA, Lesser ML. Rug shampoo and Kawasaki disease. Pediatrics 1989;84:231–234
21. Fujita Y, Nakamura Y, Sakata K, et al. Kawasaki disease in families. Pediatrics 1989;84:666–669

22. Hewitt M, Smith LJ, Joffe HS, Chambers TL. Kawasaki disease in siblings. Arch Dis Child 1989;64:398–399

23. Suzuki A, Kamiya T, Ono Y, et al. Aortocoronary bypass surgery for coronary arterial lesions resulting from Kawasaki disease. J Pediatr 1990;116:567–573

24. Suzuki A, Kamiya T, Ono Y, et al. Myocardial ischemia in Kawasaki disease: follow-up study by cardiac catheterization and coronary angiography. Pediatr Cardiol 1988;9:1–5

25. Tatara K, Kusakawa S, Itoh K, et al. Long-term prognosis of Kawasaki disease patients with coronary artery obstruction. Heart Vessels 1989;5:47–51

26. Morens DM, Anderson LJ, Hurwitz ES. National surveillance of Kawasaki disease. Pediatrics 1980;65:21–25

27. Font RL, Mehta RS, Streusand SB, et al. Bilateral retinal ischemia in Kawasaki disease: postmortem findings and electron microscopic observations. Ophthalmology 1983;90:569–577

28. Googe JM Jr, Brady SE, Argyle JC, et al. Choroiditis in infantile periarteritis nodosa. Arch Ophthalmol 1985;103:81–83

29. Landing BH, Larson EJ. Are infantile periarteritis nodosa with coronary artery involvement and fatal mucocutaneous lymph node syndrome the same? Comparison of 20 patients from North America with patients from Hawaii and Japan. Pediatrics 1977;59:651–662

30. Tanaka N, Naoe S, Masuda H, Ueno T. Pathological study of sequelae of Kawasaki disease (MCLS): with special reference to the heart and coronary lesions. Acta Pathol Jpn 1986;36:1513–1527

31. Yanagihara R, Todd JK. Acute febrile mucocutaneous lymph node syndrome. Am J Dis Child 1980;134:603–614

32. Barron K, DeCunto C, Montalvo J, et al. Abnormalities of immunoregulation in Kawasaki disease. J Rheumatol 1988;15:1243–1249

33. Kawamori J, Miyake T, Yoshida T. B cell function in Kawasaki disease and the effect of high-dose gamma-globulin therapy. Acta Paediatr Jpn [overseas ed] 1989;31:537–543

34. Leung DYM, Siegal RL, Grady S, et al. Immunoregulatory abnormalities in mucocutaneous lymph node syndrome. Clin Immunol Immunopathol 1982;23:100–112

35. Leung DYM, Chu ET, Wood N, et al. Immunoregulatory T-cell abnormalities in mucocutaneous lymph node syndrome. J Immnuol 1983;130:2002–2003

36. Kato S, Kimura M, Ysuji K, et al. HLA antigens in Kawasaki disease. Pediatrics 1978;61:252–255

37. Abe Y, Nakano S, Nakahara T, et al. Detection of serum antibody by the antimitogen assay against streptococcal erythrogenic toxins: age distributions in children and the relation to Kawasaki disease. Pediatr Res 1990;27:11–15

38. Bannister BA, Edwards S, Ibata G. Aetiology of Kawasaki disease. Arch Dis Child 1989;64:397–398

39. Brosius CL, Newburger JW, Burns JC, et al. Increased prevalence of atopic dermatitis in Kawasaki disease. Pediatr Infect Dis J 1988;7:863–866

40. Marchette NJ, Melish ME, Hicks R, et al. Epstein-Barr virus and other herpesvirus infections in Kawasaki syndrome. J Infect Dis 1990;161:680–684

41. Rauch AM, Kaplan SL, Nihill MR, et al. Kawasaki syndrome clusters in Harris County, Texas, and eastern North Carolina: a high endemic rate and a new environmental risk factor. Am J Dis Child 1988;142:441–444

42. Leung DYM. Clinical and immunologic aspects of Kawasaki disease. Immunodefic Rev 1989;1:261–271

43. Leung DYM, Geha RS, Newburger JW, et al. Two monokines, interleukin 1 and tumor necrosis factor, render cultured vascular endothelial cells susceptible to lysis by antibodies circulating during Kawasaki syndrome. J Exp Med 1986;164:1958–1972

44. Leung DY, Cotran RS, Kurt-Jones E, et al. Endothelial cell activation and high interleukin-1 secretion in the pathogenesis of acute Kawasaki disease. J Allergy Clin Immunol 1989;84:588–594

45. Salo E, Kekomaki R, Pelkonen P, et al. Kawasaki disease: monitoring of circulating immune complexes. Eur J Pediatr 1988;147:377–380

46. Savage COS, Tizard J, Jayne D, et al. Antineutrophil cytoplasm antibodies in Kawasaki disease. Arch Dis Child 1989;65:360–363

47. Furusho K, Kamiya T, Nakano H, et al. High-dose intravenous gammaglobulin for Kawasaki disease. Lancet 1984;2:1055–1058

48. Engle MA, Fatica NS, Bussel JB, et al. Clinical trial of single dose intravenous gamma globulin in acute Kawasaki disease. Am J Dis Child 1989;143:1300–1304

49. Glode MP, Joffe LS, Wiggins J Jr, et al. Effect of intravenous immune globulin on the coagulopathy of Kawasaki syndrome. J Pediatr 1989;115:469–473

50. Newburger JW, Takahashi M, Burns JC, et al. The treatment of Kawasaki syndrome with intravenous gamma globulin. N Engl J Med 1986;315:341–347

51. Bierman FZ, Gersony WM. Kawasaki disease: clinical perspective. J Pediatr 1987;111:789–793

52. Rowley AH, Duffy CE, Shulman ST, et al. Prevention of giant coronary aneurysms in Kawasaki disease by intravenous gamma globulin therapy. J Pediatr 1988;113:290–294

Congenital Corneal Opacities

■■■■■■■■ Paul R. Cotran, M.D.
■■■■■■■■ Ann M. Bajart, M.D.

The discovery of a corneal opacity in a newborn child calls for prompt diagnosis and treatment. The risk of amblyopia is high, and bilateral disease may result in a lifetime of poor vision. In addition, the corneal findings may be manifestations of an otherwise occult systemic disease. Although uncommon, congenital corneal opacities have a broad differential diagnosis of which the ophthalmologist should be aware.

■ Congenital Glaucoma

Congenital primary glaucoma presents with elevated intraocular pressure that may be unilateral or bilateral, and often with increased corneal diameter, optic nerve cupping (often reversible), and corneal opacities. The corneal findings include breaks in Descemet's membrane, which are often peripheral and arcuate or paracentral and horizontal. Corneal edema and haze may overlie the break. Although congenital glaucoma is one of the more common origins of corneal opacity in the neonate, it will not be discussed further in this chapter.

■ Birth Trauma

Traumatic rupture of Descemet's membrane and endothelium during a difficult forceps delivery is less common today than it used to be (Fig 1). Modern obstetrical practice discourages high-forceps or midforceps delivery in which the forceps are applied while the fetal head is still high in the birth canal. It is often difficult for the obstetrician to place the forceps tips accurately around the head so as to avoid the facial structures.

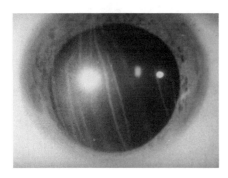

Figure 1 *Birth trauma. Multiple linear ruptures of Descemet's membrane are seen. The photograph was taken after reendotheli-alization had occurred, and the stroma is compact. (Courtesy of Dr. Kenneth R. Kenyon.)*

Inadvertent application of the blade across the orbit and globe can cause a blunt deformation injury or even rupture of the globe. The injury is usually unilateral and associated with other soft-tissue facial trauma, such as ecchymoses, contusions, and lacerations of the skin. In contrast to the type of striae present in congenital glaucoma, the tears in Descemet's membrane in forceps injuries are usually central and vertical or oblique, following the plane of application of the forceps blade across the cornea. The degree of corneal opacification and edema is variable; it may be clinically apparent several hours after birth and is located anterior to the rupture of Descemet's membrane. The edema and opacification tend to resolve, but permanent visual loss due to high astigmatic errors can occur. In these cases, the axis of the astigmatic cylinder is often oblique, and the steep meridian parallels the striae. The edges of the torn Descemet's membrane often persist as visible ridges or scrolls projecting posteriorly from the back of the cornea. Fortunately, other ocular injury, such as hyphema or retinal detachment, appears to be rarely associated.

■ Infectious Diseases

Viral diseases affecting the cornea in the neonate include rubella and herpetic keratitis. Congenital rubella is caused by transplacental infection with a togavirus in the first trimester [1]. Fifty percent of rubella infections during the first month of pregnancy lead to abnormal offspring, compared with 22% during the second month and 6% during the third month [2]. The most recent epidemic in the United States was in 1963 to 1964, prior to the introduction of the rubella vaccine, which is now routinely administered within the first 2 years of life. The ocular findings in congenital rubella syndrome include cataract, chorioretinopathy, iris hypoplasia and other iris anomalies, microphthalmos, glaucoma, and corneal haze [1]. The corneal haze, which is common and of variable severity, may occur if the lens touches the cornea, if the intraocular pressure is elevated, or if keratitis is present. In most cases, the idiopathic corneal haze has no obvious cause and tends to clear with time [2].

Herpes simplex virus (HSV) types 1 and 2 can be contracted perinatally. Of cases with ocular involvement in which virus was typed, 10 of 16 (63%) were HSV type 2 [3]. Of 297 babies infected with HSV, 51 (17%) had ocular involvement and 19 (6%) had keratitis. The keratitis can be seen within 1 or 2 days and may be bilateral. It represents a primary ocular infection, not a recurrence. Clinical findings can include diffuse opacification, ulceration, and vascularization of the cornea, spotty stromal infiltrates, or dendritic lesions of the epithelium. The keratitis usually occurs together with conjunctivitis but may be independent of skin, visceral, and central nervous system (CNS) involvement (Fig 2). Treatment is with topical antivirals such as trifluorothymidine (Viroptic) or vidarabine (adenine arabinoside); acyclovir is used systemically if evidence of other organ involvement (including skin) is noted. Any neonate with herpetic keratoconjunctivitis must be monitored carefully, as more than half will develop disseminated disease with high morbidity. Neonatal prophylaxis of eyes has been recommended in babies known to have passed through an infected birth canal [3]. Children can develop recurrent herpetic keratitis after the neonatal primary infection.

Bacterial keratitis in the newborn period is uncommon, is usually associated with corneal epithelial trauma or ophthalmia neonatorum (purulent conjunctivitis), and is caused by a variety of gram-positive and gram-negative organisms.

Neisseria gonorrhoeae acquired during passage through the birth canal causes a fulminant conjunctivitis and keratitis, usually appearing within the first week of life. The resulting corneal opacities may be dense and visually significant, and they may persist after antibacterial therapy. Topical silver nitrate or erythromycin are effective prophylactics. Currently recommended treatment of ocular and nonocular gonococcal infections in newborns is a single intramuscular dose of 125 mg ceftriaxone, or 75 mg of intramuscular kanamycin combined with either topical gentamicin or tetracycline ointment [4].

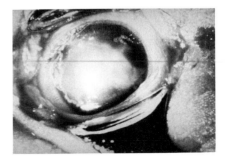

Figure 2 *Geographical epithelial defect in neonatal herpes simplex keratoconjunctivitis. (Courtesy of Dr. Kenneth R. Kenyon.)*

Syphilis can be acquired in utero or during birth. Congenital syphilis may present with ocular findings of iritis and retinitis, but the cornea is clear at birth. The interstitial keratitis of Hutchinson's triad (congenital syphilis with deafness, interstitial keratitis, and barrel-shaped central incisors) is not usually seen until the child is several years old. A pigmentary retinopathy may also be present.

Protozoal eye disease of the newborn due to *Chlamydia trachomatis* is acquired from maternal cervical infection. Infected infants usually develop chlamydial ophthalmia during the first 5 to 21 days of life and present with a mucopurulent conjunctivitis and, occasionally, a keratitis. Conjunctival scarring and neovascularization can occur if treatment is delayed, but visual loss is rare. Prophylaxis is treated with topical erythromycin; ophthalmia is treated with oral erythromycin (40 to 50 mg/kg/day for 3 weeks). The infection is systemic, and the incidence of chlamydial pneumonitis is high.

■ Developmental Anomalies

Anterior Segment Dysgenesis Syndromes

Anterior segment dysgenesis syndromes are associated with a variety of congenital corneal abnormalities. Earlier authors referred to a group of clinically overlapping anterior segment developmental anomalies as the *anterior segment cleavage syndrome* [5]; this term, however, is inaccurate, because embryologically there is no development of a cleavage plane as the anterior segment forms and differentiates and because the various anomalies never occur all together, as should occasionally be expected of a true syndrome. Development of the anterior segment [6, 7] involves first the separation posteriorly of the lens vesicle from the surface ectoderm, which then becomes the corneal epithelium. Three successive waves of neural crest–derived cells then invade the primary mesenchyme that lies behind the ectoderm. The first of these gives rise to corneal endothelium, the second to corneal stroma, and the third becomes the iris stroma. Anterior chamber angle structures are also derived from neural crest cells. At birth, the angle is incompletely differentiated, whereas the cornea is almost completely developed. The angle continues to differentiate through the first year. It is probable that the disorders described next are due to abnormalities in this developmental process.

Sclerocornea

Sclerocornea is a scleralization and vascularization of the anterior surface of the globe, associated with corneal flattening (cornea plana) and loss of limbal landmarks (Fig 3). Stromal collagen fibers are thicker than in normal cornea, and the regular lamellar orientation is absent [8]. Often there is relative clearing centrally, and the degree of opacification is vari-

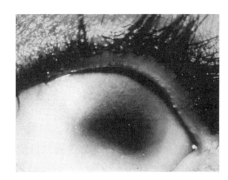

Figure 3 *Sclerocornea. In this incomplete case, there is clear cornea centrally, loss of limbal differentiation, and cornea plana.*

able. The condition is frequently bilateral, usually sporadic, and always nonprogressive. Anterior chamber angle anomalies are commonly associated [9]. Sclerocornea is associated with trisomies 13 and 18 [10].

Posterior Embryotoxon

Posterior embryotoxon is an anterior displacement and thickening of Schwalbe's line (the normal junction of Descemet's membrane, corneal endothelium, and trabecular meshwork), which is seen in approximately 10% of normals, in anterior segment dysgenesis anomalies, and in Alagille's syndrome. It is most visible in the horizontal meridian and appears as a gray, translucent, arcuate or scalloped membrane on the posterior cornea just inside the limbus.

Axenfeld's and Rieger's Anomaly

Axenfeld's and Rieger's anomaly and syndrome (*syndrome* implying the presence of glaucoma) are well defined clinically, but controversy exists regarding their pathogenesis [6, 7, 11]. Most agree that an intrauterine accident or genetically programmed abnormality occurs early in ocular development, which affects the differentiation, proliferation, or migration of the neural crest cells that form the corneal stroma, endothelium, iris, and angle structures. An anterior displacement and prominence of Schwalbe's line (*posterior embryotoxon*) with attached strands of iris is eponymically known as *Axenfeld's anomaly*. The presence, in addition, of severe iris atrophy and corectopia (sometimes with ectropion uveae or pseudopolycoria) is called *Rieger's anomaly* (Fig 4). *Iridogoniodysgenesis* is a term that has been used to describe an intermediate condition characterized by posterior embryotoxon with iris strands in the angle, malformed angle structures, and atrophy of the anterior iris stroma without corectopia. Corneal leukomas may occur peripherally in Axenfeld's or Rieger's anomaly. Glaucomatous corneal clouding may be seen in Axenfeld's or Rieger's *syndrome,* as 50% or more of these patients will develop glaucoma. Axenfeld's

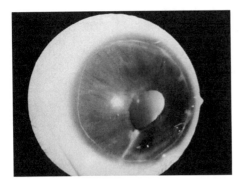

Figure 4 *Rieger's anomaly. The combination of posterior embryotoxon, iris atrophy, and corectopia is typical. (Courtesy of Dr. Kenneth R. Kenyon.)*

and, more commonly, Rieger's anomaly can often be found together with facial, dental, and skeletal abnormalities (e.g., hypertelorism [12]). A few cases have been reported in patients with chromosome 6 abnormalities [12].

Peters' Anomaly

Peters' anomaly [5] is a congenital central leukoma with central defects in the posterior stroma, Descemet's membrane, and endothelium. Iris synechiae from the collarette to the periphery of the corneal opacity are frequently present (Fig 5). Many believe that this anomaly is pathogenetically closely related to Axenfeld-Rieger's anomaly [13]. Others believe that it is distinct and due to abnormal separation of the lens vesicle from the ectoderm or to secondary atrophy of endothelium centrally due to anterior displacement of the lens [14, 15]. Keratolenticular contact is often seen, and some authors use this feature to distinguish type 1 (without lens contact) from type 2 (with lens contact) [16]. Type 1 is often consistent with good vision although, if unilateral, amblyopia may develop. Type 1 may be unilateral or bilateral, is usually sporadic, and usually is not associated

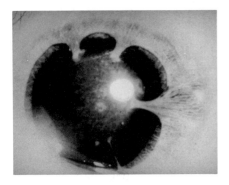

Figure 5 *Peters' anomaly, type 1. The iris has been pharmacologically dilated to demonstrate its synechial attachments to the border of a central corneal leukoma. There is no lenticular contact. (Courtesy of Dr. Kenneth R. Kenyon.)*

with other ocular or systemic pathological processes. Type 2 is visually more severe, as there is often glaucoma (>50%), dense cataract, denser corneal opacity, and bilaterality. Most cases also show other ocular malformations, such as microphthalmos and persistent hyperplastic primary vitreous, as well as other systemic anomalies. It may be that type 2 represents a more severe version of the same type of insult causing type 1, or they may have very different pathogeneses.

Corneal Staphylomas

Corneal (anterior) staphylomas are corneal ectasias accompanying, in most cases, a severely malformed anterior segment with iris adherent to posterior cornea. The cornea may protrude beyond the eyelids and be superficially keratinized. The visual prognosis is dismal. Keratolenticular contact, microphakia, and cataract are frequent. The cause is usually unknown but may be an intrauterine corneal infection and perforation or an extreme version of Peters' anomaly [16].

Corneal and Limbal Choristomas

Choristomas of the cornea and limbus are benign, nonprogressive, congenital tumors that contain epithelial, dermal, or lacrimal structures not normally found in these locations. The most common corneal choristoma, the limbal dermoid, is firm, elevated, well-demarcated, and white to tan in color (Fig 6). Limbal dermoids may be from 2 to 15 mm in diameter, single or several, and visually significant if they extend into the prepupillary cornea or cause a high degree of corneal astigmatism. Most are located inferiorly and do not respect Bowman's membrane but extend into the stroma. They are sometimes associated with eyelid colobomas (notched defects) as part of a presumed aberrant fetal lid fissure development. Ultrastructurally, they are covered by stratified squamous epithelium, are variably keratinized, and have a dense, collagenous stroma containing hair follicles and sweat and sebaceous glands. Bilateral and multiple dermoids

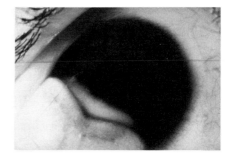

Figure 6 *Limbal dermoid. There is a bifid dermoid at the inferotemporal limbus with a cilium. The band of corneal lipid deposition anterior to the dermoid is commonly seen.*

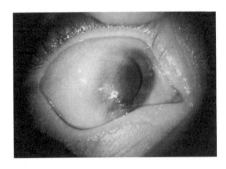

Figure 7 *Complex choristoma. The histology of this lesion revealed lacrimal gland acini as well as adipose and pilosebaceous structures.*

and dermolipomas occur in children with Goldenhar's syndrome (oculoauriculovertebral dysplasia). Due to the often deep extension into the stroma, treatment of these lesions is frequently by "shaving" rather than by complete excision.

Dermatolipomas are yellowish pink, soft, fleshy tumors usually found on the conjunctiva, often extending along the recti muscles, but they may also be limbal. They contain large amounts of adipose tissue in the stroma but otherwise look like dermoids histologically.

Complex choristomas may also contain elements of lacrimal gland, bone, cartilage, and muscle (Fig 7) [17].

Congenital corneal keloids [18] are rare lesions that are hyperproliferations of fibrous tissue derived from corneal keratocytes. These appear as glistening white corneal masses and, when congenital, are sporadic and without known cause.

Dystrophies

Congenital corneal dystrophies [14] are uncommon. Congenital hereditary endothelial dystrophy (CHED) causes diffuse bilateral corneal edema that may progress to a ground-glass appearance (Fig 8) [19]. The cornea may be very thickened by stromal edema (Fig 9). The most consistent pathological change is a severe dystrophy or absence of the endothelium

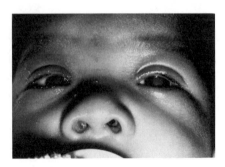

Figure 8 *Congenital hereditary endothelial dystrophy. This infant has a bilateral "groundglass" opacification of the cornea with normal intraocular pressures. (Courtesy of the Department of Ophthalmology, Children's Hospital, Boston, MA.)*

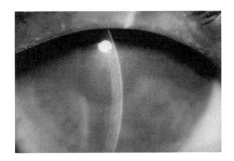

Figure 9 *Congenital hereditary endothelial dystrophy. In this adult, there is severe diffuse stromal edema. (Courtesy of Dr. Kenneth R. Kenyon.)*

[20]. The intraocular pressures are normal. Autosomal dominant and autosomal recessive pedigrees have been reported; in the former, corneal opacification is less severe and begins in the first or second year, thus not being truly congenital [21]. Since corneal endothelium is a neural crest–derived tissue, some authors believe that the endothelial dystrophies are closely related to the anterior segment dysgenesis syndromes [22].

Congenital hereditary stromal dystrophy (CHSD) is known from a small number of autosomal dominant pedigrees in which bilateral corneal clouding is noted at birth in affected patients. The stromal opacities are "feathery," nonprogressive, and associated with normal stromal thickness and a normal endothelium and Descemet's membrane [23].

Posterior polymorphous dystrophy is a familial disorder, usually inherited as an autosomal dominant trait, although some autosomal recessive families have been reported [24]. This condition is probably present at birth, although the corneal opacities have rarely been described in infants. The opacities are multiple, irregularly shaped, gray blebs at the level of Descemet's membrane; they may increase slowly in number and coalesce over years. Although usually asymptomatic, endothelial degeneration and secondary stromal edema may occur. Some affected pedigrees have had other features (e.g., endothelial cell abnormalities, iridocorneal adhesions) that suggest that this disease may also be an anterior segment dysgenesis syndrome. There have been reports [25] of families in which posterior polymorphous dystrophy was associated with Alport syndrome (hereditary nephritis and sensorineural hearing loss), suggesting a common defect in basement membrane formation.

■ Metabolic Diseases

Mucopolysaccharidoses (MPSs) cause corneal clouding by pathological accumulation of glycosaminoglycans (dermatan, heparan, or keratan sulfates) in the cells and extracellular matrix of the cornea. A number of different syndromes characterized by distinct defects in lysosomal acid hydrolases have been described. Conjunctival biopsy is frequently an important diagnostic procedure in these disorders, as is measurement of glycosaminoglycans in urine. The corneal pathological findings consist of intracytoplasmic vacuoles in stromal keratocytes, histiocytes, epithelium, and endothelium [24, 26]. MPS I-H (Hurler's syndrome) presents with early, progressive, corneal clouding, which occurs in virtually all affected children and is often severe. The cornea is diffusely involved with fine, punctate, stromal opacities (Fig 10). The epithelium and endothelium appear normal initially. MPS I-S (Scheie's syndrome) is due to the same enzymatic defect as Hurler's but has no facial, skeletal, or mental abnormality and is believed to be an allelic variant of Hurler's. MPS II A and II B (Hunter's syndrome) are X-linked disorders; all the other mucopolysaccharidoses are autosomal recessive. Corneal clouding tends to be clinically less significant or absent, particularly in II A. MPS III (A through D) are due to four distinct enzymatic defects, all causing Sanfilippo's syndrome, which can produce a mild corneal haze. MPS IV (Morquio's syndrome) has variable corneal clouding that is usually not apparent until the child is several years old. MPS VI (Maroteaux-Lamy syndrome) is similar to Hurler's, with a diffuse stromal haze frequently observed, and often is associated with increased corneal thickness. MPS VII (Sly syndrome) is due to a deficiency of beta-glucuronidase. Corneal clouding occurs in the majority of severely affected infants but has not been reported before the age of 7 months [26].

Mucolipidoses are due to a deficiency of neuraminidase and are inherited in an autosomal recessive manner. Histologically, the affected cells display vacuolization of the cytoplasm; the vacuoles contain granular or fibrillar (sometimes membranous) inclusions. Conjunctival biopsy can aid in diagnosis. Corneal opacities occur in types I, III, and IV. Type I may present with corneal clouding in all layers of the cornea, but it is rarely prominent at birth. Type IV presents with prominent corneal opacification at birth or in early infancy, affecting the epithelium and anterior stroma, especially centrally. Vision may be severely affected. Corneal changes may be the only sign of this disease in the first year of life. This disorder has been described primarily in Ashkenazi Jews [26].

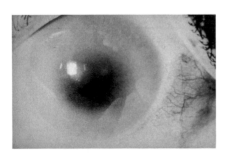

Figure 10 *Hurler's syndrome (MPS I-H). The cornea is clouded by confluent fine stromal opacities that are encroaching on the visual axis. (Courtesy of Dr. Kenneth R. Kenyon.)*

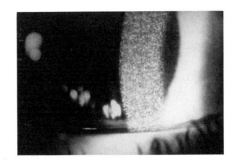

Figure 11 *Cystinosis. Refractile crystals of cystine are seen throughout the stroma. (Courtesy of Dr. Kenneth R. Kenyon.)*

Gangliosidosis type I (GM_1) is caused by a deficiency of beta-galactosidase. Mild infantile corneal opacification has been reported.

Cystinosis is a rare disorder caused by intracellular lysosomal accumulation of free cystine in a variety of tissues (Fig 11). The infantile form is associated with Fanconi's syndrome and is autosomal recessive in its inheritance. In all forms of cystinosis, refractile crystals of cystine can be noted in the cornea (especially peripherally) and conjunctiva as early as 6 months of age.

Tyrosinosis type II is an autosomal recessive disease caused by a deficiency of the enzyme tyrosine aminotransferase. Ocular symptoms and findings may present before two weeks of age as keratoconjunctivitis with bilateral superficial punctate crystalline corneal opacities, which may assume a dendritiform pattern. The irregular corneal epithelium may break down, leading to an ulcerative keratitis that may be misdiagnosed as herpetic. Dietary restriction of phenylalanine and tyrosine results in complete reversal of ocular findings [27].

■ Management of the Infant with a Corneal Opacity

Prompt diagnosis of an infantile corneal opacity is of the essence. If there is redness or discharge, one should consider infectious causes, culture appropriately, and treat. Rubella and HSV serum antibody titers may be helpful. In many cases, examination under anesthesia is necessary to measure intraocular pressures and perform slit-lamp examination, gonioscopy, or funduscopy. In the presence of a persistent central opacity or induced corneal irregularity or astigmatism, prevention of amblyopia is a major concern. In addition to frequent vision monitoring, correction of refractive errors and occlusion therapy are often involved.

Penetrating keratoplasty has a lower long-term success rate in young children than in adults [28, 29]. The technical difficulties are considerable. The patients have small eyes, low scleral rigidity, vitreous pressure and, often, associated anatomical defects or glaucoma. Postoperatively, iritis is often exuberant, rejection is a constant threat, and cataract may develop secondary to chronic steroid use. Follow-up examinations (intraocular pressures, slit-lamp examinations) are needed frequently and are difficult to perform. Patient compliance and understanding are minimal, and thus the parent or caretaker must be educated to note signs of discomfort or change in the status of the eye and must be relied on to administer medications and accompany the child on frequent visits to the doctor. A lamellar (partial-thickness) keratoplasty is particularly useful for removal of dermoids but is inadequate for most vision-threatening congenital corneal opacities because of endothelial involvement.

■ References

1. Boniuk V. Systemic and ocular manifestations of the rubella syndrome. Int Ophthalmol Clin 1972;12:67–76
2. Boniuk V, Boniuk M. The congenital rubella syndrome. Int Ophthalmol Clin 1968;8:487–514
3. Nahmias AJ, Visintine AM, Caldwell DR, et al. Eye infections with herpes simplex viruses in neonates. Surv Ophthalmol 1976;21:100–105
4. Laga M, Naamara W, Brunham RC, et al. Single-dose therapy of gonococcal ophthalmia neonatorum with ceftriaxone. N Engl J Med 1986;315:1382–1385
5. Townsend WM, Font RL, Zimmerman LE. Congenital corneal leukomas: II. Histopathologic findings in 19 eyes with central defect in Descemet's membrane. Am J Ophthalmol 1974;77:192–206
6. Waring GO III, Rodrigues MM, Laibson PR. Anterior chamber cleavage syndrome: a stepladder classification. Surv Ophthalmol 1975;20:3–27
7. Wilson ME. Congenital iris ectropion and a new classification for anterior segment dysgenesis. J Pediatr Ophthalmol Strabismus 1990;27:48–55
8. Kanai A, Wood TC, Polack FM, et al. The fine structure of sclerocornea. Invest Ophthalmol Vis Sci 1971;10:687–694
9. Friedman AH, Weingeist S, Brackup A, et al. Sclerocornea and defective mesodermal migration. Br J Ophthalmol 1975;59:683–687
10. Goldstein JE, Cogan DG. Sclerocornea and associated congenital anomalies. Arch Ophthalmol 1962;67:761–768
11. Kenyon KR. Mesenchymal dysgenesis in Peter's anomaly, sclerocornea and congenital endothelial dystrophy. Exp Eye Res 1975;21:125–142
12. Wilson FM II. Congenital anomalies. In: Smolin GA, Thoft RA, eds. The cornea: scientific foundations and clinical practice, ed 2. Boston: Little, Brown, 1987: 457–473
13. Bahn CF, Falls CF, Varley GA, et al. Classification of corneal endothelial disorders based on neural crest origin. Ophthalmology 1984;91:558–563
14. Cook CS, Sulik KK. Keratolenticular dysgenesis (Peters' anomaly) as a result of acute embryonic insult during gastrulation. J Pediatr Ophthalmol Strabismus 1988; 25:60–66
15. Stone DL, Kenyon KR, Green WR, et al. Congenital central corneal leukoma (Peters' anomaly). Am J Ophthalmol 1976;81:173–193
16. Townsend WM. Congenital anomalies of the cornea. In: Kaufman HE, Barron BA, McDonald MB, Waltmann SR, eds. The cornea. New York: Churchill Livingstone, 1988:333–360

17. Pokorny KS, Hyman BM, Jakobiec FA, et al. Epibulbar choristomas containing lacrimal tissue: clinical distinction from dermoids and histologic evidence of an origin from the palpebral lobe. Ophthalmology 1987;94:1249–1257
18. O'Grady RB, Kirk HQ. Corneal keloids. Am J Ophthalmol 1972;73:206–213
19. Waring GO III, Rodrigues MM, Laibson PR. Corneal dystrophies: II. Endothelial dystrophies. Surv Ophthalmol 1978;23:147–168
20. Kenyon KR, Maumenee AE. The histological and ultrastructural pathology of congenital hereditary corneal dystrophy: a case report. Invest Ophthalmol 1975;7: 475–500
21. Judisch GF, Maumenee IH. Clinical differentiation of recessive congenital hereditary endothelial dystrophy and dominant hereditary endothelial dystrophy. Am J Ophthalmol 1978;85:606–612
22. Waring GO III, Rodrigues MM, Laibson PR. Corneal dystrophies: I. Dystrophies of the epithelium, Bowman's layer and stroma. Surv Ophthalmol 1978;23:71–122
23. Witschel H, Fine BS, Grutzner P, McTigue JW. Congenital hereditary stromal dystrophy of the cornea. Arch Ophthalmol 1978;96:1043–1051
24. Spencer WH. Cornea. In: Font RL, Green WR, Howes EL, et al. (eds). Ophthalmic Pathology, vol 1, ed 3. New York: Saunders, 1985:229
25. Teekhasaenee C, Nimmanit S, Wutthiphan S, et al. Posterior polymorphous dystrophy and Alport syndrome. Ophthalmology 1991;98:1207–1215
26. Miller CA, Krachmer JH. Corneal diseases. In: Renie WA, ed. Goldberg's genetic and metabolic eye disease, ed 2. Boston: Little, Brown, 1986:297–367
27. Roussat B, Fournier F, Besson D, et al. A propos de deux cas de tyrosinose de type II (syndrome de Richner-Hanhart). Bull Soc Ophthal France 1988;88:751–757
28. Stulting RD, Sumers KD, Cavanagh HD, et al. Penetrating keratoplasty in children. Ophthalmology 1984;91:1222–1230
29. Waring GO III, Laibson PR. Keratoplasty in infants and children. Trans Am Acad Ophthalmol Otolaryngol 1977;83:283–296

Infantile Cataracts

Martin Arkin, M.D., Ph.D.
Dimitri Azar, M.D.
Anthony Fraioli, M.D.

The formal definitions of the terms *infantile, developmental,* and *congenital cataracts* differ somewhat. In contrast to congenital cataracts, infantile and developmental cataracts may not be present at birth. It is useful to think of congenital cataracts as those that occur within the first year of life. In this discussion, the terms *congenital* and *infantile* will be used interchangeably.

Congenital cataracts are responsible for 10% of all blindness in children worldwide [1]. One in 250 newborns has some form of congenital cataract, though some of these are not clinically significant. In the 1960s, only 26% of patients operated on for congenital cataracts were able to attend an ordinary school [2].

Several morphological classification schemes have been suggested for congenital cataracts. A simplified version adapted from Merin [3] is summarized in Table 1. This classification was chosen by the authors because the prognosis and treatment depend predominantly on the density and laterality of the cataract rather than on morphological type.

Polar cataracts involve either the anterior or posterior pole of the lens and affect the capsule and underlying lens (Fig 1) [4]. Usually unilateral and with limited visual detriment, they represent a vestigial remnant of the hyaloid artery.

Zonular cataracts involve one zone of the lens; they can be subdivided into nuclear (Fig 2), lamellar (Fig 3), sutural (Fig 4), spearlike, coralliform, floriform, and capsular cataracts. The nuclear subtype is often bilateral and is usually associated with a significant decrease in visual acuity. The lamellar subtype is characterized by an opaque layer surrounding a relatively clear nucleus. Sutural cataracts (involving the Y sutures) and capsular cataracts usually do not affect vision. In total cataracts, the entire lens is

Table 1 *Morphological Classification of Congenital Cataracts*

Polar
Zonular
   Nuclear
   Lamellar (most common)
   Sutural
   Spearlike
   Coralliform
   Floriform
   Capsular
Total
Membranous

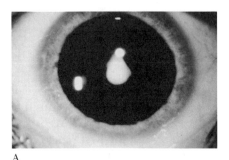
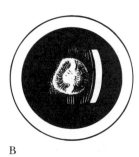

A   B

Figure 1 *(A) Congenital anterior polar cataract. (Courtesy of Dr. Craig McKeown.) (B) Diagram depicting slit-lamp view of anterior polar cataract. (Reprinted from Crawford and Morin [4] with permission.)*

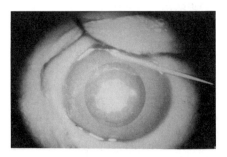

Figure 2 *Congenital nuclear cataract. (Courtesy of Dr. Craig McKeown.)*

opaque (Fig 5). These are often seen with systemic disease, as in congenital rubella, and are often associated with poor visual acuity and nystagmus.

    Membranous cataracts involve an opaque, thin, fibrotic lens that is caused by resorption of lens protein and subsequent thinning in the anteroposterior direction of the lens. The anterior and posterior capsules fuse and form a dense white membrane. This condition is usually unilateral and associated with other ocular abnormalities.

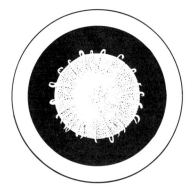

Figure 3 *Diagram of congenital lamellar cataract. (Reprinted from Crawford and Morin [4] with permission.)*

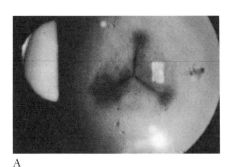

A

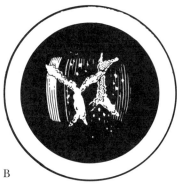

B

Figure 4 *(A) Congenital sutural cataract. (Courtesy of Dr. Craig McKeown.) (B) Diagrammatic representation of congenital sutural cataract. (Reprinted from Crawford and Morin [4] with permission.)*

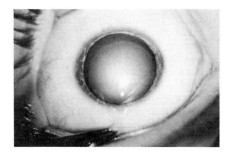

Figure 5 *Total cataract in a patient with aniridia. (Courtesy of Dr. Craig McKeown.)*

■ Etiological Features

It is important to determine whether a cataract is hereditary or sporadic and whether it is an isolated finding or part of a syndrome or systemic disease. Table 2 summarizes the classification of infantile cataracts based on etiology [1, 3–6]. Findings of the workup are negative in one-third to one-half of congenital cataracts (idiopathic).

Table 2 *Classification of Congenital Cataracts Based on Etiology*

Isolated finding
Hereditary
  Autosomal dominant
  Autosomal recessive
  X-linked
Sporadic (one-third of all congenital cataracts)
Part of syndrome or systemic disease
Hereditary
  With renal disease
    Lowe's oculocerebrorenal syndrome
    Alport's syndrome (autosomal dominant)
  With central nervous system disease
    Marinesco-Sjögren's syndrome (autosomal recessive)
    Sjögren's syndrome (autosomal recessive)
    Smith-Lemli-Opitz syndrome (autosomal recessive)
    Laurence-Moon-Bardet-Biedl syndrome
  With skeletal disease
    Conradi's syndrome (presence of cataract indicates worse prognosis)
    Marfan's syndrome
    Stippled epiphyses
  With abnormalities of head and face
    Hallermann-Streiff syndrome
    François dyscephalic syndrome
    Pierre Robin syndrome
    Oxycephaly
    Crouzon's disease
    Acrocephalosyndactyly (Apert's syndrome)
  With polydactyly
    Rubinstein-Taybi syndrome
  With skin disease
    Bloch-Sulzberger syndrome
    Congenital ectodermal dysplasia of the anhidrotic type
    Rothmund-Thomson syndrome
    Schafer's syndrome
    Siemens' syndrome
    Incontinentia pigmenti
    Atopic dermatitis
    Cockayne's syndrome
    Marshall syndrome
  With chromosomal disorders
    Trisomy 13 (usually die within 1 year)
    Trisomy 18: Edwards' syndrome
    Trisomy 21: Down's syndrome (often cataract formation delayed until
      approximately age 10)
    Turner's syndrome
    Patau's syndrome
  With metabolic disease
    Galactosemia (autosomal recessive; cataracts preventable with early dietary
      treatment; cataract secondary to galactose accumulation in the lens)
    Galactokinase deficiency (bilateral lamellar cataracts common; no other clinical
      manifestations)
    Congenital hemolytic jaundice

Table 2   *(continued)*

Part of syndrome or systemic disease (cont.)
    Fabry's disease
    Refsum's disease
    Mannosidosis
  With miscellaneous hereditary syndromes
    Norrie's disease
    Hereditary spherocytosis
    Myotonic dystrophy
Nonhereditary
  Prenatal causes
    Rubella syndrome
    Toxoplasmosis
    Varicella
    Cytomegalovirus (CMV)
    Herpes simplex virus
    Measles
    Mumps
    Vaccinia
    Intrauterine hypoxia or malnutrition
  Postnatal causes
    Retrolental fibroplasia
    Hypoglycemia
    Hypocalcemia (e.g., hypoparathyroidism; cataract secondary to altered
      permeability of lens capsule to ions)
    Radiation (often for retinoblastoma)
    Trauma
    Chronic uveitis
    Diabetes mellitus
    Wilson's disease
    Renal insufficiency
    Drug-induced
      Corticosteroids
      Immunosuppressive therapy
      Chlorpromazine
      Ergot
      Triparanol
      Dinitrophenol
      Naphthalene
    High-voltage electric shocks (e.g., lightning)
  Associated with another ocular abnormality
    Persistent hyperplastic primary vitreous
    Retinal dysplasia
    Congenital retinal detachment
    Microphthalmos
    Aniridia
    Anterior chamber cleavage
    Ectopia lentis
    Congenital retinal disinsertion syndrome
    Retinitis pigmentosa
    Norrie's disease
    Colobomas
    Lenticonus

Hereditary cataracts are usually transmitted in an autosomal dominant fashion, usually with complete penetrance. Autosomal recessive congenital cataracts are usually the result of consanguineous relationships. X-linked congenital cataracts are the least common hereditary cataracts. Fifteen percent of congenital cataracts are familial, and the rate of progression of visual loss throughout infancy is often similar within a given family.

Important historical points in relation to diagnosis include trauma, radiation exposure, systemic disease, maternal illness or exposure to drugs, and a family history of cataracts. Visual acuity measurements should be attempted; test methods may include preferential looking, optokinetic nystagmus testing, and visual evoked potentials. The extent, location, and visual significance of the cataract can be determined by slit-lamp examination, retinoscopy, and ophthalmoscopy. Glaucoma, retinal abnormalities, and refractive errors may be present. The infant or child should be examined by a pediatrician. It is often helpful to examine the child's parents and family members for subclinical cataracts. Depending on the level of suspicion of systemic disease, laboratory tests may include:

Antibody titers (rubella)
Urine testing for galactosemia
Karyotyping
Blood glucose
Urinalysis with microscopical examination
Serum calcium, phosphorus, alkaline phosphatase
Venereal Disease Research Laboratory (VDRL) test
Red blood cell (RBC) galactokinase activity and RBC galactose-1-phosphate-uridyltransferase activity (galactosemia)
Urine sodium nitroprusside test (homocystinuria)
Urine protein (Alport's syndrome), amino acid content (Lowe's syndrome), copper level (Wilson's disease)

Until recently, rubella syndrome was the most frequent single cause of congenital cataracts, accounting for 20% of cases, with epidemics in the United States in the 1950s and 1960s. The incidence was higher in developed countries where better hygiene resulted in later infection of women, though immunization has since partially offset this trend. Rubella cataracts are caused by direct invasion of the lens by virus. The syndrome includes heart defects, nerve deafness, bony lesions, intrauterine growth retardation, psychomotor retardation and, in 15% of cases, cataracts [4].

■ Treatment and Prognosis

The treatment of congenital cataracts depends on three major factors: laterality, the presence of associated ocular abnormalities, and whether the cataract is total or partial. Unilateral cataracts often carry a poor prognosis because of severe amblyopia and associated strabismus of the involved eye. Visual acuity of 20/400 or worse is common if the condition is untreated and visually significant. The prognosis for untreated partial unilateral cataracts is as poor as for untreated complete unilateral cataracts. The treatment is early surgical removal of the cataract.

Bilateral complete cataracts have a more favorable prognosis. There is little disagreement about treatment, which entails prompt surgical removal of the cataracts, operating on the second eye soon after the first.

The treatment of bilateral partial cataracts is more controversial. The difficulties encountered in measuring visual acuity early in life interfere with assessing the visual significance of the cataracts. The following are useful general rules:

Cataracts that are less than 2 mm in diameter are usually not significant.

The density of the cataract is more important than the size and type [5].

Cataracts that obstruct the examiner's view of the fundus or prevent objective refraction of the patient usually should be extracted.

Prompt surgical removal of a cataract is indicated if the contralateral cataract has been removed.

Cataracts associated with other ocular abnormalities such as microphthalmos, persistent hyperplastic primary vitreous, foveal dysplasia, and strabismus are usually associated with a very poor prognosis regardless of treatment. Congenital cataracts are associated with other ocular problems in 30 to 70% of cases [7–9]. In these cases, some authors recommend surgical treatment, often only to prevent some of the more serious complications later (for example, glaucoma or phthisis).

Surgery

Unlike in adult cataract patients, in cases of bilateral congenital cataracts it is often better to perform surgery on the better eye first [10]. Intracapsular cataract extraction is not usually done in children because children have significant Wiegert's hyaloid-lenticular adhesions that would lead to vitreous loss following intracapsular surgery.

Optical iridectomy and discission are of historical significance but are rarely used now. The object of the iridectomy is to increase pupil size to let more light in around the cataract. Mydriatics can be used as temporizing agents but are rarely tolerated over the long term [11].

Until recently, aspiration was the most commonly used surgical technique for cataract removal. It was reintroduced by Scheie in the 1960s [12, 13]. The procedure involves opening the anterior capsule with a knife,

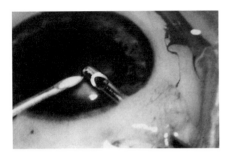

Figure 6 *Surgical technique for lensectomy with limited anterior vitrectomy through the limbal route. (Courtesy of Dr. Craig McKeown.)*

followed by irrigation and aspiration within the lens. Secondary membranes form in 18 to 73% of surgical cases and often require repeat surgery [14, 15].

The most popular current approach for pediatric cataract extraction is lensectomy with limited anterior vitrectomy [11, 16–21]. This is done with vitrectomy type cutting-aspiration instrumentation with either a limbal or pars plana entrance incision to the eye. The limbal route is favored by most surgeons (Fig 6). Phacoemulsification usually is not necessary with this procedure as the lens nucleus is generally very soft in infants. A total capsulotomy (including the posterior capsule) is done to avoid later capsular opacification and membrane formation. Some debate exists on the advisability of anterior vitrectomy in terms of the probability of postoperative cystoid macular edema [22]. The long-term incidence of retinal detachment with this technique is unknown.

Postoperative Complications

Prior to the advent of the operating microscope and cutting-aspiration instruments, postoperative complications were relatively common [23–25]. Though they occur with less frequency today, complications still arise.

Retained lens material may lead to persistent uveitis, posterior synechiae, and secondary glaucoma. Uveitis may be caused by surgical trauma or retained lens material. Vitreous loss may occur but is less likely with closed-eye surgical techniques. Glaucoma may occur secondary to peripheral anterior synechiae, posterior synechiae, or pupillary block. Retinal detachment is possible and can occur long after congenital cataract surgery [26–30]. It is difficult to repair in children due to poor visualization and retinal degeneration [26–28]. Endophthalmitis is relatively rare with modern surgical techniques in infants. Finally, posterior capsule opacification or membrane formation sometimes occurs when posterior or anterior capsules are intact.

Postoperative Therapy:
Antiamblyopia Management

Antiamblyopia treatment is an important part of patient management. It is based on experimental studies performed mostly on cats. Human infants and kittens show remarkably similar effects of visual deprivation in the critical period [31]. Current clinical antiamblyopia management includes the use of eyeglasses, contact lenses, intraocular lens (IOL) implantation, epikeratophakia, patching protocols, and strabismus surgery.

Eyeglasses Spectacles are not often used for congenital cataracts. They are not useful in monocular aphakia because of image size discrepancy between the eyes (aniseikonia). However, children adapt more easily than adults to the magnification distortions caused by eyeglasses. The visual needs in infants are limited to their immediate surroundings; thus, when spectacles are used, they are designed for near vision.

Contact Lenses Contact lenses are the mainstay of treatment of congenital aphakia. Optical correction should begin at approximately 1 week following surgery to avoid worsening amblyopia [32]. A +2-D overcorrection is included in the infant's prescription (for near vision). Children aged 4 to 5 years are given reading glasses for use over contact lenses. Hard contact lenses or daily wear soft lenses can be used with good results [33, 34], but extended-wear contact lenses are the most commonly used.

Despite common suspicion to the contrary, extended-wear lenses have been shown in research studies to be well tolerated and rarely associated with corneal damage. These lenses can be hydrogel [35] or silicone [36, 37]. Silicone lenses (Silsoft brand) have additional advantages including:

Increased oxygen permeability
Excellent thermal conductivity
Increased rigidity, which makes handling easier, with fewer lost lenses
Ability to mask up to 2 D of astigmatism
Ease of fitting, which does not require keratometry
Ability to use fluorescein patterns in fitting

In one study, only 14% of patients had significant contact lens problems resulting in discontinuation of lens wear [36]. Contact lenses seem to be better tolerated in children either younger than 18 months or older than 10 years. In all cases, parental motivation is important.

IOL Implantation IOL implantation is controversial and rarely used in infants. Possible complications include hemorrhage, prolapse of ocular contents, iris incarceration, iris sphincter erosion, anterior synechiae formation, glaucoma, iris bombé, iritis, intractable pupillary fibrotic membranes, IOL dislocation, and corneal edema [38–41]. These complications are apparently more frequent in patients younger than 12 months [38]. There are several disadvantages of IOLs in children:

The long-term safety of IOLs is not known.
Positional changes of the implant may occur as the child's eye grows.
Growth of the globe may cause changes in the axial length and, thus, the refractive power of the eye [22].
The postoperative inflammatory response in children to IOLs is greater than in adults.
Endothelial damage may occur during insertion.

Despite these problems, there are some advocates of IOL use in infants and children [42–44]. IOLs could theoretically result in better binocular vision because of decreased aniseikonia. They may be advisable in rare cases where other options such as contact lenses are not possible.

Other Management Options   Epikeratophakia is rarely used for the treatment of congenital cataracts because of inherent limitations in providing enough hyperopic power and in the haze of the graft. The latter is usually transient but interferes with vision during the critical period of visual development [22, 45, 46]. Epikeratophakia may be useful in children who are poor candidates for other forms of therapy.

Patching had long been used to increase the visual acuity of the postoperative eye after congenital cataract extraction, as some degree of amblyopia is almost always present. Although patching remains an essential part of treatment, several authors believe that poor stereoacuity and fusion are at least partially aggravated by patching [33, 47, 48].

At least 26% of pediatric cataract patients have postoperative strabismus [36]. Diplopia is more of a problem now because results of monocular cataract surgery are improving, with better final visual acuity (less amblyopia). Muscle surgery and ophthalmic prisms are used in treatment. In patients with poor fusion, the results are less than satisfactory.

Results of Treatment

The final results of surgery depend on the (1) onset of cataract, (2) delay in diagnosis, (3) patient's age at surgery, (4) presence of other ocular or systemic conditions (usually the prognosis is poor if other ocular defects are present, whether or not they are treated) [23, 49–51], and (5) compliance with postoperative treatments (patching, lenses, and so on).

Fifty-five percent of patients have a final postoperative visual acuity of 20/40 or better. Early surgery (before 2 months of age) is associated with better results [52]. A study of bilateral cataracts demonstrated that 60% of patients can achieve a visual acuity of 20/60 or better with early surgery [53].

Stereoacuity is rare after congenital cataract surgery (especially in unilateral cases) secondary to amblyopia, patching, and aniseikonia [50]. Katsumi and colleagues [54] showed that after unilateral cataract surgery in adults, where amblyopia is not a factor, stereoacuity was lost if image disparity between the 2 eyes exceeded approximately 5%. In these adult patients, stereoacuity was generally better with IOLs than with unilateral contact lenses. Since children have the problem of aniseikonia (approximately 5% with contact lens use) complicated by amblyopia as well as patching (which further decreases binocularity), it is understandable that stereoacuity is rare and strabismus is common in children postoperatively [55].

Prognosis is also dependent on the cataract type: Bilateral incomplete cataract patients do best, followed by bilateral complete cataract patients. Unilateral cataracts are associated with the worst outcome and were considered nearly hopeless until recently [39, 56, 57] (see next section).

If surgery of bilateral cataracts is delayed, profound bilateral amblyopia and permanent nystagmus may result at approximately 3 months of age, the normal time for development of fixation. The presence of nystagmus usually indicates visual acuity worse than 20/200.

■ Congenital Unilateral Cataract

Historically, congenital unilateral cataracts were considered "virtually hopeless" [1]. Subsequent improvements in prognosis have occurred with early surgery (within the first 2 months, and preferably in the first week, after birth) and early antiamblyopia treatment [47, 58–60].

A study of 38 infants showed that 53% can achieve an outcome of 20/80 or better [61]. Infants with other serious eye anomalies in addition to cataracts were excluded from the study. Poor results were found with surgery done after 2 months of age. Fellow normal (phakic) eyes developed good visual acuity despite aggressive antiamblyopia therapy. In addition, an association was shown between poor compliance (with contact lenses and patching protocols) and late surgery, where amblyopia was presumably more advanced. These authors concluded that poor compliance with therapy may, in many cases, be the *result* of amblyopia rather than the cause.

Similar results were reported by Drummond and co-workers [37] with 14 patients. Visual acuity was better than 20/50 in 43% of patients. Favorable results correlated with patient compliance, early surgery, and early antiamblyopia therapy with contact lenses and patching. Patients who exhibited excellent results had a median age at surgery of 17 days (contact lens use and patching occurred approximately 2 weeks thereafter). Aggressive patching was used, with part-time and full-time patching until age 6 to 9 years.

These studies, as well as others, demonstrate that excellent results are possible with unilateral congenital cataracts. Many patients with excellent results did indeed have dense cataracts from birth. Still, even with documented excellent results in some cases, these represent the exceptions. A great deal of work is needed to resolve continuing problems such as poor fusion and diplopia. In addition, wider implementation of current treatment recommendations is necessary.

■ References

1. Nelson LB. Diagnosis and management of cataracts in infancy and childhood. Ophthalmic Surg 1984;15:688–697
2. Grigorieva VI, Prokofieva AL. Surgical treatment of congenital cataracts in children. Oftalmol Zh 1968;23:495–498
3. Merin S. Congenital cataracts. In: Renie WA, ed. Goldberg's genetic and metabolic eye disease. Boston: Little, Brown, 1986:369–387
4. Crawford JS, Morin JD. The eye in childhood. New York: Grune & Stratton, 1983
5. Merin S, Crawford JS. Assessment of incomplete congenital cataract. Can J Ophthalmol 1972;7:56–62
6. Kohn BA. The differential diagnosis of cataracts in infancy and childhood. Am J Dis Child 1976;130:184–192
7. Falls HF. Developmental cataracts: results of surgical treatment in one hundred and thirty-one cases. Arch Ophthalmol 1943;29:210–223
8. Owens WC, Hughes WF Jr. Results of surgical treatment of congenital cataract. Arch Ophthalmol 1948;39:339–350
9. Bagley CH. Congenital cataracts: a survey of the various types of operation. Am J Ophthalmol 1948:411–419
10. Wilson FM. Glaucoma, lens, and anterior segment trauma. San Francisco: American Academy of Ophthalmology, 1990:102–150
11. Calhoun JH. Cataracts. In: Harley RD, ed. Pediatric ophthalmology, ed 2. Philadelphia: Saunders, 1983:549–567
12. Scheie HG. Aspiration of congenital or soft cataracts: a new technique. Am J Ophthalmol 1960;50:1048–1056
13. Scheie HG, Rubenstein RA, Kent RB. Aspiration of congenital or soft cataracts: further experience. Am J Ophthalmol 1967;63:3–8
14. Parks MM, Hiles DA. Management of infantile cataracts. Am J Ophthalmol 1967;63:10–19
15. Sheppard RW, Crawford JS. The treatment of congenital cataracts. Surv Ophthalmol 1973;17:340–347
16. Machemer RJ, Parel JM, Buettner H. A new concept for vitreous surgery: I. Instrumentation. Am J Ophthalmol 1972;73:1–7
17. Calhoun JH, Harley RD. The roto-extractor in pediatric ophthalmology. Trans Am Ophthalmol Soc 1975;73:292–305
18. O'Malley C, Heintz R. Vitrectomy via the pars plana: a new instrument system. Trans Pac Coast Soc Otolaryngol Ophthalmol 1972;53:121–127
19. Federman JL, Cook K, Bross R, et al. Intraocular microsurgery: I. New instrumentation (SITE). Ophthalmic Surg 1976;7(1):82–87
20. Stark WJ, Taylor HR, Michels RG, Maumenee AE. Management of congenital cataracts. Ophthalmology 1979;86:1571–1578
21. Taylor D. Choice of surgical technique in the management of congenital cataract. Trans Ophthalmol Soc [UK] 1981;101:114–117

22. Hoyt CS. Guest editorial. J Pediatr Ophthalmol Strabismus 1982;19:127–128

23. Francois J. Late results of congenital cataract surgery. Ophthalmology 1979;86: 1586–1598

24. Chandler PA. Surgery of congenital cataract. Am J Ophthalmol 1968;65:663–674

25. Cordes FC. Evaluation of the surgery of congenital cataracts. Arch Ophthalmol 1951;46:132–144

26. Taylor BC, Tasman WS. Retinal detachment following congenital cataract surgery. Tex Med 1974;70:83–87

27. Kanski JJ, Elkington AR, Daniel R. Retinal detachment after congenital cataract surgery. Br J Ophthalmol 1974;58:92–95

28. Toyofuku H, Hirose T, Schepens CL. Retinal detachment following congenital cataract surgery: I. Preoperative findings in 114 eyes. Arch Ophthalmol 1980; 98:669–675

29. Shapland CD. Retinal detachment in aphakia. Trans Ophthalmol Soc [UK] 1934; 54:176–196

30. Cordes FC. Retinal detachment following congenital cataract surgery: a study of 112 enucleated eyes. J Ophthalmol 1960;50:716–729

31. Lewis TL, Maurer D, Brent HP. Effects on perceptual development of visual deprivation during infancy. Br J Ophthalmol 1986;70:214–220

32. Enoch JM. Fitting parameters which need to be considered when designing soft contact lenses for the neonate. Contact Intraocul Lens Med J 1979;5:31–37

33. Pratt-Johnson JA, Tillson G. Hard contact lenses in the management of congenital cataracts. J Pediatr Ophthalmol Strabismus 1985;22:94–96

34. Moore B. The fitting of contact lenses in aphakic infants. J Am Optom Assoc 1985;56:180–183

35. Epstein RJ, Fernandes A, Gammon JA. The correction of aphakia in infants with hydrogel extended-wear contact lenses: corneal studies. Ophthalmology 1988; 95:1102–1106

36. Levin AV, Edmonds SA, Nelson LB, et al. Extended-wear contact lenses for the treatment of pediatric aphakia. Ophthalmology 1988;95:1107–1113

37. Drummond GT, Scott WE, Keech RV. Management of monocular congenital cataracts. Arch Ophthalmol 1989;107:45–51

38. Binkhorst CD, Gobin MH. Congenital cataract and lens implantation. Ophthalmologica 1972;164:392–397

39. Binkhorst CD. The iridocapsular (two-loop) lens and the iris-clip (four-loop) lens in pseudophakia. Trans Am Acad Ophthalmol Otolaryngol 1973;77:589–617

40. Rozenman Y, Folberg R, Nelson LB, Cohen EJ. Painful bullous keratopathy following pediatric cataract surgery with intraocular lens implantation. Ophthalmic Surg 1985;16:372–374

41. Gieser SC, Apple DJ, Loftfield K, et al. Phthisis bulbi after intraocular lens implantation in a child. Can Ophthalmol 1985;20:184–185

42. BenEzra D, Paez JH. Congenital cataract and intraocular lenses. Am J Ophthalmol 1983;96:311–314

43. Tablante TR, Lapus JV, Cruz ED, Santos AM. A new technique of congenital cataract surgery with primary posterior chamber intraocular lens implantation. J Cataract Refract Surg 1988;14:149–157

44. Aron JJ, Aron-Rosa D. Intraocular lens implantation in unilateral congenital cataract: a preliminary report. Intraocul Implant Soc J 1983;9:306–308

45. Morgan KS, Werblin TP, Asbell PA, et al. The use of epikeratophakia grafts in pediatric monocular aphakia. J Pediatr Ophthalmol Strabismus 1981;18:23–29

46. Asbell PA, Werblin TP, Loupe DN. Secondary surgical procedures after epikeratophakia. Ophthalmic Surg 1982;13:555–557

47. Pratt-Johnson JA, Tillson G. Visual results after removal of congenital cataracts before the age of 1 year. Can J Ophthalmol 1981;16:19–21

48. Uemura Y, Katsumi O. Form-vision deprivation amblyopia and strabismic amblyopia. Graefes Arch Clin Exp Ophthalmol 1988;226:193–196
49. Migdal C. Congenital cataracts—management and visual results (Cape Town, 1956–1976). J Pediatr Ophthalmol Strabismus 1981;18(3):13–21
50. Jain IS, Pillai P, Gangwar DN, et al. Congenital cataract: management and results. J Pediatr Ophthalmol Strabismus 1983;20:243–246
51. Scott WE, Drummond GT, Keech RV, Karr DJ. Management and visual acuity results of monocular congenital cataracts and persistent hyperplastic primary vitreous. Aust J Ophthalmol 1989;17:143–152
52. Rogers GL, Tishler CL, Tsou BH, et al. Visual acuities in infants with congenital cataracts operated on prior to 6 months of age. Arch Ophthalmol 1981;99:999–1003
53. Gelbart SS, Hoyt CS, Jastrebski G, Marg E. Long-term visual results in bilateral congenital cataracts. Am J Ophthalmol 1982;93:615–621
54. Katsumi O, Miyanaga Y, Hirose T, et al. Binocular function in unilateral aphakia: correlation with aniseikonia and stereoacuity. Ophthalmology 1988;95:1088–1093
55. France TD, Frank JW. The association of strabismus and aphakia in children. J Pediatr Ophthalmol Strabismus 1984;21:223–226
56. Costenbader FD, Albert DG. Conservatism in the management of congenital cataract. Arch Ophthalmol 1957;58:426–430
57. Helveston EM, Saunders RA, Ellis FD. Unilateral cataracts in children. Ophthalmic Surg 1980;11:102–108
58. Beller R, Hoyt CS, Marg E, Odom JV. Good visual function after neonatal surgery for congenital monocular cataracts. J Ophthalmol 1981;91:559–565
59. Jacobson SG, Mohindra I, Held R. Development of visual acuity in infants with congenital cataracts. Br J Ophthalmol 1981;65:727–735
60. Enoch JM, Rabinowicz IM. Early surgery and visual correction of an infant born with unilateral eye lens opacity. Doc Ophthalmol 1976;41:371–382
61. Birch EE, Stager DR. Prevalence of good visual acuity following surgery for congenital unilateral cataract. Arch Ophthalmol 1988;106:40–43

Posterior Uveitis in the Pediatric Population

Annabelle A. Okada, M.D.
C. Stephen Foster, M.D.

Uveitis is less common in children than in adults. In a 1966 clinic survey of uveitis at Moorfields Hospital in London, only 5% of the patients were children younger than 16 years, in comparison to the 20% proportion of children in the general population at that time [1]. An earlier survey by Kimura and colleagues [2] in 1954 found that of 810 cases of uveitis seen at the Proctor Foundation in San Francisco, only 5.8% were patients younger than age 16. Among pediatric uveitis patients, girls predominate with a female-to-male ratio of approximately 1.3 [1]. Furthermore, the prevalence of uveitis tends to increase with age within the pediatric group [1].

Uveitis predominating in the posterior segment comprises a relatively larger proportion in the pediatric sector than among adults. Approximately 40% of pediatric uveitis occurs in the posterior segment; the comparable figure for adults is 20% [1]. Depending on the child's age, certain diseases that cause posterior uveitis are more common than others. However, it is important that uveitis not be mistaken for other disease processes such as malignancies that occur in youth. In this chapter, a practical approach to the diagnosis of posterior uveitis in children will be emphasized. This will be followed by consideration of specific uveitis entities as they pertain to the pediatric population.

■ Clinical History

Asking the Right Questions

Younger children with uveitis are often relatively asymptomatic despite profound ocular inflammation or severely diminished vision. The reason for this is unclear but, because of it, children with posterior uveitis are often initially seen later than adults with the same disease [3]. In addition to asking the young patient questions about possible red eye, tearing, light sensitivity, rubbing of eyes, decreased vision, floaters, metamorphopsia, and prior trauma, one must also carefully query the parents with the same set of questions. If leukokoria, strabismus, or buphthalmos is present, one must attempt to identify, often with the aid of old photographs, when it first developed. The parents may also add to the clinical history by giving information as to the recent behavior of the child and the child's performance at school. A history of exposure to dogs or puppies at home or in school might lead one to suspect infection by *Toxocara canis*. Pertinent past medical history should also include birth weight and prior health of the child, vaccinations, and whether the usual developmental milestones have been achieved. Knowledge about the mother's medical history is also important, and one should elicit information regarding syphilis and other sexually transmitted diseases, intravenous drug abuse, human immunodeficiency virus (HIV) status, and intrapartum viral infections. Furthermore, maternal exposure to cats or ingestion of raw meat during pregnancy is important as it might suggest toxoplasmosis. Both parents should be asked about tuberculosis exposure and history of collagen vascular disease.

Of course, to obtain the most accurate information, older children and teenagers should be asked in confidence as to possible risk factors for HIV infection and sexually transmitted diseases, and any history of intravenous drug abuse.

Differential Diagnosis by Age

The ophthalmologist can, based on the age of the patient alone, create a short differential diagnosis list for a posterior inflammatory process (Table 1). This list can be modified further depending on the clinical history, and appropriate diagnostic tests can be obtained.

■ Clinical Examination

Characterization

The manifestations of posterior uveitis vary depending on the disease and the duration of inflammation. Specific findings are described in the latter part of this chapter under each disease heading. In general, acute inflammation might present with vitritis, peripheral retinal exudates, vasculitis, retinitis, retinal mass, retinal detachment, choroiditis, macular edema, optic disc edema, or any combination of these conditions. On the other hand, the presence of retinal pigment epithelial (RPE) changes, chorioretinal scarring, or optic atrophy would be suggestive of more long-standing disease. A significant component of anterior inflammation may be present as well and might help to refine the differential diagnosis.

Table 1   *Differential Diagnosis of Pediatric Posterior Uveitis by Age*

Pediatric Group	Diseases
Infants (age 0–2 yr)	Herpes simplex virus retinitis[a]
	Toxocara canis infection[a]
	Retinoblastoma[a,b]
	Rubella
	Congenital syphilis[b]
Toddlers, school-aged children (age 2–10 yr)	*Toxocara canis* infection[a]
	Toxoplasmosis[a,b]
	Subacute sclerosing panencephalitis
	Leukemia[b]
	Juvenile rheumatoid arthritis[b]
Adolescents (age 10–20 yr)	Toxoplasmosis[a,b]
	Intermediate uveitis[a,b]
	Presumed ocular histoplasmosis syndrome
	Acute posterior multifocal placoid pigment epitheliopathy
	Vogt-Koyanagi-Harada syndrome[b]
	Diffuse unilateral subacute neuroretinitis
	Leukemia[b]
	Juvenile rheumatoid arthritis[b]
Any childhood age	Human immunodeficiency virus retinopathy[a]
	Cytomegalovirus retinitis[a]
	Endophthalmitis[a]
	Sarcoidosis[a,b]
	Tuberculosis[b]
	Behçet's disease[b]
	Intraocular foreign body[b]
	Sympathetic ophthalmia[b]

[a]Diseases most common in each age group.
[b]Diseases in which significant anterior segment inflammation may be present.

Examination Under Anesthesia

The age and disposition of the child may preclude a proper examination in the clinical setting, and one should not hesitate to schedule an examination under anesthesia. For infants and toddlers up to the age of 3, an examination under anesthesia is almost essential for accurate diagnosis and appropriate therapy, particularly when one is excluding retinoblastoma as a possibility.

Diagnostic Tests

The ophthalmologist should cater serological tests and radiological examinations to the individual patient. For example, an otherwise healthy-appearing 5-year-old child who presents with a diffuse vitritis accompanying a retinochoroiditis might be worked up initially with *Toxoplasma gondii* and *Toxocara canis* serologies, a complete blood cell count, angio-tensin-converting enzyme level, Venereal Disease Research Laboratory (VDRL) testing, fluorescent treponemal antibody absorption (FTA-ABS) testing, purified protein derivative (PPD) skin testing, and chest x-ray. These would help to rule in or rule out toxoplasmosis, *Toxocara canis* infection, leukemia, sarcoidosis, syphilis, and tuberculosis. If the initial workup is negative, other laboratory and radiological tools might be considered. Specific diagnostic tests are discussed under each disease heading.

■ Treatment in the Pediatric Population

Risk of Amblyopia

The treatment of posterior uveitis in children is heavily influenced by the significant risk of amblyopia in the patient younger than 6 or 7 years. Certainly, if a visually impairing process is of recent onset in a young child or infant, prompt institution of appropriate medical or surgical treatment and visual rehabilitation is imperative. If the visually impairing process is long-standing and amblyopia has already developed, medical treatment might still be instituted but surgery delayed, depending on the situation. If surgery involves lens extraction, the infant or child should be fitted with aphakic correction as soon as possible, preferably a contact lens.

Drug and Dosage Considerations

The medical treatment of uveitis, toxic even to the adult, poses a much greater risk to the infant or child whose immune system, skeletal bones, and sexual organs may still not have matured. Therefore, in choosing systemic medications for the child with uveitis, the risks must be weighed carefully against the benefits.

Several common pediatric uveitis entities, such as toxoplasmosis, are treated with antimicrobial agents at doses that must be adjusted for the age and weight of the child.

Systemic corticosteroids should be prescribed if the disease is life-threatening or if, left untreated, it would lead to permanent and profound visual loss. Specific to the pediatric group, chronic corticosteroid therapy will lead to retardation of skeletal maturation and linear growth. Furthermore, peripheral antagonism of exogenous corticosteroids on growth hormone action can also hamper normal growth of a child. In patients of any age, the potential complications of systemic corticosteroid use are myriad. Central nervous system (CNS) effects include behavioral changes, insomnia, nervousness, and psychosis. Pseudotumor cerebri can occur during dosage tapering. Gastrointestinal problems include peptic ulcer disease and, rarely, intestinal perforation. Endocrine effects include sodium retention and potassium loss, arterial hypertension, cushingoid appearance, hyperlipidemia, hyperglycemia and, possibly, diabetic ketoacidosis and hyperosmolar nonketotic coma. Musculoskeletal complications include osteoporosis, aseptic necrosis, and steroid-induced myopathy. Finally, corticosteroids increase the chance of recrudescence of dormant tuberculosis, so a tuberculin test should always be performed prior to systemic corticosteroid use.

Topical corticosteroid use in children should also be carefully monitored with periodic measurement of intraocular pressure and assessment for possible cataract formation. The drug should be tapered as soon as possible.

Chemotherapeutic agents are also sometimes necessary for the effective treatment of posterior uveitis. The indications for these drugs are the same as for systemic corticosteroids. Agents used in the treatment of posterior uveitis include cyclophosphamide, cyclosporine, chlorambucil, methotrexate, and azathioprine. Each can potentiate bone marrow suppression and opportunistic infection. Furthermore, each has other specific, adverse side effects that can themselves be acutely or chronically life-threatening. Yet chemotherapy can often reduce the dependency on corticosteroids in controlling inflammation, thus playing an important role in lessening the overall morbidity related to treatment.

Laser and surgical procedures are undertaken in pediatric uveitis depending on the presumed diagnosis, degree of disease process, visual acuity, age of the patient, and potential to save or improve vision.

Although the decision to treat children with potentially harmful drugs or risky surgery is difficult, one should not be timid. The control of pediatric uveitis is often hampered by a lack of clear action on the part of the physician early on in the disease because of his or her fear of the pitfalls. However, we know that uveitis in this age group can be very aggressive, with high rates of morbidity. Therefore, mindful of the risks, the physician must take equally aggressive steps to control the disease.

Coordination of Treatment with Pediatrician and Other Services

Because the medical treatment of uveitis holds many potential hazards for the young patient, the ophthalmologist must work in close concert with the pediatrician and, if appropriate, the oncologist and the neurologist. Furthermore, social services may be crucial in providing psychological, practical, and financial aid to the family that must deal with the child who may be significantly visually impaired and, possibly, neurologically or otherwise impaired as well.

■ Specific Uveitis Entities Grouped by Etiology

Specific uveitis entities, especially as they pertain to the findings of posterior inflammation in children, are grouped here under the categories of infection, trauma, neoplasia, and autoimmune or unknown etiology. Some of the diseases that are well described in the adult literature (such as tuberculosis) or that primarily involve anterior uveitis (such as juvenile rheumatoid arthritis) are mentioned only briefly.

Infection

Toxoplasmosis Probably the most common cause of posterior uveitis in children is toxoplasmosis [1–3]. In the 1966 Perkins survey [1], approximately 40% of cases of pediatric posterior uveitis were attributable to toxoplasmosis. More recently, in 1989, Giles [3] estimated that toxoplasmosis may account for as much as 70% of pediatric posterior and generalized uveitis. The congenital form occurs in approximately 1 in 10,000 live births in the United States and is due to transmission of an acute maternal infection [4]. If this occurs in the first trimester of pregnancy, the neonate classically exhibits convulsions, cerebral calcifications, and retinitis. If transmission occurs during later trimesters, the infection is usually subclinical, with retinitis as the only observable manifestation [5]. Active toxoplasmosis seen in the clinical setting is usually reactivation of such a congenital lesion and is self-limiting. The acquired form of toxoplasmosis eventually affects up to 50% of the U.S. population by some estimates, manifested by mild, usually asymptomatic lymphadenopathy and, occasionally, an infectious mononucleosis–like syndrome but rarely associated with retinitis [5]. The exception is acute toxoplasmosis in the immunocompromised host, which is usually fatal secondary to encephalitis, necrotizing myocarditis, or pneumonitis. Such infection may be either acquired or the reactivation of a latent congenital infection [5–8]. *Toxoplasma gondii* is the causative organism, usually residing in the cat, its definitive host. It is transmitted to humans via ingestion of tissue cysts in animal meats or eggs, or by contact with oocysts in cat feces, sand, or soil.

Toxoplasmosis manifests itself in the ocular fundus as a white, fluffy, focal, necrotizing retinitis adjacent to an old chorioretinal scar (Fig 1). Choroiditis, vitritis, and anterior uveitis are believed to be a secondary hypersensitivity response. Morphological variants include punctate inner or outer retinal lesions and papillitis. Complications can include chronic iridocyclitis, cataract, glaucoma, cystoid macular edema, retinal detachment, optic atrophy, choroidal neovascular membrane, and branch retinal vessel occlusion. Diagnosis is made clinically and by measuring antibody titers by immunofluorescence assay. The specific anti–*T. gondii* IgM peaks in the first month of acute, primary infection and reverts back to negative in a few months. The specific anti–*T. gondii* IgG will rise over 2 months

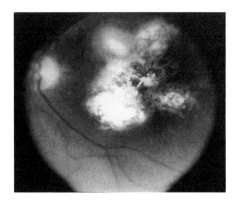

Figure 1 *Active toxoplasmosis next to an old chorioretinal scar.*

in acute primary infection or in reactivation and can remain elevated for long periods [5]. Therapy is suggested only when (1) the lesion occurs within the macula; (2) the lesion abuts the optic nerve or threatens a large retinal vessel; (3) there is a large degree of hemorrhage; (4) there is severe vitritis; or (5) the host is immunocompromised [9]. In these cases, the usual medical treatment in children involves pyrimethamine (with folinic acid), sulfadiazine, and prednisone, although clindamycin had also been shown to be effective in adults (Table 2) [6]. Topical corticosteroids and cycloplegia are added to control the anterior inflammation. Cryotherapy, photocoagulation, and vitrectomy have also been used in appropriate cases. Prognosis is generally good for patients with this self-limiting process unless the lesion is macular or the host is immunocompromised.

***Toxocara canis* Infection**   The 1966 Perkins survey [1] estimated that 20% of cases of pediatric posterior uveitis were caused by *Toxocara canis*. *T. canis* is an ascarid (roundworm) that normally completes its life cycle in puppies and dogs but can be transmitted to humans via pica of dirt or ingestion of other materials that contain the organism's eggs. After ingestion, the larvae hatch in the gut wall and migrate until they ultimately become encysted in tissues. Human infection occurs in two forms, visceral larval migrans and ocular toxocariasis. Visceral larval migrans tends to

Table 2   *Treatment of Ocular Toxoplasmosis in Children*

Drug	Dosage
Pyrimethamine	15 mg/m²/day or 1 mg/kg/day, divided into two daily oral doses, not to exceed 25 mg/day
Sulfadiazine	50 to 100 mg/kg/day, divided into two daily doses
Folinic acid	5 mg orally twice weekly during pyrimethamine therapy
Clindamycin	Has been used in adults and adolescents at 300 mg orally every 6 hours

occur in younger children, aged 2 to 4 years, and is a self-limiting, rarely lethal disease with manifestations including fever, pulmonary symptoms, hepatosplenomegaly, eosinophilia, and neurological problems such as convulsions and meningitis [10]. Ocular toxocariasis occurs in older children with an average age of 7½ years (range, 2 to 31 years), with 80% of cases presenting by age 16 [11]. Live larvae characteristically do not elicit much inflammation in the retina but, on their death, a severe uveitis can result. One study showed serological evidence of infestation in 20 to 30% of kindergarten children [12]. However, despite such prevalence of infestation, systemic or ocular disease caused by *T. canis* is relatively rare.

The typical presentation of ocular toxocariasis is a whitish, raised granuloma in the posterior pole or in the periphery, with a frequently associated intense vitritis, probably representing a reaction to released immunogenic antigens from the dead worm (Fig 2). Less commonly, a peripheral retinitis can be seen, which is believed to represent the lodging of larvae in the peripheral retinal vasculature. Other less common manifestations include optic nerve disease and branch retinal artery obstruction. Because ocular toxocariasis is perhaps the entity most often confused with retinoblastoma, accurate diagnosis is of paramount importance [13]. Diagnosis is aided by ultrasonography and computed tomographic (CT) scanning since calcifications are frequently seen with retinoblastoma and not with toxocariasis. Additionally, measurement of aqueous-to-serum lactate dehydrogenase or phosphoglucose-isomerase ratios can help to confirm retinoblastoma [14]. Although there is a high prevalence of seropositivity among children, the presence of anti–*T. canis* antibodies in the setting of typical features on clinical examination, ultrasonography, or CT scan is usually adequate for diagnosis. Periocular and systemic corticosteroid therapy aids in controlling the ocular inflammation, but treatment with antihelminthic agents, such as thiabendazole and diethylcarbamazine, has not been satis-

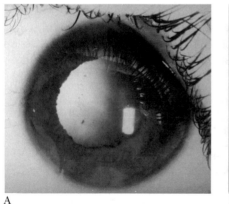 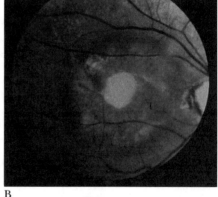

A   B

Figure 2   *(A) Leukocoria and (B) macular granuloma in ocular toxocariasis.*

factory thus far [15]. However, a new antihelminthic drug, levamisole hydrochloride (ivermectin), has been found to suppress *T. canis* infections in an experimental mouse model and may eventually be tried in humans [16]. Vitreoretinal surgery has been successfully used in a few series to stabilize or improve visual outcome [17]. Photocoagulation has been used in selected cases. Prognosis depends on the location of the granuloma and the degree of inflammation.

Diffuse Unilateral Subacute Neuroretinitis   First described by Gass and colleagues in 1977 [18], diffuse unilateral subacute neuroretinitis (DUSN) has been known as the great imitator since it can masquerade as many more common diseases. The average age at presentation is 14 years (range, 11 to 65 years) with a male-to-female ratio of 1.5 [19]. The disease is caused by a motile, white nematode (yet to be identified) that may wander in the subretinal space for years, leaving toxic byproducts and, consequently, inflammation in its wake. The two endemic areas in the United States are the Midwest, where a larger worm (1,500 to 2,000 μm) is found, and the Southeast, where a smaller worm (400 to 1,000 μm) is more common [19].

Early in the course of the disease there is visual loss, vitritis, papillitis, retinal vasculitis, and recurrent, evanescent, gray-white, outer retinal lesions. This picture can mimic acute posterior multifocal placoid pigment epitheliopathy, serpiginous choroidopathy, evanescent white dot syndrome, Behçet's disease, multifocal toxoplasmosis, and presumed ocular histoplasmosis syndrome. Later, progressive visual loss, optic atrophy, retinal vessel narrowing, and diffuse RPE degeneration ("unilateral wipeout") are seen. At this stage, DUSN can be confused with unilateral optic atrophy, unilateral retinitis pigmentosa, posttraumatic chorioretinopathy, and chorioretinal atrophy after ophthalmic artery occlusion. The worm is often difficult to find but tends to be in the vicinity of an active, deep, white, exudative lesion, most frequently outside the macula. Diagnosis is aided by fluorescein angiography, which shows disc edema and early blockage with late staining of lesions. Other diagnostic findings include a reduced electroretinogram and, rarely, peripheral eosinophilia. A negative *T. canis* titer is helpful, but a positive titer is of no diagnostic value. Oral antihelminthic therapy is ineffective in reaching the worm in the subretinal space, and the only sure cure appears to be direct destruction of the organism achieved by photocoagulation [19, 20]. Prognosis for these patients is poor unless effective treatment is instituted early.

AIDS-Related Retinopathy   Acquired immunodeficiency syndrome (AIDS) has become a major health problem in the pediatric population. It is estimated that approximately 20% of children with AIDS were infected through the transfusion of blood or blood products. The majority of the rest acquired the disease perinatally, via transplacental infection or postnatal transfer of the virus through breast milk [21]. The magnitude of the problem of perinatal HIV infection is emphasized further by studies that show seropositive rates of as high as 2% among unselected childbearing women in some inner city hospitals [21]. In female intravenous drug abusers, the seropositive rate is 30%. It is believed that 30 to 50% of children born to these seropositive women will be infected with the virus [21].

Ocular disease associated with AIDS is less common in children than in adults. In a 1989 study of 40 children seropositive for HIV, only 20% or so had ocular involvement, as compared with the published reports of 50 to 73% in adults [22]. The ocular manifestations in children, in order of prevalence, were cotton-wool spots, external infections such as molluscum contagiosum, retinal hemorrhages, cytomegalovirus retinitis, and toxoplasmosis. Other diseases, all opportunistic infections, that can involve the eye in AIDS include syphilis, tuberculosis, and *Candida* and *cryptococcus* infections.

Cotton-wool spots are a well-described AIDS-related retinopathy, occurring in approximately one-half of AIDS patients (Fig 3) [23]. Clinically, the spots appear white with feathered edges on the surface of the retina, often near the optic disc and the arcades, sometimes associated with small hemorrhages. Usually the spots resolve over a few months and are asymptomatic. Pathologically, cotton-wool spots represent focal ischemia with cytoid bodies in axons of the nerve fiber layer. They occur in a wide variety of ocular and systemic diseases, most notably diabetes mellitus and hypertension. In AIDS, their etiology remains unclear, although suggested causes include a direct toxic effect of HIV on vascular endothelium, deposition of circulating immune complexes, disseminated intravascular coagulopathy, and blood hyperviscosity.

Cytomegalovirus Retinitis Cytomegalovirus (CMV) inclusion disease in the neonate is usually congenital, characterized by a syndrome of prematurity, microcephaly, intracranial calcification, chorioretinitis. optic at-

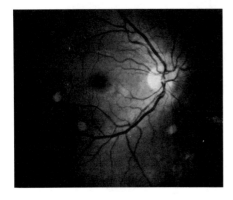

Figure 3 *Cotton-wool spots in a patient with acquired immunodeficiency syndrome. (Courtesy of Dr. Donald J. D'Amico.)*

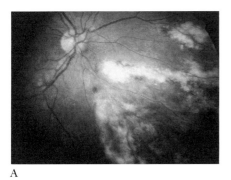 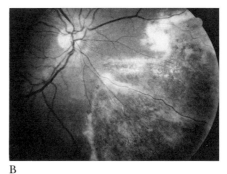

A   B

Figure 4 *(A) Active cytomegalovirus in the same patient as in Figure 3. (B) Regression 2 months later, following intravenous ganciclovir treatment. (Courtesy of Dr. Donald J. D'Amico.)*

rophy, hepatosplenomegaly, anemia, and thrombocytopenia. CMV can also represent opportunistic infection in the immunocompromised patient and is the most common cause of retinitis in the AIDS patient (Fig 4). Several series have reported that CMV retinitis eventually affects 12 to 46% of AIDS patients at some point during their disease process [24]. After spreading hematogenously to the retina, the virus spreads along the nerve fiber layer and in the corresponding deep retina. Retinal necrosis occurs in these areas, with active proliferating virus residing in the advancing edge of the lesion. Symptoms include visual loss or scotomas, depending on the location of the lesion and whether there is macular edema or papillitis. CMV retinitis rarely causes anterior inflammation or pain.

The classical hemorrhagic form of CMV retinitis involves large areas of retinal hemorrhage against a background of whitened, necrotic retina, and its appearance is often described as "crumbled cheese and ketchup" or "pizza pie." Other forms include the "brushfire" variation, which appears as a yellow-white margin of slowly advancing retinitis at the border of atrophic, whitened retina. Finally, the "granular" form is manifested by white, focal granular lesions in the peripheral retina and is sometimes seen in patients partially treated with ganciclovir. Complications of any form of CMV retinitis include central or branch retinal vein occlusion, macular edema, papillitis, and optic atrophy [25]. Diagnosis is made primarily by clinical examination, although blood and urine cultures are helpful in congenital infections. In AIDS patients, however, the overwhelming majority of patients harbor the virus or have antibodies to the virus, whether or not CMV retinitis or systemic disease such as CMV colitis has been diagnosed clinically.

Treatment is effective with systemic ganciclovir (dihydroxy propoxymethyl guanine) (see Fig 4). Ganciclovir is only virostatic, and the CMV retinitis will reactivate if therapy is discontinued; the disease recurs in up to 50% of even those patients on maintenance therapy [24]. Intravitreal ganciclovir has also been used and was found to be a successful alternative to systemic therapy when neutropenia is present or when other bone marrow–suppressing agents are being employed [24, 26]. Foscarnet (trisodium phosphonoformate hexahydrate) is a newer agent that has been used effectively for CMV retinitis [27]. Its reversible side effects include anemia without neutropenia and nephrotoxicity.

Herpes Simplex Virus Retinitis　Herpes simplex virus (HSV) is probably the most common cause of congenital ocular infection, usually the result of HSV type II. When genital herpes occurs in the pregnant mother prior to the thirty-second week of gestation, the risk of neonatal infection is approximately 10%. However, when genital herpes is present at the time of delivery, 40 to 80% of babies are affected [28]. There is also a higher rate of spontaneous abortion and prematurity in fetuses infected by HSV [29]. Signs of infection acquired during delivery in the newborn include conjunctivitis, keratitis, retinitis, papulovesicular rash, jaundice, cyanosis, encephalitis, seizure, and gastrointestinal bleeding. Mortality is high in cases of high-grade, disseminated infection. There is also evidence to support the occurrence of intrauterine, transplacental infection, with the usual outcome being fetal death, although premature births characterized by microcephaly, microphthalmos, retinal dysplasia, and intracranial calcifications have also been reported [30].

HSV retinitis caused by type I or II virus can also be acquired in the immunocompromised patient and, occasionally, in the otherwise healthy patient, often accompanied by viral encephalitis [31, 32]. Posterior pole findings include a necrotizing retinitis and an underlying choroiditis. It is also believed that HSV is one of the causes, along with varicella zoster virus, of acute retinal necrosis, which is a retinitis that can occur in both immunocompromised and immunocompetent patients [33]. The current treatment for HSV retinitis is systemic acyclovir and corticosteroids, although the true efficacy of such therapy has yet to be determined.

Rubella Retinitis　Prior to the large-scale immunization programs in 1969 and later, congenital infection by the rubella virus was an important cause of retinitis in newborns, although it is uncommon now in the United States. Eighty percent of cases are bilateral [34]. The classical finding is mottling of the RPE layers, commonly described as "salt and pepper" in appearance, which fades as the child approaches adulthood. There may also be evidence of pigment loss from the pigmented layer of the iris, manifested as transillumination defects on slit-lamp examination [35]. These ocular findings may be seen in isolation or in association with other eye findings such as cataract and microphthalmos, as well as with systemic abnormalities such as deafness and congenital heart disease [36]. In children with only the salt-and-pepper changes in the fundus, visual acuity is usually normal as are color vision, visual fields, electroretinogram, and electrooculogram. Fluorescein angiography will show mottled hyperfluorescence in the areas of pigment loss in the RPE and may aid in diagnosing early choroidal neovascularization, a known complication [35].

Congenital Syphilis The incidence of congenital syphilis, caused by the spirochete *Treponema pallidum,* has fallen more than 99% since the 1940s as a result of prenatal testing and better control of sexually transmitted diseases in the general population [37]. Transplacental transmission can occur during any stage of pregnancy, but lesions form only after the fourth month of gestation when immunological competence begins to develop. This suggests that the manifestations of congenital syphilis may represent an immune response of the host rather than a direct toxic effect of the organism. Adequate treatment of the mother prior to the fourth month can prevent fetal damage [38].

An infected fetus that survives to birth commonly has a maculopapular rash, epithelial desquamation, rhinitis, hepatosplenomegaly, and osteochondritis. The fundus characteristically shows a salt-and-pepper chorioretinitis in both eyes (Fig 5), and the condition may be confused with retinitis pigmentosa as well as with infections of the retina due to mumps, rubella, HSV, and varicella. Optic disc pallor, iritis, and glaucoma may also be present [39]. Systemic disease in untreated survivors becomes latent after 1 to 2 years but can recrudesce in approximately one-third of cases [40]. When latent disease becomes active in the eye, it usually presents as an interstitial keratitis. The stigmata of late congenital syphilis include Hutchinson's teeth, abnormal facies, deafness, meningitis, and saber shins. In newborns, serological diagnosis is most sensitive with the FTA-ABS test for IgM, since this class of immunoglobulins does not cross the placenta. The test for IgG does not differentiate between active production of antibody by the infant and passively transferred antibody from the mother [38]. In older patients, the traditional tests are the VDRL and the FTA-ABS for IgG. Treatment involves the systemic administration of penicillin and probenecid [39, 40].

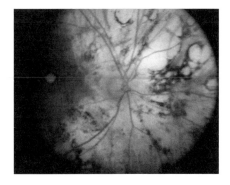

Figure 5 *Severe chorioretinal atrophy in congenital syphilis.*

Endophthalmitis Endophthalmitis in children occurs secondary to prior trauma; or as a result of hematogenous (endogenous) spread of bacteria or fungus, usually in an immunocompromised patient; or in a hospitalized patient undergoing surgical procedures elsewhere in the body or having an indwelling intravenous catheter [41–45]. Symptoms include red eye, pain, photophobia, decreased visual acuity, and headache. Examination can reveal systemic evidence of infection such as fever, lethargy, and meningism. Eye manifestations include eyelid swelling, injection of the conjunctiva, corneal edema or abscess, cells in the anterior chamber with or without hypopyon, elevated intraocular pressure, vitritis, retinal hemorrhages, and optic disc edema. Focal fluffy retinal or choroidal lesions may be seen in fungal infection. Ultrasonography is useful when the view of the fundus is inadequate.

When evidence of prior trauma is present, the cause for infection is obvious. However, when there is no history or sign of trauma, one must rule out the possibility of an endogenous source of the endophthalmitis by searching for a focus of primary infection, which may in itself be life-threatening and must be treated immediately. Most common are wound infections, meningitis, endocarditis, urinary tract infection, and infection of an indwelling intravenous catheter or a hemodialysis fistula. Specific microbial diagnosis is imperative in guiding therapy. Usually culture specimens are obtained by taps of the anterior chamber and vitreous cavity, and cultures of blood, urine, and other possible sources of infection are also obtained. The diagnosis of fungus is aided by calcofluor or Cellufluor (Polysciences, Warrington, PA) staining of the specimens [46]. Treatment may depend on the severity of the disease and include a combination of intravitreal injection of antibiotic or corticosteroid or both, vitrectomy, and systemic intravenous antibiotics. Poor visual outcome in endophthalmitis has been associated with poor initial visual acuity.

Tuberculosis Tuberculosis is a less common cause of posterior uveitis in children but can be seen in cases of miliary disease. Clinical manifestations include unifocal or multifocal choroiditis, choroidal tuberculoma, retinal periphlebitis, and sometimes subretinal neovascularization (Fig 6) [47, 48]. Occasionally, the disease can be fulminant and progress rapidly to panophthalmitis. Because it is rare to see ocular tuberculosis in otherwise healthy patients or in patients with only pulmonary tuberculosis, an underlying immunosuppressive state such as AIDS should also be considered in these children. Diagnosis is by PPD skin testing and chest x-ray. In the patient with a positive PPD and uveitis but no evidence of systemic disease, a therapeutic trial with isoniazid is recommended by some clinicians. If successful, treatment entails isoniazid, rifampin, and pyridoxine for 1 year [49]. Systemic disease mandates appropriate systemic treatment. The differential diagnosis of this disease should include sarcoidosis, syphilis, cryptococcosis, nocardiosis, and *T. canis* infection.

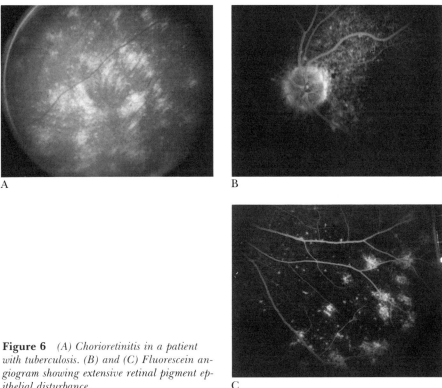

A

B

Figure 6 *(A) Chorioretinitis in a patient with tuberculosis. (B) and (C) Fluorescein angiogram showing extensive retinal pigment epithelial disturbance.*

C

Presumed Ocular Histoplasmosis Syndrome Although acute cases of ocular histoplasmosis have yet to be identified, the scarring due to this presumed syndrome is commonly seen in adults, and its prevalence increases with age. It is not commonly seen in children. The usual scenario is of asymptomatic, atrophic, punched-out, chorioretinal lesions in the periphery with peripapillary chorioretinal scarring in an otherwise healthy person in his or her twenties or thirties (Fig 7). Other manifestations that are symptomatic, however, include macular lesions, serous or hemorrhagic retinal detachment, and choroidal neovascular membrane. The endemic areas are in the eastern and central United States, particularly the Ohio and Mississippi river valleys. The presumed etiological agent is *Histoplasma capsulatum,* based on the discovery that 90 to 95% of patients with typical features of the disease show a positive reaction to histoplasmin skin testing [50].

Trauma

Intraocular Foreign Body Although most intraocular foreign bodies are inert, some can, on occasion, cause a severe uveitis—for example, plas-

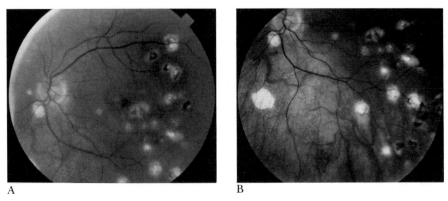

A   B

Figure 7 *(A, B) Presumed ocular histoplasmosis. (Courtesy of Dr. Robert J. Brockhurst.)*

tics such as Bakelite and casein. History of penetrating injury to the eye is important, but sometimes such history is unknown or unrecognized until months or years later when the patient experiences ocular irritation or diminished vision. The possibility of child abuse should also be kept in mind. Possible posterior manifestations of inflammation include vitritis, pigmentary degeneration of the retina, and retinal or choroidal mass [51, 52]. Of course, anterior segment signs of prior trauma, such as iridocyclitis, corneal deposits, or cataract, are helpful clues. Ultrasonography, CT scanning, and magnetic resonance imaging (MRI) can aid in diagnosis and planned surgical removal of the foreign body. The possibility of siderotic (iron) retinopathy or chalcosis (copper) maculopathy should be considered, with adjunctive visual field and electroretinography testing if appropriate [53, 54].

Sympathetic Ophthalmia With a history of penetrating ocular trauma, sympathetic ophthalmia (SO) in the "exciting" or the "sympathizing" eye is in the differential diagnosis of uveitis. In younger patients, however, an adequate history is often difficult to obtain so this possibility should always be kept in mind. Approximately 55% of cases of SO are related to prior penetrating trauma; 45% follow surgery [55]. The latency period ranges from 10 days to 50 years, with an average of 4 to 8 weeks [55, 56]. Ninety percent of trauma-related SO occurs within the first year after the trauma [57, 58]. The average age of presentation in a group of 17 patients followed at the National Institutes of Health was 39 years, with the youngest patient being 6 and the oldest 80 years of age [59]. The exact mechanism of the development of SO is not known, but an autoimmune reaction with a dominant T-cell response is suspected.

Symptoms can vary considerably, from mild photophobia, lacrimation, or conjunctival redness ("sympathetic irritation," a term coined by Marek)

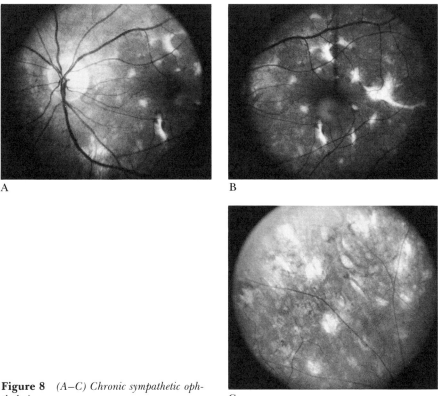

Figure 8 *(A–C) Chronic sympathetic ophthalmia.*

A

B

C

to severe visual loss [58]. Clinical features vary as well and include cell and flare, and mutton-fat keratic precipitates in the anterior segment (Fig 8). Posterior segment findings include moderate to severe vitritis, multiple white-yellow lesions at the level of the RPE (Dalen-Fuchs nodules), choroidal thickening, and papillitis. The sequelae of chronic SO include cataract, secondary glaucoma, retinal and choroidal atrophy, retinal detachment, and optic atrophy. Rarely, patients with SO can exhibit features similar to those seen in Vogt-Koyanagi-Harada syndrome: meningism with cells in the cerebrospinal fluid, hearing problems, and hair and skin changes. Histologically, the two diseases are extremely similar and probably reflect similar pathogeneses [60]. In addition, SO can mimic lesions seen in acute posterior multifocal placoid pigment epitheliopathy. Superimposed phacoanaphylaxis is seen in 23 to 46% of eyes [57, 61].

Diagnosis of SO is primarily by history and examination, although fluorescein angiography is a useful adjunct. Electroretinography is altered, but the electrooculogram is normal. Management of SO begins with the decision of whether to treat with medical therapy alone or by enucleation of the exciting eye plus medical therapy. Some evidence suggests that enucleation within 2 weeks of onset of symptoms may improve the visual outcome of the remaining eye [57, 62]. Medical treatment usually involves high-dose systemic corticosteroids and, possibly, immunosuppressive agents as well.

Neoplasia

Retinoblastoma Although retinoblastoma classically presents with leukocoria and strabismus, it can also masquerade as primary uveitis or cause a secondary uveitis. In one series from the Armed Forces Institute of Pathology in 1969 [63], 8.3% of retinoblastoma cases were misdiagnosed as primary ocular inflammations. Retinoblastoma is the most common intraocular malignancy of childhood, with an incidence of 0.99 to 10.47 cases per million children younger than 15 years [64]. Thirty-one percent of cases are diagnosed within the first year of life, with approximately 90% of cases diagnosed by age 5 [64]. Six percent of patients have a positive family history, and 20 to 35% of cases are bilateral [64, 65]. A tumor-predisposing mutation involves deletion or mutation of the retinoblastoma gene (chromosomal band 13q14) and is inherited as an autosomal dominant trait. A second mutation of the allelic pair of the gene produces a tumor [66].

Presenting clinical signs include leukocoria (61%), strabismus (22%), decreased vision (5%), orbital inflammation and proptosis (2%), red, painful eye due to secondary glaucoma (2%), spontaneous hyphema (0.5%), and heterochromia iridis (0.5%) [67]. Free-floating retinoblastoma cells in the aqueous (presenting as iritis or hypopyon) or the vitreous ("vitreous seeds") can occur, especially in advanced cases [68]. Furthermore, secondary inflammation may be a prominent feature in diffusely infiltrative tumor. In a 1965 study by Howard and Ellsworth [69] of retinoblastoma in which other diagnoses were initially invoked, uveitis accounted for 10%, larval granulomatosis for 6.5%, and endophthalmitis for 1% of the 265 cases. Diagnosis is made by clinical examination, ultrasonography, CT scanning, and examination under anesthesia. Anterior chamber paracentesis in selected cases may be useful in differentiating tumor from inflammation (by cytological evaluation of free-floating cells or by assaying the aqueous-to-serum lactate dehydrogenase ratio) [14].

Children with retinoblastoma must undergo full pediatric evaluation to rule out metastases as well as associated malignancies such as osteogenic sarcoma, fibrosarcoma, and rhabdomyosarcoma. Of patients with bilateral retinoblastoma, 10 to 20% will develop a second neoplasm within 20 years [70]. Depending on the degree of disease and the level of vision, management options include enucleation, radiotherapy, photocoagulation, cryotherapy, and chemotherapy. Relative cellular undifferentiation, optic nerve involvement, and choroidal involvement are believed to correlate with metastatic disease.

Leukemia   Approximately 82% of patients with acute leukemia and 75% of patients with chronic leukemia develop some pathological evidence of ocular disease as found in postmortem studies [71]. Clinically, however, nearly four-fifths of patients seen with eye disease related to leukemia have an acute leukemic process [72].

In acute leukemia, the retina is the most frequently involved site clinically, with cotton-wool spots, gray-white streaks along retinal vessels and, occasionally, massive leukemic infiltrates (Fig 9). On histopathological examination, however, the choroid is actually more often involved, and typically leukemic infiltrates are seen. Other ocular manifestations include leukemic infiltrates in the iris, conjunctiva, or orbit, pseudohypopyon of tumor cells, glaucoma, and hyphema [71]. The optic nerve can be involved, particularly when there is CNS involvement. Direct infiltration of the nerve by tumor cells can occur, as well as edema of the optic nerve or disc secondary to increased intracranial pressure or retrolaminar leukemic invasion [71, 73].

Treatment options for ocular disease in leukemia include local irradiation along with appropriate systemic and intrathecal chemotherapy for the underlying systemic and CNS disease. Decreased vision from leukemic

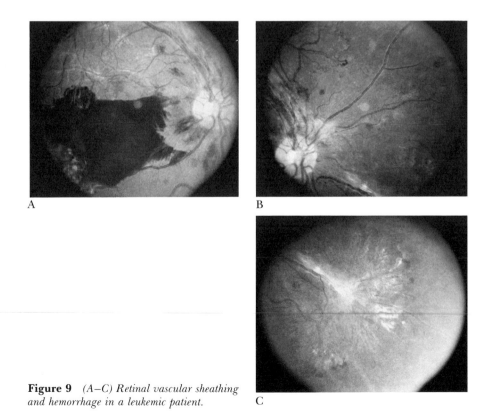

A   B   C

Figure 9   *(A–C) Retinal vascular sheathing and hemorrhage in a leukemic patient.*

infiltration of the optic nerve is an ophthalmic emergency and can be treated successfully with prompt irradiation [71]. Of course, one must also remember that with the immunosuppressive treatments given leukemic patients, opportunistic infections such as CMV retinitis and fungal endophthalmitis must be considered in the differential diagnosis of a posterior uveitis. Furthermore, intravenous injection of some chemotherapeutic agents has been known to cause a necrotizing retinal vasculitis [74].

Autoimmune or Unknown Etiology

Intermediate Uveitis   Although intermediate uveitis (also called *pars planitis* and *peripheral uveitis*) presents most commonly in the young adult, by some estimates as many as one-fifth of children presenting with uveitis have this disease [75]. There are isolated reports of familial pars planitis but no consistent HLA type association. The process is bilateral in 70 to 80% of patients, and one-third that present unilaterally progress to bilateral involvement [76, 77]. Intermediate uveitis in the pediatric group often presents as an acute anterior uveitis with red eye, pain, and photophobia, in contrast to the milder symptoms commonly seen in adults [78]. The cause of intermediate uveitis has not been determined, although an increased association has been described between intermediate uveitis and demyelinating diseases such as multiple sclerosis [79].

The classical findings are vitritis, peripheral retinal vasculitis, exudates over the pars plana, and vitreous exudates (Fig 10). The anterior inflammation can be variable but includes iritis, occasionally keratic precipitates, iris synechiae, and band keratopathy. A mild course of the disease usually does not result in any visual loss and may be treated symptomatically with topical corticosteroids and cycloplegia. More severe disease can result in significant visual loss due to vitreous hemorrhage from neovascular tufts,

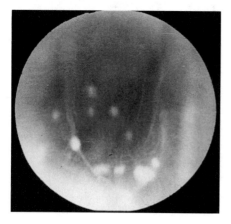

Figure 10   *Vitreous strands and clumps of white cells in the peripheral fundus of a patient with intermediate uveitis.*

Table 3 *Stepwise Treatment of Intermediate Uveitis*

1. Regional corticosteroid injection
2. Oral nonsteroidal antiinflammatory agents
3. Cryotherapy
4. Short courses of oral corticosteroids
5. Immunosuppressive agents*
6. Pars plana vitrectomy

*Agents that have been useful include cyclosporine, azathioprine, methotrexate, and colchicine.

secondary vitreous organization, macular edema, epiretinal membrane, and papillitis. In these cases, aggressive treatment should be undertaken. We recommend a modified version of the four-step approach described by Smith [80] and Kaplan [81] and shown in Table 3: Treatment would progress to a higher level if lower levels failed to control inflammation. Especially in children, cryotherapy along the pars plana is often attempted to control the inflammation and avoid chronic corticosteroid or immunosuppressive therapy [82]. Regardless, the course is usually prolonged into adulthood, and long-term complications can include cataract, tractional retinal detachment, glaucoma, and optic atrophy. Cataract extraction and intraocular lens implantation has been successfully used to rehabilitate eyes with significant secondary cataract formation [83]. The prognosis is best with control of all inflammation such that permanent ocular damage is limited and the chance for visual rehabilitation is improved. One should not accept chronic low-grade inflammation at baseline as this increases the risk of poor visual outcome. The differential diagnosis of intermediate uveitis in children includes *T. canis* infection, sarcoidosis, and Lyme disease.

Acute Posterior Multifocal Placoid Pigment Epitheliopathy Typically, this disease affects otherwise healthy young adults, the average age at presentation being approximately 25 years [84]. There is often a history of a flulike syndrome a few weeks prior to the acute onset of visual loss, eventually in both eyes [85]. Examination of the posterior pole shows multiple, postequatorial, flat, gray-white, subretinal lesions involving the RPE (Figs 11, 12). The overlying retina is usually normal in appearance. Approximately one-half of patients have an accompanying vitritis. Occasionally, there is tortuosity of the retinal veins, papillitis, optic neuritis, serous retinal detachment, episcleritis, and iridocyclitis [84–86]. The process is generally self-limiting, with resolution of lesions over weeks and a good prognosis for near-normal visual recovery. The cause of this disease is unknown.

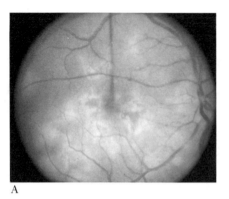 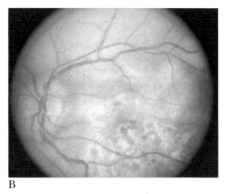

A   B

Figure 11 *(A, B) Acute posterior multifocal placoid pigment epitheliopathy. (Courtesy of Dr. John I. Loewenstein.)*

Vogt-Koyanagi-Harada Syndrome Vogt-Koyanagi-Harada syndrome (VKH, also called *uveomeningeal syndrome*) presents generally in young adults, with a mean age at onset of symptoms of approximately 40 years [87]. More common in Japan and certain parts of South America, VKH is relatively uncommon in the United States [87, 88]. Ninety-four percent of cases are bilateral [89]. The syndrome includes the extraocular manifestations of vitiligo, poliosis, and dysacousia. Often there is a prodromal stage of headache, orbital pain, stiff neck, and vertigo [89, 90]. Ocular findings include a granulomatous iridocyclitis, vitritis, optic disc edema, exudative nonrhegmatogenous retinal detachment, and peripheral, yellow-white lesions in the retina similar to the Dalen-Fuchs nodules

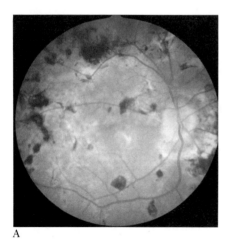 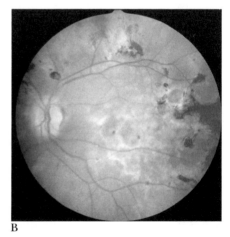

A   B

Figure 12 *(A, B) Retinal pigment epithelial hypertrophy and atrophy 10 years later in the same patient as in Figure 12. Visual acuity is normal. (Courtesy of Dr. John I. Loewenstein.)*

seen in sympathetic ophthalmia (Fig 13) [87–90]. The disease can progress to retinal and disc neovascularization and vitreous hemorrhage before spontaneous regression occurs. In regression, there is characteristic depigmentation of the RPE in the posterior pole, with the appearance of a "sunset glow" in Oriental patients or a "blond fundus" in white patients [89]. Other sequelae include subretinal fibrosis, disciform scars, and migration of RPE. The diagnosis of VKH relies heavily on the extraocular manifestations since, depending on the stage of the disease, VKH can mimic acute posterior multifocal placoid pigment epitheliopathy, sarcoidosis, sympathetic ophthalmia, and several white-dot syndromes. Treatment mainly involves systemic corticosteroids and immunosuppressive agents. Recurrences are possible, and visual prognosis depends on recurrence and on the severity of active disease.

Behçet's Disease Behçet's disease is a systemic vasculitis characterized by intraocular inflammation, oral ulcers, genital ulcers, and skin lesions. Specific diagnostic criteria are listed in Table 4. It can occur at any age, although it presents most frequently between the ages of 20 and 40 [91]. The disease is most common in the Far East and the Mediterranean basin, with the greatest prevalence in Japan [92, 93]. In the United States, the disease is relatively rare. The cause of Behçet's disease is unknown. Ocular manifestations include recurrent sterile hypopyon, iridocyclitis, retinal hemorrhages and exudates, vascular sheathing, vascular occlusions, serous retinal detachment, and optic disc edema (Fig 14) [91, 94]. It is the posterior manifestations that ultimately lead to visual loss. Treatment includes systemic corticosteroids and chemotherapeutic agents such as chlorambucil, cyclophosphamide, colchicine, azathioprine, and cyclosporine [91, 95]. Plasmapheresis has been used in medically resistant cases [96]. The prognosis is generally guarded but, with recent advances in the aggressive use

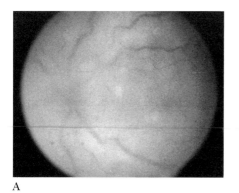 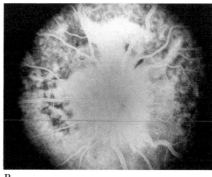

A   B

Figure 13 (A) Optic disc edema and retinal exudates in a patient with Vogt-Koyanagi-Harada syndrome. (B) Fluorescein angiogram in same patient.

Table 4 *Diagnostic Criteria for Behçet's Disease*

O'Duffy and Goldstein

Suggested criteria:
  Aphthous stomatitis, aphthous genital ulceration, uveitis, cutaneous vasculitis, synovitis, and meningoencephalitis

Diagnosis:
  At least three criteria present, one being recurrent aphthous ulceration

Incomplete form:
  Two criteria present, one being recurrent aphthous ulceration

Exclusions:
  Inflammatory bowel disease, systemic lupus erythematosus, Reiter's disease, and herpetic infections

Behçet's Disease Research Committee of Japan

Major criteria:
  Recurrent aphthous ulceration in the mouth
  Skin lesions
    Erythema nodosum–like eruptions
    Subcutaneous thrombophlebitis
    Hyperirritability of the skin
  Eye lesions
    Recurrent hypopyon, iritis, or iridocyclitis
    Chorioretinitis
  Genital ulcerations

Minor criteria:
  Arthritic symptoms and signs (arthralgia, swelling, redness)
  Gastrointestinal lesions (appendicitislike pains, melena, etc.)
  Epididymitis
  Vascular lesions (occlusion of blood vessels, aneurysms)
  Central nervous system involvements
    Brainstem syndrome
    Meningoencephalomyelitic syndrome
    Confusional type disorders

Types of Behçet's disease:
  Complete type: all four major symptoms appear in the clinical course of the patient
  Incomplete type:
    Three of four major symptoms appear in the clinical course of the patient
    Recurrent hypopyon-iritis or typical chorioretinitis and one other major symptom appear in the clinical course of the patient
  Suspect: involvement at two major sites
  Possible: involvement at one major site

Reprinted with permission from Teter MS and Hochberg MC [93].

of corticosteroids and chemotherapy, some patients have retained useful vision [97].

Juvenile Rheumatoid Arthritis   Ocular involvement in juvenile rheumatoid arthritis largely involves the anterior segment, usually producing a chronic iridocyclitis or acute, episodic, nongranulomatous anterior inflammation. Occasionally, however, the inflammation can extend to the posterior segment of the eye as well and cause vitritis, cyclitic membranes,

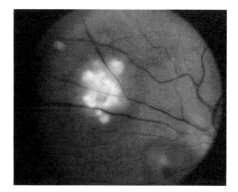

Figure 14 *Retinal exudates in Behçet's disease.*

secondary retinal traction and retinal detachment, cystoid macular edema, fixed macular cysts, and macular holes (Fig 15) [98, 99]. These, in turn, can precipitate secondary glaucoma or hypotony. The best prevention of poor visual outcome lies in the aggressive abolishment of inflammation with systemic corticosteroid and immunosuppressive therapy. Management options also include vitrectomy to clear vitreous opacities at the time of cataract extraction [100]. However, the long-term benefits of such surgery have yet to be determined.

Sarcoidosis Sarcoidosis occurs in the older pediatric population (age 8 to 15 years) at the same rate as in adults [101]. Furthermore, numerous cases (at least 17) have been reported in children younger than age 5 [102]. Sarcoidosis can occur in any ethnic group but in the United States is most common in the black population. The disease involves a chronic, granulomatous inflammatory process that can affect the mediastinal and peripheral lymph nodes, lungs, liver, spleen, skin, eyes, phalangeal bones, parotid glands, and the CNS. However, in contrast to the adult and older-child population, sarcoidosis in the very young child rarely involves the lungs but predominates in the joints, skin, and eyes [102]. The prevalence of ocular involvement in patients with sarcoidosis ranges from 15 to 50%,

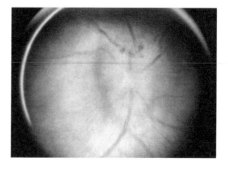

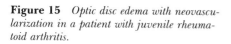

Figure 15 *Optic disc edema with neovascularization in a patient with juvenile rheumatoid arthritis.*

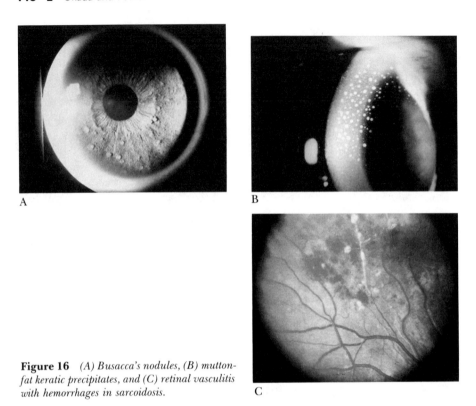

Figure 16 *(A) Busacca's nodules, (B) mutton-fat keratic precipitates, and (C) retinal vasculitis with hemorrhages in sarcoidosis.*

depending on the published series [103, 104]. The cause of the disease is not known.

Anterior segment findings, present in approximately two-thirds of patients with ocular sarcoidosis, include keratoconjunctivitis sicca, granulomatous iritis with mutton-fat keratic precipitates, iris nodules, iris synechiae, glaucoma, and cataract (Fig 16) [104]. In affected children younger than 5 years, the incidence of anterior uveitis may be higher than in adults and older children [105]. Posterior segment manifestations occur less commonly, varying from 14 to 43% of patients [103, 104]. The manifestations include vitritis, with or without focal collections of cells occurring inferiorly in the classical string-of-pearls configuration, pars planitis, retinal periphlebitis sometimes appearing as candle-wax drippings, perivenous sheathing, chorioretinal granulomas, macular edema, and optic disc edema. Other manifestations include eyelid nodules, lacrimal gland infiltration, and orbital granuloma formation [103, 104, 106].

The initial workup for sarcoidosis includes chest x-ray (which would show hilar adenopathy), angiotensin-converting enzyme (ACE) level (which is elevated in the majority of active cases), and skin testing (which often shows anergy). When the chest x-ray is negative, a gallium scan may demonstrate hilar adenopathy or parotid or lacrimal gland involvement. Definitive diagnosis is made on biopsy of lymph node, skin, or liver, showing noncaseating granulomas. Treatment for both systemic and ocular disease involves systemic corticosteroids and, rarely, chemotherapy [107]. Long-term complications of the ocular inflammation seen in sarcoidosis include retinal or disc neovascularization, choroidal neovascularization, retinal detachment, glaucoma, and cataract [103, 104].

Subacute Sclerosing Panencephalitis Subacute sclerosing panencephalitis (SSPE, also called *Dawson's encephalitis* and *inclusion body encephalitis*) is an extremely rare disease characterized by personality and behavioral changes followed by dementia, seizures, myoclonus and, usually, death. The disease occurs in children and young adults; the mean age at the time of presentation is 7 years, with 80% of cases presenting by age 11. Boys are affected between three and ten times as frequently as girls [108]. Most patients have a history of measles (rubeola infection) at a young age, and therefore SSPE is believed to be a long-term complication of measles or a slow form of measles encephalitis. SSPE may be precipitated during cytotoxic or immunosuppressive treatment or by states of immunodeficiency [109]. Measles virus or a closely related virus has been recovered from brain and retinal tissue of patients with the disease [109, 110]. Visual disturbances often precede neurological symptoms, and approximately one-half of patients eventually have unilateral or bilateral involvement of the eye or the central visual pathways [109, 111, 112].

When the disease involves the retina, small, flat, focal white lesions or larger, ragged, gray-white areas may be seen. If the macula is also involved with retinitis, a cherry-red spot may be present. The initial lesions tend to resolve into areas of RPE atrophy with gliosis and folds of the retina. The choroid and vitreous are usually minimally involved [109, 111, 112]. There is no known treatment for SSPE. Overall prognosis for this disease is grim, but there have been reports of recovery in young adults.

■ Discussion

Posterior segment inflammation in children presents a difficult diagnostic dilemma for the clinician. Based on the age of the child and a careful history, a brief differential can be constructed to guide laboratory and radiological testing. Examination of young children in the clinical setting can be inadequate and must, in many cases, be done under anesthesia. Treatment is often dictated by the risk of amblyopia. The effects of systemic corticosteroid and chemotherapeutic agents must be monitored closely in concert with pediatricians and other medical services. However, prompt and aggressive therapy is mandatory to save vision.

■ References

1. Perkins ES. Pattern of uveitis in children. Br J Ophthalmol 1966;50:169–185
2. Kimura SJ, Hogan MJ, Thygeson P. Uveitis in children. Arch Ophthalmol 1954; 51:80–88
3. Giles CL. Uveitis in childhood: III. Posterior. Ann Ophthalmol 1989;21:23–28
4. Carosi G, Filice G, Meroni V, et al. Congenital toxoplasmosis: a serologic screening of 963 mothers and their children at birth. Int J Biol Res Pregnancy 1981; 2:117–122
5. Krick JA, Remington JS. Toxoplasmosis in the adult: an overview. N Engl J Med 1978;298:550–553
6. Remington JS, Desmonts G. Toxoplasmosis. In: Remington JS, Klein JO, eds. Infectious diseases of the fetus and newborn infant. Philadelphia: Saunders, 1983:193–263
7. Boguslawska-Jaworska J, Pisarek J, Chybicka A. Toxoplasmosis in the course of neoplastic diseases of haematopoietic and lymphatic system in children. Mater Med Pol 1982;14:62–67
8. Smith RE. Toxoplasmic retinochoroiditis as an emerging problem in AIDS patients. Am J Ophthalmol 1988;106:738–739
9. Nussenblatt RB, Palestine AG. Uveitis: fundamentals and clinical practice. Chicago: Year Book, 1989:336–354
10. Schantz PM, Glickman LT. Current concepts in parasitology: toxocaral visceral larva migrans. N Engl J Med 1978;298:436–439
11. Diallo JS. Syndromes de larva migrans. In: Manifestations ophtalmologiques des parasitoses. Paris: Masson, 1985:155–161
12. Ellis GS Jr, Pakalnis VA, Worley G, et al. *Toxocara canis* infestation: clinical and epidemiological associations with seropositivity in kindergarten children. Ophthalmology 1986;93:1032–1037
13. Shields JA. Ocular toxocariasis: a review. Surv Ophthalmol 1984;28:361–381
14. Piro PA Jr, Abramson DH, Ellsworth RM, Kitchin D. Aqueous humor lactate dehydrogenase in retinoblastoma patients: clinicopathologic correlations. Arch Ophthalmol 1978;96:1823–1825
15. Wilkinson CP, Welch RB. Intraocular toxocara. Am J Ophthalmol 1971;71: 921–930
16. Carrillo M, Barriga OO. Antihelminthic effect of levamisole hydrochloride or ivermectin on tissue toxocariasis of mice. Am J Vet Res 1987;48:281–283
17. Hagler WS, Pollard ZF, Jarrett WH, Donnelly EH. Results of surgery for ocular *Toxocara canis*. Ophthalmology 1981;88:1081–1086
18. Gass JDM, Gilbert WR Jr, Guerry RK, Scelfo R. Diffuse unilateral subacute neuroretinitis. Ophthalmology 1978;85:521–545
19. Gass JDM, Braunstein RA. Further observations concerning the diffuse unilateral subacute neuroretinitis syndrome. Arch Ophthalmol 1983;101:1689–1697
20. Raymond LA, Gutierrez Y, Strong LE, et al. Living retinal nematode (filarial-like) destroyed with photocoagulation. Ophthalmology 1978;85:944–949
21. American Academy of Pediatrics Task Force on Pediatric AIDS. Perinatal human immunodeficiency virus infection. Pediatrics 1988;82:941–944
22. Dennehy PJ, Warman R, Flynn JT, et al. Ocular manifestations in pediatric patients with acquired immunodeficiency syndrome. Arch Ophthalmol 1989;107: 978–982
23. Holland GN, Pepose JS, Pettit TH, et al. Acquired immune deficiency syndrome: ocular manifestations. Ophthalmology 1983;90:859–872
24. Cantrill HL, Henry K, Melroe NH, et al. Treatment of cytomegalovirus retinitis with intravitreal ganciclovir. Ophthalmology 1989;96:367–374

25. Gass JDM. Stereoscopic atlas of macular diseases: diagnosis and treatment. St Louis: Mosby, 1987:486–487

26. Henry K, Cantrill H, Fletcher C, et al. Use of intravitreal ganciclovir (dihydroxy propoxymethyl guanine) for cytomegalovirus retinitis in a patient with AIDS. Am J Ophthalmol 1987;103:17–23

27. Jacobson MA, O'Donnell JJ, Mills J. Foscarnet treatment of cytomegalovirus retinitis in patients with the acquired immunodeficiency syndrome. Antimicrob Agents Chemother 1989;33:736–741

28. Petersdorf RB, Adams RD, Braunwald E, et al. Harrison's principles of internal medicine. New York: McGraw-Hill, 1983:1162–1167

29. Nahmias AJ, Hagler WS. Ocular manifestation of herpes simplex in the newborn (neonatal ocular herpes). Int Ophthalmol Clin 1972;12:191–213

30. Reynolds JD, Griebel M, Mallory S, Steele R. Congenital herpes simplex retinitis. Am J Ophthalmol 1986;102:33–36

31. Uninsky E, Jampol IM, Kaufman S, Naraqi S. Disseminated herpes simplex infection with retinitis in a renal allograft recipient. Ophthalmology 1983;90:175–178

32. Grutzmacher RD, Henderson D, McDonald PJ, Coster DJ. Herpes simplex chorioretinitis in a healthy adult. Am J Ophthalmol 1983;96:788–796

33. Duker JS, Blumenkranz MS. Diagnosis and management of the acute retinal necrosis (ARN) syndrome. Surv Ophthalmol 1991;35:327–343

34. Deutman AF, Grizzard WS. Rubella retinopathy and subretinal neovascularization. Am J Ophthalmol 1978;85:82–87

35. Hertzberg R. Twenty-five-year follow-up of ocular defects in congenital rubella. Am J Ophthalmol 1968;66:269–271

36. Wolff SM. The ocular manifestations of congenital rubella. Trans Am Ophthalmol Soc 1972;70:577–614

37. Schlaegel TF Jr, Kao SF. A review (1970–1980) of 28 presumptive cases of syphilitic uveitis. Am J Ophthalmol 1982;93:412–414

38. Petersdorf RB, Adams RD, Braunwald E, et al. Harrison's principles of internal medicine. New York: McGraw-Hill, 1983:1034–1045

39. Folk JC, Weingeist TA, Corbett JJ et al. Syphilitic neuroretinitis. Am J Ophthalmol 1983;95:480–486

40. Goldman J. Clinical experience with ampicillin and probenecid in the management of treponeme-associated uveitis. Trans Am Acad Ophthalmol Otolaryngol 1970; 74:OP509–514

41. Bohigian GM, Olk RJ. Factors associated with a poor visual result in endophthalmitis. Am J Ophthalmol 1986;101:332–341

42. Greenwald MJ, Wohl LG, Sell CH. Metastatic bacterial endophthalmitis: a contemporary reappraisal. Surv Ophthalmol 1986;31:81–101

43. Parke DW II, Jones DB, Gentry LO. Endogenous endophthalmitis among patients with candidemia. Ophthalmology 1982;89:789–796

44. Puliafito CA, Baker AS, Haaf J, Foster CS. Infectious endophthalmitis: review of 36 cases. Ophthalmology 1982;89:921–929

45. Rowsey JJ, Newsom DL, Sexton DJ, Harms WK. Endophthalmitis: current approaches. Ophthalmology 1982;89:1055–1066

46. Sutphin JE, Robinson NM, Wilhelmus KR, Osato MS. Improved detection of oculomycoses using induced fluorescence with Cellufluor. Ophthalmology 1986;93: 416–417

47. Cangemi FE, Friedman AH, Josephberg R. Tuberculoma of the choroid. Ophthalmology 1980;87:252–258

48. Inoue S, Ubuka M. A case of choroidal miliary tuberculosis as studied by fluorescence fundus photography. Folia Ophthalmol Jpn 1972;23:256–259

49. Schlaegel TF Jr, O'Connor GR. Tuberculosis and syphilis. Arch Ophthalmol 1981; 99:2206–2207

50. Gass JDM. Stereoscopic atlas of macular diseases: diagnosis and treatment. St Louis: Mosby, 1987:112–129

51. Brown A. Intraocular foreign bodies: nature of injury. Int Ophthalmol Clin 1968;8:147–152

52. Khan MD, Kundi N, Mohammed Z, Nazeer AF. A 6½–7 years' survey of intraocular and intraorbital foreign bodies in the Northwest Frontier Province, Pakistan. Br J Ophthalmol 1987;71:716–719

53. Cibis PA, Yamashita T, Rodriguez F. Clinical aspects of ocular siderosis and hemosiderosis. Arch Ophthalmol 1959;62:180–187

54. Felder KS, Gottlieb F. Reversible chalcosis. Ann Ophthalmol 1984;16:638–641

55. Gass JDM. Sympathetic ophthalmia following vitrectomy. Am J Ophthalmol 1982; 93:552–558

56. Liddy N, Stuart J. Sympathetic ophthalmia in Canada. Can J Ophthalmol 1972; 7:157–159

57. Lubin JR, Albert DM, Weinstein M. Sixty-five years of sympathetic ophthalmia: a clinicopathologic review of 105 cases (1913–1978). Ophthalmology 1980;87: 109–121

58. Marak GE Jr. Recent advances in sympathetic ophthalmia. Surv Ophthalmol 1979; 24:141–156

59. Nussenblatt RB, Palestine AG. Uveitis: fundamentals and clinical practice. Chicago: Year Book, 1989:257–273

60. Rao NA, Marak GE. Sympathetic ophthalmia simulating Vogt-Koyanagi-Harada's disease: a clinicopathologic study of four cases. Jpn J Ophthalmol 1983;27: 506–511

61. Blodi FC. Sympathetic uveitis as an allergic phenomenon. Trans Am Acad Ophthalmol Otolaryngol 1959;63:642–649

62. Reynard M, Riffenburgh RS, Maes EF. Effect of corticosteroid treatment and enucleation on the visual prognosis of sympathetic ophthalmia. Am J Ophthalmol 1983;96:290–294

63. Stafford WR, Yanoff M, Parnell BL. Retinoblastomas initially misdiagnosed as primary ocular inflammations. Arch Ophthalmol 1969;82:771–773

64. Pendergrass TW, Davis S. Incidence of retinoblastoma in the United States. Arch Ophthalmol 1980;98:1204–1210

65. Carlson EA, Letson RD, Ramsay NKC, et al. Factors for improved genetic counseling for retinoblastoma based on a survey of 55 families. Am J Ophthalmol 1979; 87:449–459

66. Yandell DW, Campbell TA, Dayton SH, et al. Oncogenic point mutations in the human retinoblastoma gene: their application for genetic counseling. N Engl J Med 1989;321:1689–1695

67. Howard GM, Ellsworth RM. Differential diagnosis of retinoblastoma: a statistical survey of 500 children. II. Factors relating to the diagnosis of retinoblastoma. Am J Ophthalmol 1965;60:618–621

68. Binder PS. Unusual manifestations of retinoblastoma. Am J Ophthalmol 1974; 77:674–679

69. Howard GM, Ellsworth RM. Differential diagnosis of retinoblastoma: a statistical survey of 500 children. I. Relative frequency of the lesions which simulate retinoblastoma. Am J Ophthalmol 1965;60:610–618

70. Abramson DH, Ronner HJ, Ellsworth RM. Second tumors in nonirradiated bilateral retinoblastoma. Am J Ophthalmol 1979;87:624–627

71. Kincaid MC, Green WR. Ocular and orbital involvement in leukemia. Surv Ophthalmol 1983;27:211–232

72. Allen RA, Straatsma BR. Ocular involvement in leukemia and allied disorders. Arch Ophthalmol 1961;66:490–508

73. Brown GC, Shields JA, Augsburger JJ, et al. Leukemic optic neuropathy. Int Ophthalmol 1981;3:111–116

74. Anderson B, Anderson B Jr. Necrotizing uveitis incident to perfusion of intracranial malignancies with nitrogen mustard or related compounds. Trans Am Ophthalmol Soc 1960;58:95–104

75. Schlaegel TF. Ocular toxoplasmosis and pars planitis. New York: Grune & Stratton, 1978

76. Henderly DE, Haymond RS, Rao NA, et al. The significance of the pars plana exudate in pars planitis. Am J Ophthalmol 1987;103:669–671

77. Smith RE, Godfrey WA, Kimura SJ. Chronic cyclitis: course and visual prognosis. Trans Am Acad Ophthalmol Otolaryngol 1973;77:OP760–768

78. Giles CL. Pediatric intermediate uveitis. J Pediatr Ophthalmol Strabismus 1989; 26:136–139

79. Giles CL. Peripheral uveitis in patients with multiple sclerosis. Am J Ophthalmol 1970;70:17–19

80. Smith RE. Pars planitis. In: Ryan SJ, ed. Retina. St Louis: Mosby, 1989:637–645

81. Kaplan HJ. Intermediate uveitis (pars planitis, chronic cyclitis)—a four-step approach to treatment. In: Saari KM, ed. Uveitis update. Amsterdam: Excerpta Medica, 1984:169–172

82. Aaberg TM, Cesarz TJ, Flickinger RR Jr. Treatment of pars planitis: I. Cryotherapy. Surv Ophthalmol 1977;22:120–125

83. Foster CS, Fong LP, Singh G. Cataract surgery and intraocular lens implantation in patients with uveitis. Ophthalmology 1989;96:281–288

84. Gass JDM. Acute posterior multifocal placoid pigment epitheliopathy: a long-term follow-up study. In: Fine SL, Owens SL, eds. Management of retinal vascular and macular disorders. Baltimore: Williams & Wilkins, 1983:176–181

85. Savino PJ, Weinberg RJ, Yassin JG, Pilkerton AR. Diverse manifestations of acute posterior multifocal placoid pigment epitheliopathy. Am J Ophthalmol 1974;77: 659–662

86. Fishman GA, Rabb MF, Kaplan J. Acute posterior multifocal placoid pigment epitheliopathy. Arch Ophthalmol 1974;92:173–177

87. Snyder DA, Tessler HH. Vogt-Koyanagi-Harada syndrome. Am J Ophthalmol 1980;90:60–75

88. Sugiura S. Vogt-Koyanagi-Harada disease. Jpn J Ophthalmol 1978;22:9–35

89. Nussenblatt RB, Palestine AG. Uveitis: fundamentals and clinical practice. Chicago: Year Book, 1989:274–290

90. Perry HD, Font RL. Clinical and histopathologic observations in severe Vogt-Koyanagi-Harada syndrome. Am J Ophthalmol 1977;83:242–254

91. James DG, Spiteri MA. Behcet's disease. Ophthalmology 1982;89:1279–1284

92. Ohno S. Behcet's disease in the world. In: Lehner T, Barnes CG, eds. Recent advances in Behcet's disease. London: Royal Society of Medicine Services, 1986: 181–186

93. Teter MS, Hochberg MC. Diagnostic criteria and epidemiology. In: Plotkin GR, Calabro JJ, O'Duffy JD. Behcet's disease: a contemporary synopsis. Mount Kisco, NY: Futura Publishing, 1988:9–28

94. Atmaca LS. Fundus changes associated with Behcet's disease. Graefes Arch Clin Exp Ophthalmol 1989;227:340–344

95. BenEzra D, Cohen E. Treatment and visual prognosis in Behcet's disease. Br J Ophthalmol 1986;70:589–592

96. Raizman MB, Foster CS. Plasma exchange in the therapy of Behcet's disease. Graefes Arch Clin Exp Ophthalmol 1989;227:360–363

97. Baer JC, Raizman MB, Foster CS. Ocular Behcet's disease in the United States: clinical presentation and visual outcome in 29 patients. In: Usui M, Ohno S, Aoki K, eds. Ocular immunology today. Amsterdam: Elsevier Science, 1990:383–386

98. Key SN III, Kimura SJ. Iridocyclitis associated with juvenile rheumatoid arthritis. Am J Ophthalmol 1975;80:425–429
99. Smiley WK. The eye in juvenile rheumatoid arthritis. Trans Ophthalmol Soc UK 1974;94:817–829
100. Diamond JG, Kaplan HJ. Uveitis: effect of vitrectomy combined with lensectomy. Ophthalmology 1979;86:1320–1327
101. Giles CL, Handleman I. Panuveitis: presenting symptom of systemic sarcoidosis in a child. J Pediatr Ophthalmol 1976;13:189–191
102. Cohen KL, Peiffer RL Jr, Powell DA. Sarcoidosis and ocular disease in a young child: a case report and review of the literature. Arch Ophthalmol 1981;99: 422–424
103. James DG, Neville E, Langley DA. Ocular sarcoidosis. Trans Ophthalmol Soc UK 1976;96:133–139
104. Crick RP, Houle C, Smellie H. The eyes in sarcoidosis. Br J Ophthalmol 1961;45: 461–481
105. Hoover DL, Khan JA, Giangiacomo J. Pediatric ocular sarcoidosis. Surv Ophthalmol 1986;30:215–228
106. Gass JDM, Olson CL. Sarcoidosis with optic nerve and retinal involvement. Arch Ophthalmol 1976;94:945–950
107. Nussenblatt RB, Palestine AG. Uveitis: fundamentals and clinical practice. Chicago: Year Book, 1989:198–211
108. Petersdorf RB, Adams RD, Braunwald E, et al. Harrison's principles of internal medicine. New York: McGraw-Hill, 1983:2096
109. Haltia M, Tarkkanen A, Vaheri A, et al. Measles retinopathy during immunosuppression. Br J Ophthalmol 1978;62:356–360
110. Landers MB III, Klintworth GK. Subacute sclerosing panencephalitis (SSPE): a clinicopathologic study of the retinal lesions. Arch Ophthalmol 1971;86:156–163
111. Robb RM, Watters GV. Ophthalmic manifestations of subacute sclerosing panencephalitis. Arch Ophthalmol 1970;83:426–435
112. Nelson DA, Weiner A, Yanoff M, De Peralta J. Retinal lesions in subacute sclerosing panencephalitis. Trans Am Neurol Assoc 1970;95:334

New Techniques for Evaluating Pediatric Retinal Disease: Molecular Genetics

Elias Reichel, M.D.
Eliot L. Berson, M.D.

Most children who present with decreased vision can have their visual loss corrected with eyeglasses. Some have asymmetrical loss and, in these cases, amblyopia and strabismus must be suspected. Some children have congenital cataracts that can be removed; a few have retinal detachments that can also be repaired. However, it is important for pediatricians to recognize that some children can present with bilateral reduction in vision due to hereditary diseases affecting the retina, choroid, or optic nerve for which no treatments are known.

Hereditary diseases of the retina, choroid, and optic nerve should be suspected in children or adolescents who present with profound light sensitivity, a color deficiency, night deficiency, a tendency to bump into objects, or a propensity to hold objects very close to the face. A careful family history may reveal similarly affected relatives, thereby helping to establish a diagnosis. A family history of consanguinity should also increase the index of suspicion that the patient is suffering from a hereditary disease, but it should be borne in mind that many of these hereditary diseases involving the retina and optic nerve are recessively inherited so that the family history can be negative.

An ophthalmoscopic examination of the disc, macula, and near mid-periphery can sometimes help to establish the diagnosis of a hereditary disease involving the retina, choroid, or optic nerve. However, some of these diseases may show minimal, if any, changes on ophthalmoscopic examination in the early stages. Retinal or choroidal diseases may show changes only in the far periphery, thereby making it difficult to establish a diagnosis in a child or adolescent.

Recent advances in molecular genetic techniques can now aid in the diagnosis of some hereditary diseases that affect the retina, choroid, and optic nerve. This chapter provides an overview of six diseases affecting these tissues for which precise gene defects have recently been discovered through analysis of DNA extracted from peripheral blood. These diseases, discussed in the order in which the gene abnormalities were found, are gyrate atrophy of the choroid and retina, Leber's hereditary optic neuropathy, blue-cone monochromacy, X-linked cone degeneration, dominant forms of retinitis pigmentosa, and choroideremia.

■ Gyrate Atrophy of the Choroid and Retina

Gyrate atrophy of the choroid and retina is a rare autosomal recessive disorder. The condition has been observed in children in the United States but the number affected is probably fewer than 100. Patients usually present in adolescence with myopia and night blindness. Ocular findings include chorioretinal atrophy that appears scalloped in the far peripheral fundus. The visual field is constricted, dark adaptation thresholds are elevated, and the electroretinogram (ERG) is reduced [1]. As the disease progresses, the chorioretinal atrophy proceeds toward the posterior pole, and eventually the macula becomes involved. Patients are usually completely blind by the fifth or sixth decade.

Patients affected with gyrate atrophy have a tenfold to twentyfold elevation of the amino acid ornithine in their serum, hypolysinemia, hyperornithinuria, and absence of the enzyme ornithine-∂-aminotransferase (OAT) in cultured skin fibroblasts. Extracts of cultured skin fibroblasts from obligate heterozygotes have shown a 50% reduction in OAT activity.

Pyridoxine (vitamin B_6) is known to be a cofactor for the OAT enzyme in normal individuals. Some patients with gyrate atrophy have been found to be biochemically responsive to pyridoxine (B_6 responders) in doses of 300 to 500 mg/day, with lowering of serum ornithine levels toward normal. Others with gyrate atrophy have not responded to vitamin B_6 but have responded biochemically to a low-protein, low-arginine diet, reducing protein intake to 0.2 gm/kg/day while supplying by capsule essential amino acids, minerals, and vitamins. A low-protein, low-arginine diet in these patients has led to lowering of serum ornithine levels toward normal. However, it remains to be established whether lowering of serum ornithine levels with vitamin B_6 or a low-protein, low-arginine diet will substantially alter the course of the chorioretinal degeneration over the long term.

The gene encoding OAT has been mapped to the long arm of chromosome 10. The normal OAT gene contains 11 exons and is approximately 21 kilobases in length, with 1,400 bases of coding sequences. This gene was identified after the enzyme defect was identified; that is, synthetic DNA probes were made after the amino acid sequence of the enzyme was determined. Using various cloning and sequencing strategies, several investigators have discovered many different mutations in the OAT gene [2–5]. Defining these mutations and how they affect the function of OAT enzyme should allow us to understand the basis of OAT deficiency in gyrate atrophy. Interestingly, those patients who have responded to vitamin B_6 appear to have different mutations of the OAT gene than those who have not responded.

■ Leber's Hereditary Optic Neuropathy

Leber's hereditary optic neuropathy (LHON) is a rare, maternally inherited disease that usually manifests itself as acute or subacute severe bilateral visual loss in otherwise healthy male adolescents. Affected young men present with reduced visual acuity, and fundus examination usually reveals pallor of both optic discs. In contrast to optic neuritis, this condition does not result in discomfort on extraocular movements, and no inflammation can be seen in the vitreous. Patients typically have large cecocentral scotomas. Visual acuity can be reduced from 20/200 to 20/400. Patients will try to compensate by holding print close to the face or by seeking magnifiers to alleviate the difficulty with reading.

A young man who presents with LHON may appear to have a family history of X-linked disease, but closer inspection will reveal that affected men have not transmitted the condition to their children whereas affected women, even though they are asymptomatic, have had affected children of either sex. Some women may show visual symptoms later in life. The maternal pattern of inheritance pointed to the possibility that the gene defect for LHON was located in mitochondrial DNA, which is itself strictly maternally inherited.

A point mutation in mitochondrial DNA was identified in LHON [6]. This mutation is a guanine-to-adenine substitution at position 11,778 corresponding to a substitution of histidine for arginine. This mutation affects the fourth subunit of nicotinamide adenine dinucleotide dehydrogenase. Using restriction enzymes that specifically cut at the altered DNA sequence has provided a test that is 100% specific (no false positives) but only 50% sensitive (50% false negatives). The false-negative rate has been established by knowing that only 50% of individuals with LHON have the 11,778 mutation. Recently, a new technique has been described for identifying the 11,778 mutation with 100% specificity and sensitivity [7]. This entails using a restriction enzyme called (*Mae*III) that cuts at a new restriction cutting site in the DNA created by the point mutation causing LHON.

Analyses of mitochondrial DNA isolated from a peripheral blood sample can now provide a diagnosis of LHON. Moreover, by knowing what part of the protein subunit is affected, new insight is provided into the pathogenesis of this condition, with possible implications for therapy.

■ Blue-Cone Monochromacy

Blue-cone monochromacy is a rare X-linked disorder. Patients with this condition typically present with 20/60 to 20/200 vision early in life, nystagmus, photophobia, a scotopic axis of confusion on the Farnsworth D15 color panel, and a macula that is granular in the early stages with atrophy ensuing in the more advanced stages. Psychophysical testing shows a peak sensitivity in the blue-green region of the visible spectrum (near 504 nm) in the dark due to the remaining rod function and a peak sensitivity in the blue region of the spectrum (near 440 nm) in the light due to remaining blue-cone function and loss of red- and green-cone function [8, 9]. Young male patients with this condition can perform the blue-cone monochromat color vision plate test, while young men with autosomal recessive complete achromatopsia fail these plates [10]. ERGs show normal rod function and reduced cone responses (less than 2 μV) to 30-Hz white flicker (lower norm, 50 μV), again due to loss of red- and green-cone function and the persistence of some blue-cone function. The ERGs of female carriers of this X-linked disorder show a partial loss of red- and green-cone function [11].

Two different types of mutations have been discovered in men with blue-cone monochromacy [12]. The red and green pigment genes lie in a tandem array on the long arm of the X chromosome. In one class of mutation, there is a deletion that occurs 4 kilobases upstream of the red pigment gene that defines a 579 base pair region that appears to be essential for the transcriptional activity of both red and green pigment genes. The second type of mutation exists in individuals with only one cone pigment gene. Loss of function of this single cone pigment gene occurs because of a point mutation in the gene that results in an inability to maintain a disulfide bond that is critical for the structure of the only remaining cone opsin protein. Molecular genetic tests, therefore, can aid in distinguishing X-linked blue-cone monochromacy from autosomal recessive complete achromatopsia.

Once blue-cone monochromacy is recognized, the pediatrician can assure a parent that his or her son would be expected to retain rod function, and possibly some blue-cone function as well, for his entire life. With the rod system, such patients can read fine print (sometimes requiring magnification) and can use telescopes to see the blackboard in school. Because of their light sensitivity, they may benefit from dark sunglasses with side shields, which may allow them to maintain some rod function under daylight conditions. These sunglasses might well be worn not only outdoors but also indoors under room light conditions.

■ X-Linked Cone Degeneration

X-linked cone degeneration, protan type, is a rare condition characterized by a mutation in the red-cone pigment gene [13]. In some ways, it can be considered as related to blue-cone monochromacy. However, there are significant clinical differences between the two. Patients who have X-linked cone degeneration have visual acuity of approximately 20/30 in early life, a protan axis of confusion on the Farnsworth D15 color panel, and normal extraocular movements with no evidence of nystagmus. The macula appears to be normal or granular in early life; however, atrophy ensues in later life, and visual acuity declines to 20/200. Patients have normal rod dark-adaptation thresholds and normal rod ERGs throughout life. Full-field cone ERGs are partially reduced in childhood and become nondetectable in later life due to gradual diminution in red- and green-cone function. ERGs from a young man with this disease have revealed a cone response of approximately 25 μV, significantly greater than what is found in blue-cone monochromats [13]. Southern blot analysis of individuals from one family affected with X-linked cone degeneration has shown a deletion of part of the red-cone pigment gene. It has been postulated that a 6.5-kilobase deletion between exons 1 and 4 of the red pigment gene occurs. No altered restriction fragments have been discovered in the green pigment gene in this family, although point mutations or small deletions in the green pigment gene have not been excluded.

Once X-linked cone degeneration, protan type, is diagnosed, the pediatrician can reassure the parents that the child would be expected to retain normal rod function but have a gradual loss of cone function over life. As in the case of blue-cone monochromacy, these patients can use their remaining rod function for reading and mobility. They too will express a preference for sunglasses outdoors and sometimes indoors as well.

■ Autosomal Dominant Retinitis Pigmentosa

Retinitis pigmentosa is another hereditary retinal disease that affects children. This condition is among the more common hereditary diseases in the United States, with an estimated 50,000 to 100,000 people affected. The incidence at birth is estimated to be 1 in 3,500 [14]. Patients with retinitis pigmentosa may have difficulty with dark adaptation, night blindness, and light sensitivity in childhood or adolescence. As the disease progresses, they lose midperipheral visual field and, eventually, central vision as well. Signs on fundus examination in more advanced stages include narrowed retinal vessels, intraretinal bone spicule pigment around the periphery, and waxy pallor of the optic discs. In the early stages, fundus changes may be minimal or absent, but the disease can be detected on the basis of an abnormal ERG. Most patients with retinitis pigmentosa are legally blind by age 40. The condition can be inherited by an autosomal dominant, autosomal recessive, or X-linked mode [14].

A restriction fragment length polymorphism called CRI-C17 was found to be strongly linked to the disease trait in a large family with dominant retinitis pigmentosa in Ireland [5]. CRI-C17 was known to be located on the long arm of chromosome 3. Since the rhodopsin gene mapped to chromosome 3 and since rhodopsin is expressed in rod photoreceptors that are affected early in this condition, it was likely that the rhodopsin gene was defective in individuals with some forms of dominant retinitis pigmentosa (candidate gene approach). Using the polymerase chain reaction to amplify selected portions of the rhodopsin gene and directly sequencing these regions, it has been possible to identify point mutations in the rhodopsin gene sequence [15, 16]. Oligomer-specific hybridization, restriction endonuclease digestion, and analysis of single-strand conformation polymorphisms have also been used to detect point mutations. More than twenty different mutations have been reported to exist in the rhodopsin gene in clinically affected patients with autosomal dominant retinitis pigmentosa [17–19]. None of these mutations has been observed in clinically unaffected relatives.

The first reported mutation was in codon 23 of the rhodopsin gene. In this case, a cytosine is changed to an adenine. This change corresponds to a substitution of histidine for proline in the twenty-third amino acid of the rhodopsin protein. Other mutations have been observed in codons 58 and 347 of the rhodopsin gene. Patients with the proline-23-histidine mutation appear to have a milder disease than those with the proline-347-leucine mutation [20, 21]. Among patients with the proline-23-histidine mutation, interfamilial as well as intrafamilial variability with respect to severity of their ocular disease has been observed. These findings imply that some factor(s) other than the gene defect itself is involved in the expression of the severity of this form of retinitis pigmentosa [20, 21]. Therefore, children identified with rhodopsin gene mutations should have an ocular examination, including ERGs, to help determine the severity of their disease.

■ Choroideremia

Choroideremia is an X-linked chorioretinal degeneration that is more common than gyrate atrophy but considerably less common than retinitis pigmentosa. In the outpatient Electroretinography Service of the Massachusetts Eye and Ear Infirmary, choroideremia accounts for approximately 3% of the individuals affected with chorioretinal degeneration, and from this it can be estimated that the condition affects a few thousand male individuals in the United States. Young men with this condition are often asymptomatic, and the condition is suspected only when there is a family history of affected male relatives who have become blind from ages 30 to 60 due to this condition. The symptoms of night deficiency and loss of side vision become evident in late adolescence or early adulthood, even though the condition can be seen clinically with the ophthalmoscope early in life. Affected men show granularity and depigmentation of the retinal pigment epithelium, initially visible around the periphery with the ophthalmoscope. As the condition advances, clumped pigment and chorioretinal atrophy are visible around the periphery. Affected men usually retain little, if any, central vision after the age of 60 years. Female carriers of this condition may be asymptomatic but demonstrate patchy depigmentation of the retinal pigment epithelium, coarse pigment granularity, or even pigment clumps in the periphery. Affected men show grossly reduced ERGs early in life, whereas female carriers may show normal or reduced ERGs [22].

The gene for choroideremia has been localized to the long arm of the X chromosome [23]. With the use of strategies by which the protein defect is not known (reverse genetics), the gene that corresponds to this condition was found to encompass a cDNA of 948 base pairs [24]. Small deletions of genetic material were identified in individuals with choroideremia. By focusing on the region of the X chromosome where the deletion that caused choroideremia was found, highly conserved fragments were isolated. Highly conserved fragments are often believed to represent functional genes because they have been maintained throughout evolution. One gene was found that is expressed in the retina, choroid, and retinal pigment epithelium. The gene also appears to be expressed in HeLa cells and in Epstein-Barr virus–immortalized B cells. The sequence of this gene bears no significant homology to any genes or protein sequences that have been isolated thus far [25].

Again, it is important to recognize that intrafamilial and interfamilial variability exists with respect to the severity of the disease at a given age in patients with choroideremia. The reason for this variability is not known. Patients detected through analysis of leukocyte DNA should have regular ocular examinations, including ERGs, to help define the severity of their disease.

■ Conclusion

Hereditary diseases involving the retina, choroid, or optic nerve represent a significant cause of visual loss to children in the United States. These conditions should be suspected in patients who present with light sensitivity, night deficiency, color deficiencics, or poor vision not correctable with eyeglasses. In some cases, the diagnosis can be easily established by a careful ophthalmoscopic examination but, in some of these conditions, the findings on ophthalmoscopy may be minimal or absent in the early stages.

Advances in molecular biology have revealed precise gene defects in gyrate atrophy of the choroid and retina, Leber's hereditary optic neuropathy, blue-cone monochromacy, X-linked cone degeneration, dominant forms of retinitis pigmentosa and, most recently, choroideremia. Knowing the exact gene defect in these conditions provides new opportunities to understand the pathogenesis of these diseases. Treatment modalities can now be considered since we know the exact biochemical abnormalities. Technology is in hand to create transgenic mice that carry these human gene abnormalities. Different pharmacological agents can be tried in transgenic models in an attempt to find methods to ameliorate these conditions. Transplantation of specific cell types and even gene therapy may be attempted in transgenic animals.

Clinical variability exists in hereditary diseases of the retina, choroid, and optic nerve among patients with the same mutation. Children suspected of having these conditions should have their leukocyte DNA analyzed with molecular genetic techniques to confirm the mutations. Children identified with retinal and choroidal diseases should have a complete ocular examination with electroretinography to determine the severity of their disease and as an additional guide with respect to establishing long-term prognoses. Risk factor analyses of patients with the same gene mutation and varying severity of disease may reveal factors other than the gene itself that may be contributing to the course of the disease, with possible implications for therapy.

This work was supported in part by a grant from the National Retinitis Pigmentosa Foundation, Baltimore, MD.

■ References

1. Berson EL, Schmidt SY, Shih VE. Ocular and biochemical abnormalities in gyrate atrophy of the choroid and retina. Ophthalmology 1978;85:1018–1027
2. Inana G, Chambers C, Hotta Y, et al. Point mutation affecting processing of the ornithine aminotransferase precursor protein in gyrate atrophy. J Biol Chem 1989; 264:17432–17436
3. McClatchey AI, Kaufman DL, Berson EL, et al. Splicing defect at the ornithine aminotransferase (OAT) locus in gyrate atrophy. Am J Hum Genet 1990;47: 790–794
4. Mitchell GA, Brody LC, Sipila I, et al. At least two mutant alleles of ornithine ∂-aminotransferase cause gyrate atrophy of the choroid and retina in Finns. Proc Natl Acad Sci USA 1989;86:197–201
5. Ramesh V, McClatchey AI, Ramesh N, et al. Molecular basis of ornithine aminotransferase deficiency in B-6-responsive and -non-responsive forms of gyrate atrophy. Proc Natl Acad Sci USA 1988;85:3777–3780
6. Wallace DC, Singh G, Lott MT, et al. Mitochondrial DNA mutation associated with Leber's hereditary optic neuropathy. Science 1988;242:1427–1430
7. Johns DR. Improved molecular genetic diagnosis of Leber's hereditary optic neuropathy. N Engl J Med 1990;323:1488–1489
8. Alpern M, Lee GB, Spivey BE. π_1 Cone monochromatism. Arch Ophthalmol 1965;74:334–337
9. Blackwell HR, Blackwell OM. Blue mono-cone monochromacy: a new color vision defect (Abstract). J Opt Soc Am 1957;47:338
10. Berson EL, Sandberg MA, Rosner B, Sullivan PL. Color plates to help identify patients with blue cone monochromatism. Am J Ophthalmol 1983;95:741–747

11. Berson EL, Sandberg MA, Maguire A, et al. Electroretinograms in carriers of blue cone monochromatism. Am J Ophthalmol 1986;102:254–261
12. Nathans J, Davenport CM, Maumenee IH, et al. Molecular genetics of human blue cone monochromacy. Science 1989;245:831–838
13. Reichel E, Bruce AM, Sandberg MA, Berson EL. An electroretinographic and molecular genetic study of X-linked cone degeneration. Am J Ophthalmol 1989;108: 540–547
14. Berson EL. Ocular findings in a form of retinitis pigmentosa with a rhodopsin gene defect. Trans Am Ophthalmol Soc 1990;88:355–388
15. McWilliam P, Farrar GJ, Kenna P, et al. Autosomal dominant retinitis pigmentosa (ADRP): localization of an ADRP gene to the long arm of chromosome 3. Genomics 1989;5:619–622
16. Dryja TP, McGee TL, Reichel E, et al. A point mutation of the rhodopsin gene in one form of retinitis pigmentosa. Nature 1990;343:364–366
17. Bhattachyra SS, Inglehearn CF, Keen J, et al. Identification of novel rhodopsin mutations in patients with autosomal dominant retinitis pigmentosa. Invest Ophthalmol Vis Sci 1991;32(suppl):890
18. Dryja TP, Hahn LB, McGee TL, et al. Mutation spectrum of the rhodopsin gene among patients with autosomal dominant retinitis pigmentosa. Invest Ophthalmol Vis Sci 1991;32(suppl):890
19. Stone EM, Khadini P, Kimura AE, Sheffield VC. A rapid denaturing gradient gel method of screening for rhodopsin gene mutations in patients with retinitis pigmentosa. Invest Ophthalmol Vis Sci 1991;32(suppl):891
20. Berson EL, Rosner B, Sandberg MA, Dryja TP. Ocular findings in patients with autosomal dominant retinitis pigmentosa and a rhodopsin gene defect (pro 23 his). Arch Ophthalmol 1991;109:92–101
21. Dryja TP, McGee TL, Hahn LB, et al. Mutations within the rhodopsin gene in patients with autosomal dominant retinitis pigmentosa. N Engl J Med 1990;323: 1302–1307
22. Berson EL, Rosner B, Sandberg MA, et al. Ocular findings in patients with autosomal dominant retinitis pigmentosa and rhodopsin, proline-347-leucine. Am J Ophthalmol 1991;111:614–623
23. Sieving PA, Niffenegger JH, Berson EL. Electroretinographic findings in selected pedigrees with choroideremia. Am J Ophthalmol 1986;101:361–367
24. McCulloch C. Choroideremia: a clinical and pathologic review. Trans Am Ophthalmol Soc 1969;67:142–195
25. Pameyer JK, Waardenburg PJ, Henkes HE. Choroideremia. Br J Ophthalmol 1960;44:724–738

Retinopathy of Prematurity: Pathogenesis, Diagnosis, and Treatment

David G. Hunter, M.D., Ph.D.
Shizuo Mukai, M.D.

Retinopathy of prematurity (ROP) is a proliferation of abnormal retinal blood vessels that occurs in newborn infants. The condition was first described as retrolental fibroplasia by Terry in 1942 [1], who noted the presence of a fibroblastic mass behind the lens in 100 premature infants. Over the following decade, the disease reached epidemic proportions and, at its peak, was responsible for 30% of all blindness in preschool children in the United States. In 1952, Patz and colleagues [2] identified the link between ROP and high concentrations of oxygen. This was followed by restriction of oxygen administration to premature neonates and a dramatic decrease in the incidence of the disease in the 1950s and 1960s. The withdrawal of oxygen therapy, however, led to an increase in neurologic sequelae and death from prematurity, and oxygen use was judiciously increased in the 1970s.

Advances in neonatology have led to an increase in the survival of very young premature infants over the past 20 years, with a corresponding resurgence of ROP. This has renewed interest in the pathogenesis, prevention, and treatment of ROP [3–6]. In this chapter, we will review the clinical presentation of ROP and recent advances in our understanding of this potentially blinding disease.

■ Epidemiological Features

Incidence

The first studies of the incidence of ROP considered only the most severe forms of the disease (retrolental fibroplasia), as indirect ophthalmoscopy was not widely available [7–17]. Still, approximately 25% of all premature infants were diagnosed with the condition. By the late 1950s, the incidence had plummeted to fewer than 5% of premature infants following

163

admonitions that no infant be subjected to higher than a 40% concentration of oxygen. Nonetheless, by the time the epidemic had passed, as many as 20,000 infants had been affected.

In the mid-1960s, the reported incidence of ROP again began to rise. At least three factors contributed to this increase. First, rising mortality and neurologic morbidity prompted a cautious relaxation of the strict 40% oxygen rule [18]. Second, indirect ophthalmoscopy allowed diagnosis of milder forms of ROP. Finally, advances in neonatology resulted in survival of more neonates at high risk for developing ROP [17]. Thus, in the 1980s the incidence of all forms of ROP had risen to approximately 25% of premature infants. Flynn and co-workers [5] reported an 89% incidence of ROP in infants having a birth weight of less than 900 gm.

Eighty percent of the less severe cases of ROP (stages 1 and 2) regress. Therefore, despite the high incidence of mild forms of the disease, the incidence of severe (stage 3 or worse) ROP in the past decade has remained at approximately 5 to 10%. In 1979, it was estimated that approximately 600 infants in the United States went blind annually from ROP [19]. As the survival rate of very low birth weight preterm infants continues to improve, the number of children blinded by ROP may increase.

Risk Factors

The most important risk factor for development of ROP is immaturity, as determined by gestational age or birth weight. Infants larger than 1,500 gm rarely develop the disease, and infants smaller than 1,000 grams are at highest risk for severe ROP. The second most important factor is oxygen supplementation. Both the level (percentage) and duration of oxygen therapy correlate with the severity of ROP. However, ROP does occur in the absence of oxygen supplementation [20]. Other factors that correlate with ROP severity include sepsis and intraventricular hemorrhage. A recent prospective study suggested that acidosis may be an additional risk factor [21]. Retrospective studies have suggested numerous other potential risk factors [22], but no cause-and-effect relationship has been demonstrated.

▪ Clinical Features and the International Classification

ROP typically develops gradually, with the earliest stages appearing 6 to 8 weeks after delivery. The clinical pattern of the disease can be divided into acute ROP and chronic (scarring, or cicatricial) disease [3–6].

Mild Acute ROP

In the uninvolved premature eye, the division between vascular and avascular retina is not clinically apparent. Fine branches of retinal vessels extend toward but do not reach the ora serrata. The earliest manifestation of acute ROP is the formation of a demarcation line between vascular (*rearguard*) and avascular (*vanguard*) retina. The vessels adjacent to the line are abnormally branched and tortuous. The demarcation line is thin, white, and flat, remaining within the plane of the retina. Avascular retina is present anterior to this line. In clinical studies, this early stage of ROP is the most variably reported, as it may be transient.

If ROP progresses, the demarcation line develops into the *ridge* (also known as the *shunt* or *mesenchymal shunt*), a thickened white or pink structure that extends out of the plane of the retina. Vessels from the posterior retina enter the ridge, and isolated tufts of vessels are also seen in this region. Spontaneous regression with minimal residual scarring occurs in more than 80% of patients with mild acute ROP.

Severe Acute ROP

With further progression, the posterior surface of the ridge develops a ragged appearance due to fibrovascular proliferation. The proliferative vessels extend into the vitreous. Severe forms of ROP can regress spontaneously, though not as frequently as the mild forms. Severe forms are more likely than mild forms to progress to retinal detachment or to leave scarring after they regress.

As ROP progresses, the peripheral retinal vessels become dilated and tortuous. Dilatation and tortuosity of vessels in the posterior pole is a particularly significant development. This can occur at any stage and correlates with a progressive course of ROP. Other indicators of advancing disease include iris vascular engorgement, retinal hemorrhage, and vitreous haze [23].

With continued progression of ROP, vitreoretinal traction develops and causes retinal detachment with secondary exudative fluid accumulation. Vitreoretinal traction develops when myofibroblasts migrate into the vitreous from the ridge and form a contractile fibrovascular mass. The myofibroblasts pull in a purse-string configuration. Peripheral tractional detachments can proceed to total retinal detachment within a day, and complete detachments can form funnels within a week. When the funnel closes, cellular proliferation continues between the apposed layers of retina, resulting in an apparent mass behind the lens.

Exudative detachment with collection of subretinal fluid can occur in ROP in the absence of traction [24]; however, this mechanism is rare. Retinal detachments can also be rhegmatogenous, but this mechanism too is rare during acute ROP. Rhegmatogenous detachments usually occur during surgery at this early stage. After infancy, rhegmatogenous detachments are the most common type seen in ROP patients.

Rush Disease

There are reports of patients who develop ROP earlier than usual (appearing at age 3 to 5 weeks). These patients have an extremely low birth weight (less than 1,000 gm). Some progress rapidly to severe ROP and retinal detachment. This unusually aggressive pattern of ROP development has been termed *rush* disease [25, 26].

Scarring

The mildest permanent anatomical alterations in the eye from ROP include high myopia (often greater than 6 D), vitreoretinal membranes in the periphery, and small areas of peripheral irregular pigmentation. More significant changes include optic nerve pallor and a characteristic straightening and dragging of vessels to the periphery. The macula may also be dragged. The macula is usually pulled temporally in zone 2 disease; in zone 1 disease, however, the traction can be in any direction. Areas of avascular peripheral retina may be present. Lattice degeneration with retinal holes is frequently observed. In more severe cases, falciform retinal folds are seen [15].

In the most severe cases of end-stage scarring, the totally detached retina becomes a thickened mass posterior to the lens. The term *retrolental fibroplasia*, originally applied to the entire disease process, now refers only to this form of scarring.

Classification

The international classification of ROP was developed in 1984 in an attempt to make studies of the natural history and response to treatment more comparable. This widely adopted classification considers the scarring sequelae independently from the acute disease process [27, 28]. The classification scheme provides a standardized framework that can be used to follow clinical progression of the disease. The classification is based on three clinical parameters: the stage of vascular proliferation, the location of the disease, and the extent of involvement.

Stage   The stage of disease indicates the degree of vascular proliferation (Table 1). A "plus" designation is added if vascular dilation and tortuosity involve the vessels in the posterior pole. Stage 3 (Fig 1) has been informally subdivided into mild (3a), moderate (3b), and severe (3c) in some publications. In stage 5, retinal detachment is subdivided by configuration of the detachment.

Table 1 *Stages of Disease in the International Classification of Retinopathy of Prematurity*

Stage	Characteristics		
1	Demarcation line		
2	Ridge		
3	Ridge with extraretinal fibrovascular proliferation		
4	Subtotal retinal detachment		
a	Extrafoveal		
b	Including fovea		
5	Total retinal detachment		
	Funnel:	*Anterior*	*Posterior*
		Open	Open
		Narrow	Narrow
		Open	Narrow
		Narrow	Open

Source: From the International Committee for the Classification of Retinopathy of Prematurity [27, 28].

Location and Extent   The location of disease is plotted in relation to the progression of normal retinal vascularization anteriorly from the optic disc (Fig 2). Thus, zone 1 is a circle surrounding the optic disc that extends to twice the distance from the optic disc to the fovea. This is approximately the most posterior 60 degrees of the fundus. Zone 2 is concentric and anterior to zone 1 and extends nasally to the ora serrata but does not reach the temporal ora. Zone 3 is the remaining temporal crescent of anterior retina. The extent of disease activity is measured in clock hours.

■ Pathogenesis

Retinal Vascular Development

In the human, ocular vascular development occurs in the hypoxic in utero environment [29, 30]. At a gestational age of 6 weeks, the hyaloid artery enters the eye and begins to fill the vitreous cavity with vessels. The retina, however, remains avascular until at least 16 weeks, when mesenchymal spindle cells arise from the adventitia of the hyaloid artery. The spin-

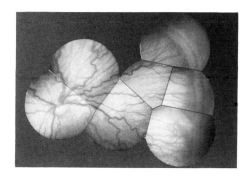

Figure 1   *Montage of fundus photographs from optic disc to avascular retina of an eye with mild stage 3 ROP. There is mild fibrovascular proliferation posterior to the ridge. (Courtesy of Drs. Frank Kretzer and Helen Mintz-Hittner.)*

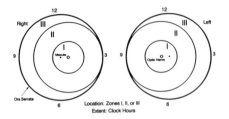

Figure 2 *Disease location and extent in the international classification of acute retinopathy of prematurity. Location is expressed in terms of a numbered zone (I, II, or III). Extent is described in terms of clock hours. (Modified from the Committee for the Classification of Retinopathy of Prematurity [27].)*

dle cells migrate peripherally through cystoid spaces as the outer plexiform layer differentiates. The migrating spindle cells are interconnected and form a circumferential apron that advances peripherally toward the ora serrata. Behind the advancing apron, the spindle cells form solid cords that canalize and metamorphose into capillary endothelial cells. Spindle cells reach the temporal ora serrata by 29 weeks' gestational age, but inner retinal vasoformation does not reach the ora serrata until term.

Early Models of ROP Pathogenesis

The most widely accepted early theory of the pathogenesis of ROP was proposed by Ashton [31] and Patz [15] and co-workers and was based on experimental models of kitten and puppy retinal neovascularization. This theory proposed that elevated oxygen levels led to retinal vasoconstriction which, if prolonged, led to permanent closure of the vessels. Following return to room air, the endothelial cells adjacent to closed capillaries proliferated, leading to new vessel growth.

There are problems with this vasoconstriction-vasoobliteration theory. First, it fails to explain how ROP can develop in infants exposed to minimal supplemental oxygen. Second, the hypothesis cannot explain the efficacy of cryoablation of the avascular peripheral retina. Third, these animal models are not identical to human disease in that the vasoproliferation does not progress to retinal detachment and the retinal vasculature in the species studied does not develop via spindle cells.

The kitten retinal vasculature studied by Ashton and colleagues [31] was almost completely obliterated by elevated oxygen. To study this model in humans, Kretzer and associates [32] used electron microscopy to study vascular development in eyes from preterm infants exposed to supplemental oxygen. These infants were at high risk for developing ROP, but there was no indication of retinal vasoobliteration or endothelial cell destruction, nor any evidence of inner retinal hypoxia or ischemia.

Spindle Cell Model of Neovascularization

Kretzer and colleagues [32, 33] have proposed that the pathogenesis of ROP is due to the presence of spindle cells in the periphery of the immature retina. When developing spindle cells are removed from the hypoxic in utero environment at birth, they are bombarded with oxygen free radicals. The reduced free-radical scavenging capability of preterm infants allows the free radicals to induce extensive plasma membrane lipid peroxidation. The injured spindle cells react by forming massive intercellular linkages via gap junctions. The gap junction–linked spindle cells lose their ability to migrate and to canalize into normal vessels. Instead, they become "activated"—that is, bloated with rough endoplasmic reticulum. Activated spindle cells may secrete an angiogenic factor that promotes vasoproliferation at the border between vascular and avascular retina [34].

The spindle cell hypothesis explains many of the clinical features of ROP [35]. Immaturity is a key component to the development of ROP, as no undifferentiated spindle cells are present at term. Gap junction formation is a documented biological response to cell damage, environmental stress, low pH, and lipid peroxidation. Thus, markedly elevated oxygen tension is not the exclusive requirement for ROP initiation. Immature infants have larger expanses of spindle cells, which makes them more susceptible to developing ROP. Properly administered cryotherapy destroys the peripheral apron of spindle cells, removing the source of the angiogenic factor. According to this model of pathogenesis, delivery of adequate levels of antioxidants to the retina should slow or prevent disease progression.

Animal Models

Animal models of ROP have been developed in the kitten, puppy, rabbit, baboon, and rat [36–38]. In these models, the degree of retinal vascular development in the newborn animals is equivalent to that seen in preterm infants. The newborn animals are exposed to high oxygen tension and the retinal vascular response is studied. Unfortunately, none of the models parallel the human situation. New vessel growth has not been documented in the rabbit. The kitten, puppy, and baboon vasculature does not develop via spindle cells. Rat and mouse retinas contain spindle cells but are very immature at birth compared with humans. Thus, although much can be learned about retinal vascular development through studying animal models, the clinical applicability of the data will be limited until a model more comparable to human disease is developed.

■ Prevention and Treatment

Vitamin E

With ROP closely linked to oxygen administration in the premature infant, it is logical to explore the effect of antioxidants, such as vitamin E, on the incidence and progression of the disease. The preterm infant is deficient in vitamin E at birth owing to a 4:1 placental permeability factor and low plasma lipid and lipoprotein levels. This results in plasma levels of 0.4 mg/dl, compared with normal levels of 1 to 3 mg/dl. Furthermore, vitamin E levels drop quickly in unsupplemented preterm newborns owing to the lack of adipose tissue for storage. In 1949, Owens and Owens [39] presented a controlled clinical trial that suggested that vitamin E supplementation prevented the development of severe ROP. Other investigators were unable to confirm these results. Shortly after publication of this work, oxygen was identified as an etiological agent and interest in vitamin E waned. With the resurgence of ROP in the 1970s came a renewed interest in vitamin E supplementation; controversy regarding its efficacy has continued over the past decade.

In 1981, Hittner and associates [35] reported on a double-blind, controlled study of the efficacy of vitamin E in preventing ROP in preterm infants. Plasma levels of vitamin E were supplemented up to the adult levels of 1.2 mg/dl or greater using low doses of oral vitamin E, which were administered continuously from birth until retinal vascularization extended to the ora serrata. There was a statistically significant decrease in the incidence of severe ROP in the treated infants; the overall incidence of ROP was not affected. Vitamin E was most efficacious in infants of between 1,000- and 1,500-gm birth weight. The study was supported by ultrastructural evidence that spindle cells in the retinas of treated infants did not develop the extensive gap junction linkages seen in control eyes [32]. The vitamin E presumably prevented free radical–induced lipid peroxidation of spindle cell plasma membranes. The decreased efficacy in infants of less than 1,000 gm corresponded with a deficiency of vitamin E transport mechanisms in the developing retina [40]. In two other controlled clinical trials, vitamin E given continuously from the first day of life resulted in a statistically significant decrease in the development of severe ROP [41, 42]. Finer and colleagues [41, 43] used oral and intramuscular supplementation. Johnson and co-workers [42] had a high target plasma level of 5 mg/dl, which led to an increase in vitamin E toxicity.

Three controlled clinical trials have failed to show efficacy of vitamin E; however, each was flawed in design or execution. In one study, the *control* group received supplemental vitamin E to a therapeutic level of 1.1 mg/dl [44]. In another, vitamin E was discontinued in the treated group after only 6 weeks [45]. In the third study, by Phelps and colleagues [46], very high doses of vitamin E were given by rapid intravenous infusion. This route of administration increases the toxicity of the vitamin when given rapidly. In many of the infants in the treatment group, the therapy was interrupted for unspecified reasons, which may have allowed vitamin E levels to drop to a nonefficacious range.

The clinical trials do not suggest that vitamin E eliminates ROP from the neonatal intensive care unit. However, a decrease in the incidence of severe ROP has been observed in three properly conducted studies. Even if vitamin E supplementation is considered efficacious, questions have been raised about its risk-benefit ratio. Most reports of vitamin E toxicity, however, have involved the use of intravenous, pharmacological megadoses or unapproved formulations rather than continuously administered vitamin E supplementation within the upper physiological range.

In 1986, the Institute of Medicine of the National Academy of Sciences [47] concluded that there was no definite evidence of either benefit or harm from prophylaxis with vitamin E against ROP. They also concluded that the risks of giving vitamin E seemed minimal for premature infants as long as the blood concentration was kept below 3 mg/dl. As the controversy over vitamin E continues, multivitamin formulations in general use in neonatal intensive care units now contain sufficient vitamin E to maintain plasma levels close to the adult physiological range. Combining these preparations with a single intramuscular dose of 10 mg/kg/dl alpha-tocopherol (in water) given within 24 hours of birth should be a safe and sufficient way to obtain the maximum benefit of vitamin E [30, 48]. If intravenous multivitamin formulations are not used, the optimal dose suggested by Kretzer and Hittner [30] is a 100 mg/kg/day oral supplement (in a medium-chain triglyceride solution) from the first days of life until retinal vascularization is complete. When oral feedings are interrupted, 10 mg/kg intramuscularly every 3 days (or 3 mg/kg/day intravenously over 8 hours) can be given.

Surfactant

Artificial lung surfactant is now being used with increasing frequency to prevent or treat respiratory distress in preterm infants [49, 50]. The impact of surfactant administration on the incidence of ROP is not yet known. The increasing use of surfactant in neonatal intensive care units will make it more difficult to perform a randomized, masked, controlled trial to investigate its effect on the incidence of ROP.

Cryotherapy

Cryotherapy for ablation of the peripheral retina and treatment of ROP was first used in Japan in 1971 [51] and has been advocated by Ben-Sira [52] and Hindle [53]. Many authors have reported promising results of treatment [52–54], with vascular dilatation and tortuosity sometimes regressing within hours. Complications have been reported, including bleeding following treatment of the ridge (shunt) and late retinal detachment [55]. The effectiveness of cryotherapy is predicted by the spindle cell model, since destruction of spindle cells in the avascular retina is presumed to remove the angiogenic stimulus.

Despite many encouraging reports, widespread acceptance of cryotherapy had been limited by the lack of a controlled study conclusively demonstrating efficacy. Therefore a multicenter, double-blind, controlled

Table 2 *Threshold and Prethreshold ROP as Defined in the Cryotherapy-ROP Study [56]*

Stage	Zone	Extent	Definition
<3+	1	Any	Prethreshold
2+ or 3	2	Any	Prethreshold
3+	1 or 2	5 Contiguous	Threshold
3+	1 or 2	8 Cumulative	Threshold

ROP = retinopathy of prematurity.
Source: From the Cryotherapy for Retinopathy of Prematurity Cooperative Group [56].

study of cryotherapy for ROP was conducted, and the 1-year outcome was released in 1990 [56]. In this study, threshold and prethreshold for development of blinding consequences of ROP were defined as described in Table 2. Only threshold eyes were eligible for treatment. Treatment was applied contiguously to the entire avascular retina anterior to the ridge. The ridge itself was not treated. At most, a single eye was treated. If plus disease persisted, the treatment was repeated. Forty-seven percent of control eyes had an unfavorable outcome at 1 year (retinal detachment, posterior retinal fold, or retrolental tissue obscuring the posterior pole). In contrast, 26 percent of treatment eyes had an unfavorable outcome. The authors recommended treatment of patients with threshold ROP. However, because of uncertainty about long-term sequelae, they refrained from advocating treatment of both eyes, except in cases of bilateral stage 3+, zone 1 retinopathy. Instead, they suggested that each case be considered individually.

The design and recommendations of the cryotherapy study are considered overly conservative by Hindle and others [57, 58]. The ultrastructural studies of Kretzer and Hittner [34] indicate that in stage 3b (moderate) eyes, myofibroblasts are emerging from the ridge. These myofibroblasts migrate into the vitreous and will contract, leading to retinal detachment even if the avascular retina has been destroyed. Therefore, they recommend a final ring of cryotherapy directly to the ridge in any patient with stage 3b ROP [59]. They also recommend that in stage 3a, cryotherapy to the avascular retina is sufficient as ultrastructural studies do not suggest the presence of myofibroblasts. Mintz-Hittner (personal communication, May 1991) recommends cryotherapy (or photocoagulation) in infants of less than 600-gm birth weight with disease in the posterior part of zone 1 ("small" zone 1 disease) before threshold is reached, as these infants progress rapidly and have disappointing visual outcomes despite cryotherapy at threshold.

Whether to treat both eyes in patients who have symmetrical zone 2, stage 3 disease is also subject to debate and depends on the definition of disease severity and on the potential for unrecognized late complications of cryotherapy that may emerge [57, 60, 61]. Ben-Sira and colleagues [62] have followed cryotherapy-treated patients for 8 years and found only a higher incidence of myopia and a trend toward increased astigmatism compared with age- and birth weight–matched controls. Seiberth and associates [63] found no evidence of increased refractive errors 2 to 7 years after cryotherapy. Greven and Tasman [64] described 3 cases of rhegmatogenous retinal detachment at the junction of treated and untreated areas 1 to 4 years following cryotherapy. Topilow and Ackerman [65] followed 25 preterm infants treated with cryotherapy for an average of 2 years and had only 1 case of retinal detachment.

Laser Photocoagulation

Early attempts at peripheral retinal ablation in ROP involved the use of light photocoagulation. Photocoagulation subsequently fell out of favor because of the relative ease of performing cryotherapy in the nursery. With the advent of indirect ophthalmoscope–mounted laser delivery systems, interest in the use of peripheral photocoagulation has increased [66]. Photocoagulation is particularly advantageous in zone 1 disease, where cryotherapy is technically difficult and often requires conjunctival resection.

McNamara and associates [67] performed a prospective, randomized clinical trial of argon green laser photocoagulation of the peripheral retina for threshold ROP. They found that the outcome of laser-treated infants was at least equal to that of cryotherapy-treated infants. The authors stated that laser treatment was technically easier to perform than cryotherapy, with more discrete scars and less discomfort for the infant.

Vitreoretinal Surgery

Scleral Buckling Scleral buckling is an accepted treatment for ROP patients with rhegmatogenous retinal detachment [68], but the timing of its use in nonrhegmatogenous detachment is more controversial. Satisfactory anatomical results have been reported in 50 to 100% of patients [24, 65, 69–71]; however, partial nonrhegmatogenous detachments often reattach spontaneously in ROP patients [70].

In the scleral buckling procedure, an encircling silicone band is placed at the site of the highest ridge elevation. Scleral buckling is frequently combined with cryotherapy at the time of surgery. Drainage of subretinal fluid may be necessary. Scleral dissection is usually not performed, although Greven and Tasman [64] recommend this in some cases.

The timing of reattachment is important because the retina may become dysplastic if not reattached promptly [70]. If surgery is delayed too long, there may be successful anatomical reattachment but no vision. Thus, most authorities agree that prompt surgery is indicated when the macula is detached (stage 4b). Some cases of stage 5 ROP can be treated by scleral buckling alone. By avoiding vitrectomy, the lens can be left in place and visual rehabilitation is less complex.

When tractional detachment does not involve the posterior pole, there is less agreement about when to proceed with surgery. A randomized, controlled trial of scleral buckling surgery in early ROP would help determine the optimal timing. Until such a study is complete, the risk of progression to macular detachment must be weighed on an individual basis against the risk of performing surgery.

Mintz-Hittner and Kretzer [72] advocate the use of a prophylactic scleral buckle in zone 1 eyes that have progressed to threshold, before retinal detachment has occurred. The rationale is that the buckle prevents the development of macular detachment or ectopia induced by the anterior ocular growth that occurs after cryotherapy. Figure 3 demonstrates the tremendous amount of ocular growth that occurs following premature birth.

One potential problem with scleral buckling in such small eyes is globe constriction by the band as ocular growth proceeds. McPherson and colleagues [70] and Orellana [24] state that the band should be transected 3 to 6 months postoperatively in most cases. They report no detachments following buckle transection. Greven and Tasman [64] and Machemer and deJuan [71] generally leave the buckle in place unless there is clinically apparent retardation of ocular growth.

Vitrectomy   When retinal detachment progresses beyond early stage 5, scleral buckling is not sufficient to reattach the retina, and vitrectomy may be necessary. Although surgery may be extremely difficult in cases where a retrolental mass has formed, anatomical reattachment of the retina can be achieved in an apparently unsalvageable eye by meticulous removal of proliferative membranes during vitrectomy surgery [70, 73–77].

There are two major approaches to vitrectomy in advanced ROP: closed and open-sky. There is disagreement in the literature as to which technique gives superior results. Charles [73] developed the closed technique for management of ROP in 1977. In the closed technique, the

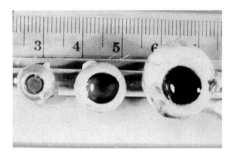

Figure 3 *Demonstration of ocular growth that occurs in preterm infants between gestational ages of 19 weeks (left), 24 weeks (center), and 37 weeks (right). The anterior segments have been removed from the 19-week and 24-week eyes. (Courtesy of Dr. Frank Kretzer.)*

marked anterior displacement of the retina necessitates pars plicata or corneal entry sites. After lensectomy the anterior plate of cellular proliferation is removed. The posterior hyaloid face and epiretinal membrane are then removed by delamination, followed by infusion of fluid or gas. Charles reports an anatomical success rate of 45%.

The technical difficulties with closed vitrectomy led Schepens to propose the open-sky technique [76]. In open-sky vitrectomy, the cornea is removed and stored in culture media during surgery [6]. The lens is then removed, revealing a transparent anterior hyaloid and the fibrous white retrolental membrane. The membrane and the fibrous mass filling the funnel of detached retina are removed as a block, and hyaluronic acid is placed into the funnel to improve exposure of the posterior pole. The corneal button is replaced at the end of the procedure. Open-sky vitrectomy allows good visualization of the entire retrolental mass. It also facilitates maneuvering vitrectomy instruments within the small closed space of the premature infant eye. Hirose and Schepens [78] reported a 38% anatomical success rate in 1984 using this technique. McPherson and colleagues [79] had a 22% anatomical success rate with open funnels and an 11% success rate with closed funnels. Potential disadvantages of the open-sky technique include prolonged hypotony with choroidal detachment, corneal clouding, and prolonged operating time. Hirose [80] reports that these complications are rare in experienced hands and that operating times are typically less than 2 hours.

Because of the risk of recurrent proliferation, vitrectomy surgery is not normally performed until after the retinopathy is quiescent. Trese [81] performs cryotherapy prior to vitrectomy in patients with stage 5 retinal detachment. This promotes quiescence of the acute process, allowing earlier vitrectomy surgery. Chong and co-workers [82] also recommend operating early—as soon as "plus" disease has regressed—while the detachment is still an open funnel. Using either technique, an open-funnel detachment has a better prognosis than does a closed funnel. However, surgery may be more difficult technically when performed earlier, with an increased chance of developing secondary membranes. The presence of a persistent hyaloid artery can complicate surgery and worsen the prognosis [83].

No matter what the technique, vision remains poor despite anatomical reattachment [65, 82, 84]. In stage 4 cases, anatomical success of 64% and functional success of 43% have been reported by Machemer and deJuan [71]. Their results for stage 5 ROP remain disappointing (anatomical, 40%; functional, 16%). Infants enrolled in the cryotherapy-ROP study who underwent vitrectomy for stage 5 retinal detachment had similarly disappointing results (anatomical, 28%; functional, 3%). This led the authors of the study to emphasize the importance of preventing retinal detachment in ROP [84].

■ Diagnosis

Examination Technique

Examination of premature infants is not entirely without risk [85], and steps must be taken to prevent complications. Dilating drops should be used with caution. Phenylephrine 10% (which causes tachycardia and hypertension) and cyclopentolate greater than 1% (which can cause vomiting or ileus) are too concentrated to be safe in preterm infants. Phenylephrine 2.5% and cyclopentolate 0.5% or tropicamide 0.5% are probably safe, especially when used with punctal occlusion. Eyelid specula should be used at the examiner's discretion. Care should be taken to watch for oculocardiac reactions to examinations, as resuscitative measures are sometimes necessary.

Technical difficulties interfere with examination of the youngest premature infants. Corneal clouding, transient cataract, and the tunica vasculosa lentis can prevent a good view of the retina, as can postpartum intraretinal hemorrhage.

Screening

With increasing acceptance of the efficacy of cryotherapy for the treatment of advanced ROP, more attention is being paid to optimal screening protocols [9, 86, 87].

Selection of Infants   All infants with a birth weight of less than 1,250 to 1,500 gm should be screened, although Brown and colleagues [88] recommended 1,600-gm birth weight be the cutoff. Larger premature infants should be examined if they have had more than 50 days of supplemental oxygen. Trese and Batton [89] noted that infants with artificially elevated birth weights (e.g., fetal hydrops) should also be screened.

Timing of Examination   The authors of the cryotherapy-ROP study recommended that eye examinations begin at 4 to 6 weeks of age [56]. In very young premature infants, earlier and more frequent examinations may be required to detect and treat *rush* disease. At times, the health of the child may interfere with this timing; however, a less thorough screening for plus disease or for zone 1 location may be possible even in very sick infants. If disease is detected, biweekly examinations are the minimum necessary to identify eyes that cross over the threshold for treatment, and more frequent examinations may be required as threshold is approached. If there is no disease, the timing of follow-up examinations depends on individual risk factors. Weekly examinations may be necessary in many infants, especially if vascularization has not proceeded beyond the equator at the time of first examination. Examinations should continue until vascularization has extended to the ora serrata.

Differential Diagnosis

The differential diagnosis of advanced ROP includes all of the entities in the differential for leukokoria, including persistent hyperplastic primary vitreous, retinal dysplasia, Coats' disease, and especially retinoblastoma [90]. Familial exudative vitreoretinopathy can resemble earlier stages of ROP, with temporal dragging of the retina leading to retinal detachment. Norrie's syndrome, the Walker-Warburg syndrome (agyria), and incontinentia pigmenti have all been confused with early stages of ROP.

■ Prognosis and Complications

Much of the emphasis on the morbidity of ROP is placed on the number of infants who are blind or suffer severe visual impairment. A much larger number of patients suffer significant, but less catastrophic, functional or cosmetic disability. Ophthalmological problems may develop in 55% of patients with regressed ROP followed over 6 to 10 years [91]. These complications are not always considered when risk-benefit ratios of cryotherapy are calculated [60]. The most common nonneovascular complications of ROP are poor acuity, myopia, strabismus, and amblyopia.

Visual Acuity

Visual acuity is difficult to study in ROP, as many years elapse between the time of disease onset and the time the child is mature enough for accurate acuity measurement. The refinement of visual evoked potentials [92] and acuity card procedures [93] may allow earlier and more accurate assessment in these infants. Unfortunately, these procedures do not grade macular acuity well.

One-third of infants with advanced ROP had less than 20/200 vision in their better eye [4]. Twenty-six percent of eyes of infants with stage 3 disease had this level of acuity. Macular dragging was a frequent cause of decreased acuity in these cases. Children with only moderate ROP changes in the retinal periphery often have poor acuity. The mechanism behind this is not understood, but myopia may be an associated factor.

Despite successful surgical intervention for threshold ROP, the macula may not develop normally. Hittner and colleagues [94] found an abnormal foveal reflex, a poorly developed foveal avascular zone, and a prolonged pattern electroretinogram. Ultrastructural analysis of the eyes of such patients indicated that the macula failed to differentiate. They proposed that surgical intervention, while successful in preventing the devastating consequences of ROP, brings the process of macular differentiation to a halt. This arrest of differentiation is a serious problem in infants with a birth weight of less than 1,000 gm, who often require cryotherapy early in macular development.

The long-term adverse consequences of ROP on visual acuity may be underestimated. Tasman and Brown [95, 96] recently presented 2 disturbing cases of patients with mild to moderate ROP sequelae who developed unexplained visual loss to 20/400 or worse years after the acute phase of the disease.

Myopia

Myopia is a frequent complication of ROP, occurring in up to 80% of patients with scarring sequelae [97]. When ROP regresses completely, there is no increase in refractive error [98]. However, if even minimal retinal sequelae such as peripheral vitreal changes are present, myopia, astigmatism, and anisometropia are increased when compared with premature infants who had no retinal disease [99]. ROP myopia can be the result of abnormal lens power or axial length. Gordon and Donzis [100] found a statistically significant increase in lens power in 4- to 9-year-old patients; however, they did not specify whether their age-matched control population consisted of former preterm infants. They noted a close correlation of severity of myopia with lens power. There was a weaker correlation of myopia severity with keratometry readings and axial length. Since lens power normally diminishes during development, the data support the concept that normal development of the lens may be arrested by the disease process in ROP.

Strabismus and Amblyopia

Strabismus and amblyopia are commonly observed in ROP patients. Between 23% and 47% of infants with ROP develop strabismus, compared with 10 to 20% of premature infants with no ROP [91]. Approximately one-half of these patients are amblyopic [4, 101]. Management is complicated by high refractive errors, nystagmus, and the asymmetrical potential acuity of the 2 eyes in some patients. When acuity remains asymmetrical, any alignment achieved by surgery may be difficult to maintain [99].

Dragging of the retina by peripheral proliferative tissue can lead to an ectopic location of the macula and resultant pseudostrabismus. This macular ectopia (or *heterotopia*) also has been termed the *Annette von Droste-Hulshoff syndrome* [102]. ROP is the most common cause of macular ectopia, and up to 20% of ROP patients develop macular ectopia [4].

Glaucoma

Narrow-angle glaucoma is emerging as a late complication of nonblinding forms of ROP [103–105]. The mechanism is usually pupillary block secondary to a large lens. As ROP patients from the first epidemic of ROP reach their forties, many more cases may occur. The glaucoma usually responds to iridotomy, but lensectomy may be necessary [106, 107]. In more severe cases of ROP, narrow angles develop earlier and may require lensectomy for definitive treatment.

Other Late Complications

Other complications of mild to moderate ROP include nystagmus, cataract, peripheral retinal breaks, microcornea, band keratopathy, and optic atrophy [4, 108]. Six percent of all eyes studied by Biglan and co-workers [4] developed phthisis bulbi.

Patients with ROP are at increased risk for nonophthalmic complications from their immaturity. In Biglan's study [4], 80% of patients with stage 4 or 5 disease had a seizure disorder, and 50% had other neurological complications.

■ Comments

With the reappearance of ROP in the nursery has come renewed interest in the disease. This has led to advances in our understanding of the risk factors and pathogenesis of retinopathy of prematurity, a widely accepted classification of the disease process, and new approaches to its prevention and treatment. However, the incidence of ROP continues to increase, and the magnitude of long-term complications is only now beginning to emerge.

Drs. Helen Mintz-Hittner, Tatsuo Hirose, Frank Kretzer, Robert Petersen, and Michael Repka all shared their clinical experiences and provided helpful insights.

■ References

1. Terry TL. Extreme prematurity and fibroblastic overgrowth of persistent vascular sheath behind each crystalline lens: I. Preliminary report. Am J Ophthalmol 1942;25:203–204
2. Patz A, Hoeck LE, DeLaCruz E. Studies on the effect of high oxygen administration in retrolental fibroplasia. Nursery observations. Am J Ophthalmol 1952; 35:1248–1253
3. Ben-Sira I, Nissenkorn I, Kremer I. Retinopathy of prematurity. Surv Ophthalmol 1988;33:1–16
4. Biglan AW, Cheng KP, Brown DR. Update on retinopathy of prematurity. Int Ophthalmol Clin 1989;29:2–9
5. Flynn JT, Bancalari E, Bachynski BN, et al. Retinopathy of prematurity: diagnosis, severity, and natural history. Ophthalmology 1987;94:620–629

6. Hirose T, Lou PL. Retinopathy of prematurity. Int Ophthalmol Clin 1986;26(2): 1–23

7. Archambault P, Gomolin JES. Incidence of retinopathy of prematurity among infants weighing 2000 g or less at birth. Can J Ophthalmol 1987;22:218–220

8. Cats BP, Tan KEWP. Retinopathy of prematurity: review of a four-year period. Br J Ophthalmol 1985;69:500–503

9. Clemett RS, Darlow BA, Hidajat RR, Tarr KH. Retinopathy of prematurity: review of a five-year period, examination techniques and recommendations for screening. Aust NZ J Ophthalmol 1986;14:121–125

10. Gibson DL, Sheps SB, Schechter MT, et al. Retinopathy of prematurity: a new epidemic? Pediatrics 1989;83:486–492

11. Harden AF. Retinopathy of prematurity—a long term follow-up. Trans Ophthalmol Soc UK 1986;105:717–719

12. Hoon AH, Jan JE, Whitfield MF, et al. Changing pattern of retinopathy of prematurity: a 37-year clinic experience. Pediatrics 1988;82:344–349

13. Keith CG, Doyle LW, Kitchen WH, Murton LJ. Retinopathy of prematurity in infants of 24–30 weeks' gestational age. Med J Aust 1989;150:293–296

14. Ng YK, Fielder AR, Shaw DE, Levene MI. Epidemiology of retinopathy of prematurity. Lancet 1988;2:1235–1238

15. Payne JW, Patz A. Current status of retrolental fibroplasia: the retinopathy of prematurity. Ann Clin Res 1979;11:205–221

16. Schulenburg WE, Prendiville A, Ohri R. Natural history of retinopathy of prematurity. Br J Ophthalmol 1987;71:837–843

17. Valentine PH, Jackson JC, Kalina RE, Woodrum DE. Increased survival of low birth weight infants: impact on the incidence of retinopathy of prematurity. Pediatrics 1989;84:442–445

18. Avery ME, Oppenheimer EH. Recent increase in mortality from hyaline membrane disease. J Pediatr 1960;57:553–559

19. Phelps DL. Retinopathy of prematurity: an estimate of vision loss in the United States—1979. Pediatrics 1981;67:924–925

20. Lucey JF, Dangman B. A reexamination of the role of oxygen in retrolental fibroplasia. Pediatrics 1984;73:82–96

21. Todd D, Kennedy J, Roberts V, John E. Risk factors in progression beyond stage 2 retinopathy of prematurity. Aust NZ J Ophthalmol 1990;18:57–60

22. Ackerman B, Sherwonit E, Williams J. Reduced incidental light exposure: effect on the development of retinopathy of prematurity in low birth weight infants. Pediatrics 1989;83:958–962

23. Bachynski BN, Kincaid MC, Nussbaum J, Green WR. A hemorrhagic form of zone 1 retinopathy of prematurity. J Pediatr Ophthalmol Strabismus 1989;26:56–60

24. Orellana J. Scleral buckling in acute retinopathy of prematurity stages 4 and 5. In: Eichenbaum JW, Mamelok AE, Mittl RN, Orellana J, eds. Treatment of retinopathy of prematurity. Chicago: Year Book, 1990:194–213

25. Majima A. Studies on retinopathy of prematurity: I. Statistical analysis of factors related to occurrence and progression in active phase. Jpn J Ophthalmol 1977; 21:404–420

26. Nissenkorn I, Kremer I, Gilad E, et al. 'Rush' type retinopathy of prematurity: report of three cases. Br J Ophthalmol 1987;71:559–562

27. Committee for the Classification of Retinopathy of Prematurity. An international classification of retinopathy of prematurity. Arch Ophthalmol 1984;102:1130–1134

28. International Committee for the Classification of Retinopathy of Prematurity. An international classification of the late stages of retinopathy of prematurity: II. The classification of retinal detachment. Arch Ophthalmol 1987;105:906–912

29. Fielder AR, Moseley MJ, Ng YK. The immature visual system and premature birth. Br Med Bull 1988;44:1093–1118
30. Kretzer FL, Hittner HM. Retinopathy of prematurity: clinical implications of retinal development. Arch Dis Child 1988;63:1151–1167
31. Ashton N, Ward B, Serpell G. Effect of oxygen on developing retinal vessels with particular reference to the problem of retrolental fibroplasia. Br J Ophthalmol 1954;38:397–432
32. Kretzer FL, Mehta RS, Johnson AT, et al. Vitamin E protects against retinopathy of prematurity through action on spindle cells. Nature 1984;309:793–795
33. Kretzer FL, Hunter DG, Mehta RS, et al. Spindle cells as vasoformative elements in the developing human retina: vitamin E modulation. In: Coates PW, Markwald RR, Kenney AD, eds. Developing and regenerating vertebrate nervous systems. New York: Alan R Liss, 1983:199–210
34. Kretzer FL, Hittner HM. Spindle cells and retinopathy of prematurity: interpretations and predictions. Birth Defects 1988;24:147–168
35. Hittner HM, Godio LB, Rudolph AJ, et al. Retrolental fibroplasia: efficacy of vitamin E in a double-blind clinical study of preterm infants. N Engl J Med 1981;305:1365–1371
36. Gole GA. Animal models of retinopathy of prematurity. In: Silverman WA, Flynn JT, eds. Retinopathy of prematurity. Boston: Blackwell, 1985:53–96
37. Kretzer FL, Mehta RS, Goad D, Hittner HM. Animal models in research on retinopathy of prematurity. In: McPherson AR, Hittner HM, Kretzer FL, eds. Retinopathy of prematurity—current concepts and controversies. Toronto: BC Decker, 1986:79–88
38. Penn JS, Thum LA. The rat as an animal model for retinopathy of prematurity. Prog Clin Biol Res 1989;314:623–642
39. Owens WC, Owens EU. Retrolental fibroplasia in premature infants: II. Studies on the prophylaxis of the disease: the use of alpha tocopheryl acetate. Am J Ophthalmol 1949;32:1631–1637
40. Johnson AT, Kretzer FL, Hittner HM, et al. Development of the subretinal space in the preterm human eye: ultrastructural and immunocytochemical studies. J Comp Neurol 1985;233:497–505
41. Finer NN, Grant G, Schindler RF, et al. Effect of intramuscular vitamin E on frequency and severity of retrolental fibroplasia: a controlled trial. Lancet 1982; 1:1087–1091
42. Johnson L, Quinn GE, Abbasi S, et al. Effect of sustained pharmacologic vitamin E levels on incidence and severity of retinopathy of prematurity: a controlled clinical trial. J Pediatr 1989;114:827–838
43. Finer NN, Peters KL, Hayek Z, Merkel CL. Vitamin E and necrotizing enterocolitis. Pediatrics 1984;73:387–393
44. Puklin JE, Simon RM, Ehrenkranz RA. Influence on retrolental fibroplasia of intramuscular vitamin E administration during respiratory distress syndrome. Ophthalmology 1982;89:96–102
45. Milner RA, Bell E, Blanchette V, et al. Vitamin E supplement in under 1500 gram neonates. Retinopathy of prematurity conference, December 4–6, 1981. Columbus, OH: Ross Laboratories, 1981:703–716
46. Phelps DL, Rosenbaum AL, Isenberg SJ, et al. Tocopherol efficacy and safety for preventing retinopathy of prematurity: a randomized, controlled, double-masked trial. Pediatrics 1987;79:489–500
47. Committee of the Institute of Medicine. Report of a study—vitamin E and retinopathy of prematurity. IOM-86-02. Washington, DC: National Academy Press, 1986
48. Ehrenkranz RA. Vitamin E and retinopathy of prematurity: still controversial. J Pediatr 1989;114:801–803

49. Kendig JW, Notter RH, Cox C, et al. A comparison of surfactant as immediate prophylaxis and as rescue therapy in newborns of less than 30 weeks' gestation. N Engl J Med 1991;324:865–871

50. Merritt TA, Hallman M, Berry C, et al. Randomized, placebo-controlled trial of human surfactant given at birth versus rescue administration in very low birth weight infants with lung immaturity. J Pediatr 1991;118:581–594

51. Yamashita Y. Studies on retinopathy of prematurity: III. Cryocautery for retinopathy of prematurity. Jpn J Clin Ophthalmol 1972;26:385–393

52. Ben-Sira I, Nissenkorn I, Gurnwald E, Yassur Y. Treatment of acute retrolental fibroplasia by cryopexy. Br J Ophthalmol 1980;64:758–762

53. Hindle NW. Cryotherapy for retinopathy of prematurity to prevent retrolental fibroplasia. Can J Ophthalmol 1982;17:207–212

54. Tasman W, Brown GC, Naidoff M, et al. Cryotherapy for active retinopathy of prematurity. Graefes Arch Clin Exp Ophthalmol 1987;225:3–4

55. Brown GC, Tasman WS, Naidoff M, et al. Systemic complications associated with retinal cryoablation for retinopathy of prematurity. Ophthalmology 1990;97:855–858

56. Cryotherapy for Retinopathy of Prematurity Cooperative Group. Multicenter trial of cryotherapy for retinopathy of prematurity: one year outcome—structure and function. Arch Ophthalmol 1990;108:1408–1416

57. Hindle NW. Cryotherapy for retinopathy of prematurity [letter]. Surv Ophthalmol 1988;33:134–135

58. Hindle NW. Cryotherapy for retinopathy of prematurity [letter]: none, one, or both eyes. Arch Ophthalmol 1990;108:1375

59. Kretzer FL, McPherson AR, Hittner HM. An interpretation of retinopathy of prematurity in terms of spindle cells: relationship to vitamin E prophylaxis and cryotherapy. Graefes Arch Clin Exp Ophthalmol 1986;224:205–214

60. Phelps DL, Phelps CE. Cryotherapy in infants with retinopathy of prematurity: a decision model for treating one or both eyes. JAMA 1989;261:1751–1756

61. Teller J, Nissenkorn I, Ben-Sira I, Abraham FA. Ocular dimensions following cryotherapy for active stage of retinopathy of prematurity. Metab Pediatr Syst Ophthalmol 1988;11:81–82

62. Ben-Sira I, Nissenkorn I, Weinberger D, et al. Long-term results of cryotherapy for active stages of retinopathy of prematurity. Ophthalmology 1986;93:1423–1428

63. Seiberth V, Knorz MC, Trinkmann R. Refractive errors after cryotherapy in retinopathy of prematurity. Ophthalmologica 1990;201:5–8

64. Greven CM, Tasman W. Rhegmatogenous retinal detachment following cryotherapy in retinopathy of prematurity. Arch Ophthalmol 1989;107:1017–1018

65. Topilow HW, Ackerman AL. Cryotherapy for stage 3 + retinopathy of prematurity: visual and anatomic results. Ophthalmic Surg 1989;20:864–871

66. Landers MB III, Semple HC, Ruben JB, Serdahl C. Argon laser photocoagulation for advanced retinopathy of prematurity. Am J Ophthalmol 1990;110:429–431

67. McNamara JA, Tasman W, Brown GC, Federman JL. Laser photocoagulation for stage 3 + retinopathy of prematurity. Ophthalmology 1991;98:576–580

68. Sneed SR, Pulido JS, Blodi CF, et al. Surgical management of late-onset retinal detachments associated with regressed retinopathy of prematurity. Ophthalmology 1990;97:179–183

69. Greven C, Tasman W. Scleral buckling in stages 4B and 5 retinopathy of prematurity. Ophthalmology 1990;97:817–820

70. McPherson AR, Hittner HM, Kretzer FL. Treatment of acute retinopathy of prematurity by scleral buckling. In McPherson AR, Hittner HM, Kretzer FL, eds.

Retinopathy of prematurity—current concepts and controversies. Toronto: BC Decker, 1986:179–192

71. Machemer R, deJuan E. Retinopathy of prematurity: approaches to surgical therapy. Aust NZ J Ophthalmol 1990;18:47–56

72. Mintz-Hittner HA, Kretzer FL. The rationale for cryotherapy with a prophylactic scleral buckle for zone 1 threshold retinopathy of prematurity. Doc Ophthalmol 1990;74:263–268

73. Charles S. Vitrectomy with ciliary body entry for retrolental fibroplasia. In McPherson AR, Hittner HM, Kretzer FL, eds. Retinopathy of prematurity—current concepts and controversies. Toronto: BC Decker, 1986:225–234

74. deJuan E Jr, Machemer R. Retinopathy of prematurity: surgical technique. Retina 1987;7:63–69

75. Jabbour NM, Eller AE, Hirose T, et al. Stage 5 retinopathy of prematurity: prognostic value of morphologic findings. Ophthalmology 1987;94:1640–1646

76. Schepens CL. Clinical and research aspects of subtotal open-sky vitrectomy. Am J Ophthalmol 1981;91:143

77. Zilis JD, deJuan E, Machemer R. Advanced retinopathy of prematurity: the anatomic and visual results of vitreous surgery. Ophthalmology 1990;97:821–826

78. Hirose T, Schepens CL. Open-sky vitrectomy in total retinal detachment in cicatricial retinopathy of prematurity. Ophthalmology 1984;91(academy suppl):73

79. McPherson AR, Hittner HM, Moura RA, Kretzer FL. Treatment of retrolental fibroplasia with open-sky vitrectomy. In McPherson AR, Hittner HM, Kretzer FL, eds. Retinopathy of prematurity—current concepts and controversies. Toronto: BC Decker, 1986:225–234

80. Hirose T, Schepens CL, Katsumi O, Mehta MC. Open-sky vitrectomy in severe retinal detachment caused by advanced retinopathy of prematurity. In press

81. Trese MT. Surgical therapy for stage V retinopathy of prematurity: a two-step approach. Graefes Arch Clin Exp Ophthalmol 1987;225:266–268

82. Chong LP, Machemer R, deJuan E. Vitrectomy for advanced stages of retinopathy of prematurity. Am J Ophthalmol 1986;102:710–716

83. Eller AW, Jabbour NM, Hirose T, Schepens CL. Retinopathy of prematurity: the association of a persistent hyaloid artery. Ophthalmology 1987;94:444–448

84. Quinn GE, Dobson V, Barr CC, et al. Visual acuity in infants after vitrectomy for severe retinopathy of prematurity. Ophthalmology 1991;98:5–13

85. Bates JH, Burnstine RA. Consequences of retinopathy of prematurity examinations: case report. Arch Ophthalmol 1987;105:618–619

86. Stannard KP, Mushin AS, Gamsu HR. Screening for retinopathy of prematurity in a regional neonatal intensive care unit. Eye 1989;3:371–378

87. Tan KE, Cats BP. Timely incidence of retinopathy of prematurity and its consequences for the screening strategy. Am J Perinatol 1989;6:337–340

88. Brown DR, Biglan AW, Stretavsky MAM. Screening criteria for the detection of retinopathy of prematurity in patients in a neonatal intensive care unit. J Pediatr Ophthalmol Strabismus 1987;24:212–215

89. Trese MT, Batton DG. Ocular examination schedule for infants with fetal hydrops. Am J Ophthalmol 1989;108:459

90. Hittner HM. Retinal and central nervous system abnormalities: syndromes which resemble retrolental fibroplasia. Metab Pediatr Syst Ophthalmol 1985;8(2): 5–10

91. Cats BP, Tan KEWP. Prematures with and without regressed retinopathy of prematurity: comparison of long-term (6–10 years) ophthalmological morbidity. J Pediatr Ophthalmol Strabismus 1989;26:271–275

92. Mintz-Hittner HA, Prager TC, McGee JK, Kretzer FL. Correlation of pattern VER latency with visual acuity, vessel traction, macular ectopia, ROP stage, and

refraction in preterm infants <1500 grams birth weight with untreated ROP. Invest Ophthalmol Vis Sci 1991;32(suppl):1147

93. Dobson V, Quinn GE, Biglan AW, et al. Acuity card assessment of visual function in the cryotherapy for retinopathy of prematurity trial. Invest Ophthalmol Vis Sci 1990;31:1702–1708

94. Hittner HM, Mehta RS, Brown ES, et al. Macular structure and function following surgical intervention for threshold retinopathy of prematurity (ROP). Invest Ophthalmol Vis Sci 1989;30(suppl):317

95. Tasman W, Brown GC. Progressive visual loss in adults with retinopathy of prematurity (ROP). Graefes Arch Clin Exp Ophthalmol 1989;227:309–311

96. Tasman W, Brown GC. Progressive visual loss in adults with retinopathy of prematurity (ROP). Trans Am Ophthalmol Soc 1988;86:367–379

97. Tasman W. Late complications of retrolental fibroplasia. Ophthalmology 1979; 86:1724–1740

98. Schaffer DB, Quinn GE, Johnson L. Sequelae of arrested mild retinopathy of prematurity. Arch Ophthalmol 1984;102:373–376

99. Kushner BJ. The sequelae of regressed retinopathy of prematurity. In: Silverman WA, Flynn JT, eds. Retinopathy of prematurity. Boston: Blackwell, 1985:239–248

100. Gordon RA, Donzis PB. Myopia associated with retinopathy of prematurity. Ophthalmology 1986;93:1593–1598

101. Snir M, Nissenkorn I, Sherf I, et al. Visual acuity, strabismus, and amblyopia in premature babies with and without retinopathy of prematurity. Ann Ophthalmol 1988;20:256–258

102. Alfieri MC, Magli A, Chiosi E, De Crecchio G. The Annette von Droste-Hulshoff syndrome: pseudostrabismus due to macular ectopia in retinopathy of prematurity. Ophthalmic Paediatr Genet 1988;9:13–16

103. Hittner HM, Rhodes LM, McPherson AR. Anterior segment abnormalities in cicatricial retinopathy of prematurity. Ophthalmology 1979;86:803–818

104. Pollard ZF. Secondary angle-closure glaucoma in cicatricial retrolental fibroplasia. Am J Ophthalmol 1980;89:651–653

105. Ueda N, Ogino N. Angle-closure glaucoma with pupillary block mechanism in cicatricial retinopathy of prematurity. Ophthalmologica 1988;196:15–18

106. Pollard ZF. Lensectomy for secondary angle-closure glaucoma in advanced cicatricial retrolental fibroplasia. Ophthalmology 1984;91:395–398

107. Smith J, Shivitz I. Angle-closure glaucoma in adults with cicatricial retinopathy of prematurity. Arch Ophthalmol 1984;102:371–372

108. Kelly SP, Fielder AR. Microcornea associated with retinopathy of prematurity. Br J Ophthalmol 1987;71:201–203

Albinism

M. Lisa McHam, M.D.
Anne Fulton, M.D.

The term *albinism* describes a heterogeneous group of genetically determined disorders of the melanin pigmentary system, resulting in hypopigmentation of the eye and integument. The estimated prevalence is 1 in 20,000 worldwide but is significantly higher in many subgroups. Albinism is found throughout the animal kingdom, with several presumed homologues to human forms. Accounts describing probable albinos are found as early as the *Old Testament*. In modern times, the entity was initially recognized among darkly pigmented races, owing to the stark contrast in skin color. Called "moon-ey'd" because of their preference for the night, albinos were believed to have supernatural powers [1]. All forms of true albinism demonstrate foveal hypoplasia, congenital nystagmus, decreased visual acuity, and decussation defects at the optic chiasm. They also share some degree of relative hypopigmentation of the eye and integument and a high incidence of refractive errors and strabismus. *Albinoidism* refers to congenital hypomelanosis without the visual system abnormalities.

■ Normal Melanogenesis

The primary sites of melanogenesis are the skin (including hair bulbs), the uvea, and the ocular pigment epithelium. Melanocytes of the skin and uveal tract are of neural crest origin, whereas the cells of the retinal, ciliary, and iris pigment epithelium originate from the outer layer of the optic vesicle, which is neuroectoderm. In uveal melanocytes, melanogenesis begins at approximately 20 weeks' gestation in humans and ceases several months after birth, leading to the darkening of iris color often noted. Unlike in the skin, there is no lifelong melanogenesis and no transfer of melanin-filled organelles to adjacent cells. In the pigment epithelium, melanogenesis is evident at 4 weeks' gestation and is complete shortly after birth. There is no apparent capacity to resume melanogenesis, the hyper-pigmentation seen after stimuli such as cryotherapy being attributable to pigment clumping [2].

In both neural crest–derived melanocytes and the ocular pigment epithelium, melanogenesis occurs in specialized membrane-bound organelles called *melanosomes*. By electron microscopy, melanosomes from brown and black hair, known as eumelanosomes, are ellipsoidal with evenly distributed, heavy melanization. Eumelanosomes are larger in the RPE and more spherical in the iris pigment epithelium. Melanosomes from red and yellow hair, known as pheomelanosomes, are spherical with spotty pigmentation and are not found in the pigment epithelium. In stage 1 of maturation, eumelanosomes and pheomelanosomes are identical. Alignment of structural filaments is found in stage 2, with melanization beginning in stage 3 and completed in stage 4 (Fig 1) [1].

Melanin synthesis begins with the amino acid substrate tyrosine, which is hydroxylated to L-3,4-dihydroxyphenylalanine (dopa) and then oxidized to dopaquinone. Both steps are catalyzed by the copper-containing enzyme tyrosinase. The pathway then branches to produce either eumelanin or pheomelanin, the latter of which requires cysteine (Fig 2). The mechanism for controlling this branch step is unknown, but the pheomelanin pathway has a higher affinity for dopaquinone than does the eumelanin pathway [3]. This may explain why pheomelanin predominates in forms of albinism in which small amounts of pigment are produced. Tyrosinase activity is assessed via the hair bulb incubation test, in which intact hair bulbs from patients are incubated in tyrosine and examined under light or electron

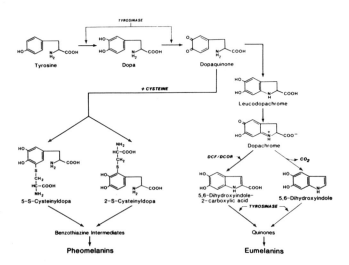

Figure 1 *Stages of eumelanosome formation. (Reprinted from Witkop et al [1] with permission.)*

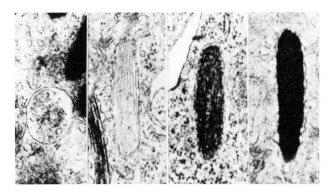

Figure 2 *The melanin pathway. (Reprinted from Witkop et al [1] with permission.)*

microscopy for the degree of melanosome maturation [4]. This technique has led to a more biochemically based classification of albinism.

Melanin has a growing list of functions, the most well-known being photoprotection from the harmful effects of ultraviolet radiation. This is accomplished by dissipation of light as heat and by free-radical scavenger activity [1]. Melanin also serves in thermoregulation and camouflage. There is now evidence that melanin has a role in neurodevelopment, possibly via axonal guidance [5, 6].

■ Clinical Features

All forms of true albinism have in common foveal hypoplasia, congenital nystagmus, decussation defects at the optic chiasm, and some degree of decreased visual acuity. Although not invariably present, there is a high incidence of refractive errors and strabismus. Overall, the visual system abnormalities are the most constant feature in albinism.

The albino pigmentary phenotype is variable and cannot be used as the sole diagnostic criterion for albinism. Hypopigmentation of the skin and hair ranges from complete absence of pigment, as in tyrosinase-negative oculocutaneous albinism, to a mild diminution within the range of normal in forms of ocular albinism. In the eye, uveal hypopigmentation ranges from complete translucency of the iris stroma and choroid to brown irides and moderately pigmented choroid. There is less variation in hypopigmentation of the ocular pigment epithelium, probably because melanogenesis ceases shortly after birth rather than continuing for several months as in the uveal tract. Because of the ocular hypopigmentation, some degree of photophobia is usually present.

■ Classification

Traditionally, albinism has been divided into oculocutaneous (OCA) and ocular (OA) forms. It is now known, however, that some degree of relative cutaneous pigmentary dilution occurs in all forms of albinism, with so-called ocular albinism being least affected. For clinical purposes, this general grouping will be maintained here.

Oculocutaneous Albinism

Tyrosinase-Negative OCA   The classical form of albinism and the second most common type is tyrosinase-negative OCA. There is no measurable tyrosinase activity via the hair bulb incubation test and, thus, melanin is absent [4], despite normal numbers of stage 1 and 2 melanosomes [1]. The skin is pink and the hair white, with complete transillumination of the irides and severe photophobia. Visual acuity is usually 20/200 or worse, with marked nystagmus. Strabismus is present in approximately 90% of patients, most being esotropic [1].

Tyrosinase-negative OCA has long been recognized as autosomal recessive. Recent isolation of a human tyrosinase cDNA clone has led to the discovery that there are multiple mutant alleles at the tyrosinase locus. One study [7] found a proline-for-leucine substitution in codon 81, at an important copper-binding site, present in 20% of alleles in a group of unrelated tyrosinase-negative albinos. There has also been a frameshift mutation found among the Japanese albino population [8].

Heterozygotes for tyrosinase-negative OCA may show clinical differences in iris transillumination from normals, but this is not consistent. Using a quantitative variation of the hair bulb incubation test, which measures free, unbound tyrosinase, heterozygotes have shown little or no tyrosinase activity [9]. Presumably this is because all existing enzyme is bound and being utilized in melanin synthesis [1]. This method can be used in carrier detection.

Yellow Mutant and Platinum OCA   In the yellow mutant and platinum forms of OCA, tyrosinase activity as measured by the quantitative hair bulb assay is very low and melanosomes are mostly stage 2 [10]. Children resemble tyrosinase-negative albinos at birth but go on to develop some pigmentation with age. In the yellow mutant form of albinism, hair becomes yellow-red and the skin a yellow-cream color. In platinum OCA, the hair has a platinum sheen and the skin a creamy color. The fundus and iris usually show small amounts of pigment. Visual acuity averages 20/200 but can be significantly better, especially in yellow mutant albinos. As in all forms of true albinism, nystagmus is present and strabismus is common.

Yellow mutant and platinum OCA are autosomal recessive and are now believed to be allelic variations of the tyrosinase-negative form. Presumably these mutations result in either very low-activity tyrosinase or reduced tyrosinase production. The mating of a tyrosinase-negative heterozygote and a probable yellow mutant heterozygote produced 3 daughters with clinical and laboratory features of yellow mutant albinism [11].

Tyrosinase-Positive OCA   Tyrosinase-positive OCA is the most common form of albinism, with normal tyrosinase activity. Incubation in tyrosine of hair bulbs from a tyrosinase-positive albino results in fully melanized stage 4 melanosomes. However, pathological examination of tyrosinase-positive skin reveals melanosome maturation only to early stage 3. There is a high degree of phenotypical variation, especially among persons of different racial backgrounds. In general, tyrosinase-positive infants are indistinguishable from tyrosinase-negative albinos but, with age, acquire pigmentation in accordance with their constitutive pigmentary background. African tyrosinase-positive albinos may have skin and hair color darker than normal blonde Caucasians. The iris typically shows a cartwheel pattern of transillumination and varies from gray-blue to light brown in color. The fundus develops pigmentation usually consistent with the skin color. Visual acuity tends to be better than in tyrosinase-negative, yellow mutant, or platinum forms, ranging from 20/70 to 20/200. Tyrosinase-positive albinism is autosomal recessive, and studies suggest that the block in melanogenesis may be in the distal eumelanin pathway [1]. Heterozygotes are not clinically or biochemically identifiable at this time. There is no allelism with tyrosinase-negative OCA.

Brown OCA   Brown OCA has been observed in Africans, Afro-Americans, and natives of New Guinea. Tyrosinase activity is normal, with a mixture of fully melanized stage 4 melanosomes and immature stage 1 and 2 melanosomes. There is a light brown tinge to hair, skin, and irides, and vision ranges from 20/60 to 20/200. Inheritance is autosomal recessive, with the presumed block in the eumelanin pathway. This condition may be similar to autosomal recessive ocular albinism in the white population [1].

Red or Rufous OCA   The red (or rufous) form of OCA is seen in natives of Africa and New Guinea [12]. Patients have a reddish tint to the hair, skin, and irides, as well as the fundus. Vision can be close to 20/20 or reduced to 20/100. Nystagmus is present but often mild. Tyrosinase activity is normal, and transmission is autosomal recessive.

Hermansky-Pudlak Syndrome   Hermansky-Pudlak syndrome (HPS) is the third most common type of albinism and consists of a triad of tyrosinase-positive OCA, a mild bleeding diathesis, and an accumulation of ceroidlike material in tissues. It is found throughout the world but is especially prevalent in Puerto Rico.

The pigment defect in HPS has a variable phenotypical expression. Cutaneous pigmentation can range from nearly amelanotic, resembling tyrosinase-negative OCA, to nearly normal, as in ocular albinism. The uveal tract is also variable but, as in all forms of albinism, the pigment epithelium is consistently hypopigmented. Visual acuity ranges widely but averages 20/200 and is accompanied by the other albinotic visual system abnormalities [13]. Hair bulb incubation reveals low to normal tyrosinase activity. Electron micrography demonstrates mostly stage 2 melanosomes with some irregularly pigmented pheomelanosomes resembling those from normal red hair. In HPS, thioredoxin reductase activity in skin is markedly reduced [14]. The thioredoxin–thioredoxin reductase system present in melanocytes and keratinocytes may function as a regulatory mechanism for ultraviolet-generated pigmentation. A decrease in membrane-bound thioredoxin reductase activity causes increased intracellular ultraviolet-generated free radicals, which inhibit tyrosinase and decrease melanogenesis [1]. This mechanism may explain the variation in tyrosinase activity and cutaneous pigmentary dilution found among HPS albinos. It is not clear, however, how this could account for the visual system abnormalities, which are presumably related to decreased melanogenesis in early embryonic development.

A mild hemorrhagic diathesis is present in all patients with HPS and usually manifests with easy bruisability, epistaxis, gingival bleeding, and prolonged bleeding following minor surgical procedures. There have been cases of massive postpartum and gastrointestinal hemorrhage resulting in death, often associated with the ingestion of acetylsalicylic acid [15]. Examination of platelets consistently reveals a marked reduction in the number of dense bodies, which are storage organelles for serotonin, adenine nucleotides, and calcium. This results in abnormal platelet aggregation and an increased bleeding time [1]. Thus, it is advisable to elicit a careful bleeding history from all albino patients, especially before childbirth or surgical procedures, and to measure bleeding time in suspicious cases. Avoidance of aspirin is generally recommended before all surgical procedures.

A ceroid-lipofuscin material accumulates in the tissues of HPS patients. The most clinically significant sites of deposition are the lung, resulting in pulmonary fibrosis; the gastrointestinal tract, resulting in granulomatis colitis; and the kidneys, resulting in renal failure. One study found that among Puerto Rican HPS patients surviving beyond 1 year of age, pulmonary fibrosis was the most common cause of death and usually occurred between the ages of 35 and 48 years [16]. Significant amounts of the ceroid-like material also accumulate in the liver, spleen, and bone marrow macrophages, and trace amounts have been found in almost all tissues tested, including brain [1].

HPS is autosomal recessive. The three features of the disease consistently segregate as a unit trait, and thus it is likely that a single gene mutation is responsible. The current evidence suggests that the underlying defect may be in the processing of lysosomal membranes [1]. Heterozygotes cannot be reliably identified by platelet studies, but reduced thioredoxin reductase activity in skin may prove useful [14].

Chédiak-Higashi Syndrome   The Chédiak-Higashi syndrome (CHS), a rare form of albinism, is characterized by a tyrosinase-positive pigmentary dilution, marked susceptibility to infection, a progressive peripheral neuropathy, and giant peroxidase-positive lysosomal granules in leukocytes and in cells of other tissues. Young children often succumb to infection, usually by gram-positive organisms. Those surviving develop neurological manifestations at approximately age 5. Eventually, they contract a terminal lymphohistiocytic proliferation known as the *accelerated phase,* which may be virus-associated [17]. Few patients survive to adulthood.

As in HPS, the phenotype in CHS can be highly variable. In general, the uveal pigmentation tends to be relatively greater than that of the skin, with iris color ranging from light blue to brown. Some authors have classified CHS as a form of ocular albinism [2]. The hair often has a metallic sheen and the skin may have patches of slate-gray coloration. The hair bulb incubation test shows normal to high tyrosinase activity, and most melanosomes tend to be abnormally large. Visual system derangements typical of albinism are present, including foveal hypoplasia and decussation defects [18].

Immunodeficiency accounts for the early mortality of CHS patients. Neutrophils containing giant peroxidase-positive granules show defective chemotaxis in vitro and decreased migration into inflammatory sites in vivo [1, 10]. It appears that the reduced chemotaxis is largely due to the mechanical impediment of the giant granules [19]. In addition, there is a derangement of lysosome function and reduced bactericidal activity [1]. Cellular immunity is also abnormal. Studies in the beige mouse, a presumed homologue for CHS, as well as studies in humans have shown a profound impairment in natural killer cell activity [20, 21]. There may also be a platelet abnormality, with decreased storage pool constituents [22]. The underlying defect in CHS is unknown, but present evidence suggests an abnormality in organelle membranes. Defective microtubule assembly and cyclic nucleotide metabolism have also been postulated but appear less likely [1]. High-dose ascorbic acid therapy has been advocated to improve resistance to infection in CHS patients, but the data are conflicting [23, 24]. There is one report of successful bone marrow transplantation in a 3-year-old child with CHS [25]. Inheritance is autosomal recessive, with heterozygotes occasionally showing giant granules in peripheral leukocytes, but not with sufficient reliability for identification [1]. Any albino child with possible manifestations of immunodeficiency should undergo peripheral blood examination, searching for the giant peroxidase-positive granules in leukocytes.

Autosomal Dominant OCA   Autosomal dominant OCA has been reported in only two kindreds [1, 26]. Tyrosinase activity as well as melanosome number and structure are normal. Phenotype and degree of visual dysfunction are similar to autosomal recessive tyrosinase-positive albinos.

Conditions with Reduced Melanocytes   Black locks albinism with deafness of the sensorineural type (BADS syndrome) and hypopigmentation with microphthalmos (Cross syndrome) display the clinical features of OCA, including the visual system abnormalities. These conditions appear to be due to failure of melanocyte migration rather than a defect in melanogenesis and thus are not strictly forms of albinism. Inheritance is autosomal recessive [10].

Ocular Albinism

Nettleship-Falls X-linked OA   Nettleship-Falls X-linked OA is a classical form of ocular albinism in which there is significant ocular and mild cutaneous pigmentary dilution. The hair and skin color are within the normal range but are somewhat decreased relative to nonaffected siblings. The irides are usually pale blue to green, becoming darker with age, and are frequently diaphanous on transillumination (Fig 3). The fundus shows considerable hypopigmentation of both the choroid and RPE, except in blacks in whom the diagnosis of ocular albinism is often missed. In these patients, hypopigmented patches on the skin and lack of a well-defined fovea can be important clues. Tyrosinase activity is normal, but overall there are reduced numbers of melanosomes. Melanocytes throughout the body of affected men possess abnormal giant melanosomes known as *macromelanosomes* [27].

Heterozygous female patients show a mosaic pattern of fundal pigmentation described as "splashes of mud" [10]. This is secondary to lyonization

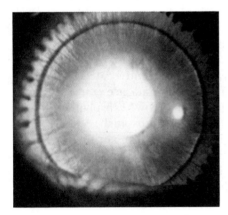

Figure 3   *Diaphanous iris in transillumination. (Reprinted with permission from RM Lewen, Ocular albinism. Arch Ophthalmol 1988;106:121.)*

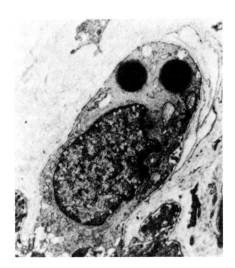

Figure 4 *Macromelanosomes from the skin of a woman heterozygous for Nettleship-Falls X-linked ocular albinism. (Reprinted from Witkop et al [1] with permission.)*

of the X chromosome, with some melanocytes transcribing the albino allele and others the normal allele (Fig 4). The iris may show cartwheel transillumination defects, but this is variable. The typical fundus appearance can be used for carrier detection.

Hemizygous men display the typical albino visual system disturbances, with photophobia, nystagmus, and visual acuity ranging from 20/50 to 20/200. Heterozygous women are usually without visual abnormalities, but severely affected carriers have been reported [28]. There are three known kindreds in which ocular albinism and late-onset sensorineural deafness were inherited as X-linked traits [1, 29].

The underlying cause of X-linked ocular albinism is unknown but is believed to be related to abnormal melanosome formation. Macromelanosomes have been found in melanocytes in CHS, HPS, albinism lentigines deafness syndrome, neurofibromatosis, nevus spilus, and xeroderma pigmentosum [1, 10]. Their occurrence in these disorders is variable, whereas it is a necessary finding for the diagnosis of X-linked ocular albinism. The significance of macromelanosomes is unclear. Genetic linkage has been demonstrated between X-linked OA and the Xg blood group [1].

Autosomal Recessive Ocular Albinism Patients with autosomal recessive ocular albinism (AROA) display the typical phenotypical features described for men with X-linked OA. There is marked ocular hypopigmentation and visual system changes consistent with albinism. Skin and hair pigmentation is in the range of normal but is usually decreased relative to nonaffected siblings. The hypopigmented macules sometimes found in blacks with X-linked OA are not present. Tyrosinase activity is positive, and melanosomes appear normal in number and structure. There are no macromelanosomes, and the basic defect is unknown. No allelism exists between AROA and either X-linked OA or tyrosinase-negative OCA [10]. It appears that AROA is at least as frequent as X-linked OA and probably more so.

Autosomal Dominant Ocular Albinism with Lentigines and Deafness One family has been described with the typical OA phenotype and visual findings inherited in an autosomal dominant manner [30]. These patients also possessed multiple cutaneous lentigines in which the melanocytes contained macromelanosomes, along with congenital sensorineural deafness and vestibular abnormalities.

Developmental Ocular Defects in Albinism

Ocular defects associated with albinism include mesodermal dysgenesis of the Axenfeld type, minor color vision abnormalities, and foveal hypoplasia. Axenfeld's anomaly consists of peripheral iris strands attached to a prominent anterior Schwalbe's line. It occurs with an increased incidence in tyrosinase-negative and tyrosinase-positive OCA, ocular albinism, and probably other forms as well [31, 32]. Progression to congenital glaucoma is rare but has been reported [33]. Advanced color vision testing reveals a mild red defect in a higher-than-expected proportion of patients.

By far the most important developmental ocular abnormality in albinism is foveal hypoplasia. It is believed to be present in all true albinos and can be appreciated clinically by an absent or decreased foveal light reflex and loss of normal foveal vascular wreathing on ophthalmoscopy. Often, a loss of the macula lutea pigment and a diminution of the relative foveal retinal pigment epithelium (RPE) hyperpigmentation can also be noted on examination. On histological evaluation, no foveal pit is evident. Rather, all retinal layers are present throughout the fovea, with the nuclear layers being relatively thinned and the ganglion cell layer thickened. The parafoveal radial nerve fiber pattern is absent, the fibers running among the ganglion cells instead of being in a distinct layer. No rod-free area is present, and spacing of the central cones is similar to that seen in normal parafoveal cones. In addition, the structure of albino central cone outer segments more closely resembles that of parafoveal cones. Thus, in the albino, the central macula never fully differentiates into a specialized fovea. However, the RPE phagocytic function appears normal, as does the peripheral retina [34]. Some studies have shown a supernormal scotopic electroretinogram (ERG), but generally the ERG is normal when one accounts for light transmission through the hypopigmented anterior eye wall [35].

■ Visual Pathway Abnormalities

In normal humans, approximately 45% of ganglion cell axons from each eye remain uncrossed as they pass through the optic chiasm and project to the ipsilateral lateral geniculate nucleus (LGN). These uncrossed axons originate in the temporal half of the retina, with the greatest number serving the central 20 degrees of temporal retina. In albinos, ganglion cell axons from the central temporal retina abnormally decussate at the chiasm and synapse in the contralateral LGN. Most axons from the peripheral temporal retina remain ipsilateral. In all, only 10 to 20% of axons from each retina remain uncrossed, as opposed to 45% in normals. As a result, in albinos each occipital cortex receives a monocular representation of the entire central visual field rather than corresponding images of the contralateral field. This accounts for the asymmetry between the hemi- spheres found with monocular visual evoked potentials in albinos of all types [36, 37].

The abnormal projections cause a disruption of the normal retinotopic representation of the visual field in the LGN and, consequently, its laminar arrangement is altered [38, 39]. The anomalous field representations reach the cortex via the geniculostriate tracts and, without modification, result in noncorrespondence and inversion between adjacent cortical layers. In Siamese cats, two methods of compensation have been found (Fig 5). In the midwestern modification, anomalous cortical input from the contralateral temporal retina via the geniculostriate tract is suppressed [38]. In the Bos- ton modification, axons in the geniculostriate tract are rerouted such that the inversion of adjacent parts of visual field is corrected [40]. Studies in primate albinos suggest they most resemble the midwestern modification in that there is no axonal rerouting [39]. Despite these compensations, each occipital cortex receives a monocular representation of the central visual field, and thus the neuroanatomical basis for binocular vision is lost.

Alterations in afferent visual pathways are also believed to be involved in the oculomotor system abnormalities seen in albinism. Studies in albino animals have shown that visual stimulation of the temporal retina produces optokinetic nystagmus (OKN) in a direction opposite, or sometimes oblique to, the motion. Stimulation of the nasal retina produces normal OKN in the direction of the motion [41, 42]. It is postulated that there is an inversion of directional selectivity at the level of the retina. This misdirection of oculomotor reflexes may contribute to nystagmus and the high incidence of strabismus seen in albinism [1, 43].

■ Pathogenesis of Visual System Abnormalities

Studies of the normal development of the optic stalk in rodents and cats have shown that the dorsal tier of the distal stalk is pigmented early. In mice and rats, pioneering retinal axons grow preferentially through the melanin-free ventral area of the stalk [5]. In cats, the dorsal pigmented cells are shed, again with growing retinal axons entering the ventral part of the stalk [6]. In albino animals, the dorsal tier of the optic stalk lacks melanin, and the pioneering retinal axons grow into this normally pro-

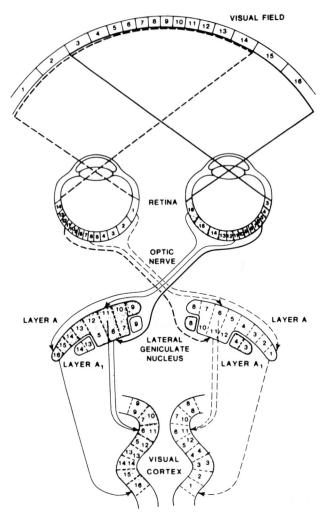

Figure 5 *Abnormal visual pathways in Siamese cat. (Reprinted from Guillery [38] with permission.)*

tected area. This abnormal early axonal guidance may result in an altered retinotopic representation in the optic stalk and, subsequently, may lead to the decussation defects previously discussed [5, 6]. It is not known whether melanin itself has an inhibitory effect on the ingrowth of ganglion cell axons or whether the cell type in which the melanin is being produced is more important. Melanin does bind calcium and, in this way, may influence the intracellular and extracellular milieu, particularly with regard to gap junction formation [44].

The etiology of the foveal hypoplasia present in all albinos is unknown.

It is postulated that relative hyperpigmentation of the RPE in the area of the fovea may be necessary to induce its differentiation.

■ Visual Disability in Albinism

Many factors lead to visual disability in albinism. The decreased foveal cone spacing limits the potential acuity of most patients to that found in the parafoveal area, 20/50 to 20/100. Other histological derangements in the fovea further limit the acuity, as does the image destabilization caused by nystagmus. Light entry through the hypopigmented anterior eye and light scatter in the hypopigmented fundus cause photophobia and may also contribute to decreased acuity. Light transmission filters are useful, and many albinos in whom there is increasing pigmentation with age will report a subjective improvement in vision.

For unknown reasons, there is a high incidence of refractive errors of all types in albinism, and good correction is important to maximize acuity. Because of the white reflex of the albinotic fundus as well as nystagmus, subjective methods of refraction are generally preferable if possible.

Strabismus is also a common finding, probably related to the absent cortical framework for binocularity and the neuroanatomical miswiring of oculomotor centers. There is evidence that some albinos may be capable of limited stereopsis [45] but, in general, early strabismus surgery to achieve stereopsis is not indicated in albinism.

As discussed, congenital nystagmus is present in all cases of true albinism. It is likely multifactorial, with oculomotor miswiring, altered directional selectivity, and foveal hypoplasia all contributing. Many patients will have a null point, often in an abnormal head position. Surgery to normalize head position by adjusting the null point is controversial but may be indicated in extreme cases.

Overall, visual functioning in albinism is often better than the acuity alone would suggest. In particular, with proper correction the near vision tends to be superior to distance vision, and most young albinos can read fairly small print unaided. Some benefit from a strong reading addition and, occasionally, telescopic low-vision aids are useful. Most albino children do well in the public school setting, and a disproportionately large number enter professional careers [1]. Parents should be warned that in the first weeks of life, albino infants may behave as if they are not seeing, but visual attentiveness usually develops within 2 to 3 months [10].

■ Skin Protection

Patients with oculocutaneous albinism have an increased incidence of neoplastic skin lesions, usually in sun-exposed areas. This is especially true in tropical climates, where solar keratoses and squamous cell carcinomas of the skin are very common and may be lethal [1]. Both cutaneous and ocular melanomas can occur in albinos, but they are probably less common than in normally pigmented persons [1, 46]. Basal cell carcinomas are rare. Skin protection with clothing and barrier creams, as well as regular self-examinations and a yearly dermatological evaluation, are indicated.

■ Genetic Counseling

Reliable prenatal diagnosis is currently available for tyrosinase-negative OCA only, using scalp biopsy at 20 weeks' gestational age [47]. Identification of the carrier state is possible in tyrosinase-negative OCA, HPS, and X-linked ocular albinism, with implications for prevention through genetic counseling.

■ References

1. Witkop CJ, Quevedo WC, Fitzpatrick TB, King RA. Albinism. In: Scriver CR et al, eds. The metabolic basis of inherited disease. New York: McGraw-Hill, 1989: 2905–2940
2. O'Donnell FE Jr, Green WR. The eye in albinism. In: Tasman W, Jaeger EA, eds. Duane's clinical ophthalmology, vol 4. Philadelphia: Lippincott, 1990: chap 385, 1–24
3. Prota G. Recent advances in the chemistry of melanogenesis in mammals. J Invest Dermatol 1980;75:127
4. Kugelman TP, Van Scott EJ. Tyrosinase activity in melanocytes of human albinos. J Invest Dermatol 1961;37:73–76
5. Silver J, Sapiro J. Axonal guidance during development of the optic nerve: the role of pigmented epithelia and other extrinsic factors. J Comp Neurol 1981;202: 521–538
6. Webster MJ, Shatz CJ, Kliot M, Silver J. Abnormal pigmentation and unusual morphogenesis of the optic stalk may be correlated with retinal axon misguidance in embryonic Siamese cats. J Comp Neurol 1988;269:592–611
7. Giebel LB, Strunk KM, King RA, et al. A frequent tyrosinase gene mutation in classic, tyrosinase-negative (type IA) oculocutaneous albinism. Proc Natl Acad Sci USA 1990;87:3255–3258
8. Tomita Y, Takeda A, Okinaga S, et al. Human oculocutaneous albinism caused by single base insertion in the tyrosinase gene. Biochem Biophys Res Commun 1989;164:990–996
9. King RA, Witkop CJ. Detection of heterozygotes for tyrosinase-negative oculocutaneous albinism by hairbulb tyrosinase assay. Am J Hum Genet 1977;29:164–168
10. Kinnear PE, Jay B, Witkop CJ Jr. Albinism. Surv Ophthalmol 1985;30:75–101
11. Hu F, Hanifin JM, Prescott GH, Tongue AC. Yellow mutant albinism: cytochemical, ultrastructural, and genetic characterization suggesting multiple allelism. Am J Hum Genet 1980;32:387–395
12. Hornabrook RW, McDonald WI, Carroll RL. Congenital nystagmus among the Red-skins of the Highlands of Papua New Guinea. Br J Ophthalmol 1980;64: 375–380

13. Summers CG, Knobloch WH, Witkop CJ Jr, King RA. Hermansky-Pudlak syndrome: ophthalmic findings. Ophthalmology 1988;95:545–554

14. Schallreuter KU, Witkop CJ. Thioredoxin reductase activity in Hermansky-Pudlak syndrome: a method for identification of putative heterozygotes. J Invest Dermatol 1988;90:372–377

15. Witkop CJ, White JG, King RA. Oculocutaneous albinism. In: Nyhan WL, ed. Heritable disorders of amino acid metabolism: patterns of clinical expression and genetic variation. New York: Wiley, 1974:177–261

16. Witkop CJ, White JG, Townsend D, et al. Ceroid storage disease in Hermansky-Pudlak syndrome: induction in animal models. In: Nasy ZS, ed. Lipofuscin—1987: state of the art. Amsterdam: Elsevier, 1988:413

17. Rubin CM, Burke BA, McKenna RW, et al. The accelerated phase of Chediak-Higashi syndrome: an expression of the virus-associated hemophagocytic syndrome? Cancer 1985;56:524–530

18. Pettit RE, Berdal KG. Chediak-Higashi syndrome: neurologic appearance. Arch Neurol 1984;41:1001–1002

19. Clawson CC, White JG, Repine JE. The Chediak-Higashi syndrome: evidence that defective leukotaxis is primarily due to an impediment by giant granules. Am J Pathol 1978;92:745–753

20. Haliotis T, Roder J, Klein M, et al. Chediak-Higashi gene in humans: I. Impairment of natural-killer function. J Exp Med 1980;151:1039–1048

21. Klein M, Roder J, Haliotis T, et al. Chediak-Higashi gene in humans: II. The selectivity of the defect in natural-killer and antibody-dependent cell-mediated cytotoxicity function. J Exp Med 1980;151:1049–1058

22. Clawson CC, White JG. Chediak-Higashi syndrome. In: Buyse M, ed. Birth defects (compendium), ed 3. New York: Alan R Liss, 1982

23. Boxer LA, Watanabe AM, Rister M, et al. Correction of leukocyte function in Chediak-Higashi syndrome by ascorbate. N Engl J Med 1976;295:1041–1045

24. Gallin JI, Elin RJ, Hubert RT, et al. Efficacy of ascorbic acid in Chediak-Higashi syndrome (CHS): studies in humans and mice. Blood 1979;53:226–234

25. Griscelli C, Virelizier JL. Bone marrow transplantation in a patient with Chediak-Higashi syndrome. Birth Defects 1983;19:333–334

26. Witkop CJ. Depigmentations of the general and oral tissues and their genetic foundations. Ala J Med Sci 1979;16:330–343

27. O'Donnell FE Jr, Hambrick GW Jr, Green WR, et al. X-linked ocular albinism: an oculocutaneous marcomelanosomal disorder. Arch Ophthalmol 1976;94:1883–1892

28. Morison WL. What is the function of melanin? Arch Dermatol 1985;121:1160–1163

29. Winship I, Gericke G, Beighton P. X-linked inheritance of ocular albinism with late-onset sensorineural deafness. Am J Med Genet 1984;19:797–803

30. Lewis RA. Ocular albinism and deafness. Am J Hum Genet 1978;30:57A

31. Witkop CJ. Albinism. In: Harris H, Hirschhorn K, eds. Advances in human genetics, vol 25. New York: Plenum, 1971:61

32. Van Dorp DB, Delleman JW, Loewer-Sieger DH. Oculocutaneous albinism and anterior chambre cleavage malformations: not a coincidence. Clin Genet 1984; 26:440–444

33. Larkin DFP, O'Donoghue HN. Developmental glaucoma in oculocutaneous albinism. Ophthalmic Paediatr Genet 1988;9:1–4

34. Fulton AB, Albert DM, Craft JL. Human albinism: light and electron microscopy study. Arch Ophthalmol 1978;96:305–310

35. Wack MA, Peachey NS, Fishman GA. Electroretinographic findings in human oculocutaneous albinism. Ophthalmology 1989;96:1778–1785

36. Creel D, O'Donnell FE Jr, Witkop CJ Jr. Visual system anomalies in human ocular albinos. Science 1978;201:931–933
37. Apkarian P, Reits D, Spekreijse H, Van Dorp D. A decisive electrophysiological test for human albinism. Electroencephalogr Clin Neurophysiol 1983;55:513–531
38. Guillery RW. Visual pathways in albinos. Sci Am 1974;230:44–54
39. Guillery RW, Hickey TL, Kaas JH, et al. Abnormal central visual pathways in the brain of an albino green monkey (*Cercopithecus aethiops*). J Comp Neurol 1984;226: 165–183
40. Hubel DH, Wiesel TN. Aberrant visual projections in the Siamese cat. J Physiol (Lond) 1971;218:33–62
41. Collewijn H, Winterson BJ, Dubois MFW. Optokinetic eye movements in albino rabbits: inversion in anterior visual field. Science 1978;199:1351–1353
42. Winterson BJ, Collewijn H. Inversion of direction selectivity to anterior fields in neurons of nucleus of optic tract in rabbits with ocular albinism. Brain Res 1981; 220:31–49
43. Drager UC. Albinism and visual pathways. N Engl J Med 1986;314(25):1636–1638
44. Drager UC. Calcium binding in pigmented and albino eyes. Proc Natl Acad Sci USA 1985;82:6716–6720
45. Apkarian P, Reits D. Global stereopsis in human albinos. Vision Res 1989;29: 1359–1370
46. Casswell AG, McCartney ACE, Hungerford JL. Choroidal malignant melanoma in an albino. Br J Ophthalmol 1989;73:840–845
47. Eady RAJ, Gunner DB, Garner A, Rodeck CH. Prenatal diagnosis of oculocutaneous albinism by electron microscopy of fetal skin. J Invest Dermatol 1983; 80:210–212

Pediatric Orbital Tumors

■■■■■■■ Nicholas J. Volpe, M.D.
■■■■■■■ Frederick A. Jakobiec, M.D.

Proptosis in children occurs rarely and can be caused by a wide spectrum of disease processes. It is essential that the ophthalmologist be familiar with the different clinical features of the various orbital lesions capable of producing proptosis. Prompt diagnosis must be made in all situations to expedite treatment and prevent loss of ocular function and, in certain cases, to increase the likelihood of patient survival.

The eye and its adnexa are situated snugly within the confines of the bony orbit. The space is used so efficiently that nearly all space-occupying lesions will induce signs and symptoms of disease. Because it is not firmly attached, the eye is nearly always caused to protrude by the various disease processes that occupy orbital volume. The entire spectrum of disease pathogenesis has been recognized in orbital abnormalities in both children and adults: That is, congenital lesions, infections, inflammatory disorders, tumors (benign and malignant), and vascular lesions all occur in the orbit. Each can present with relatively acute onset of exophthalmos, making it difficult to distinguish these entities based on clinical and radiological criteria.

Several unique aspects are involved in the evaluation of pediatric patients with orbital tumors. First is the increased frequency of congenital lesions as the cause of orbital signs and symptoms. Second is the increased frequency of sinusitis with orbital cellulitis and proptosis in the pediatric population. Third, the benign and malignant tumors as well as the primary and secondary tumors involving the orbit in children are different from those in the adult. The proper management of these orbital tumors requires a thorough knowledge of not only the differential diagnosis but also of investigative modalities and treatment options.

■ Frequency and Differential Diagnosis of Space-Occupying Orbital Lesions in Children

In reported series, the incidence of the various orbital tumors in children varies according to the type of study (clinical, histopathological, or radiological) and whether the series comes from a primary or tertiary facility (Table 1) [1–8]. Although there are significant differences among the studies, certain patterns are clear. The vast majority (approximately 90% in these series) of orbital space-occupying lesions in children and adolescents are benign. Among the most common benign lesions are the orbital dermoids, vascular tumors (particularly capillary hemangioma), and inflammatory processes.

In Rootman's series [5], inflammatory lesions were the most common orbital disease encountered in children, but this was skewed by the fact that the author's series included clinically diagnosed disease as well as biopsied cases. In addition, there was a 3:2 ratio of the number of infectious cases to the number of cases of acute and subacute idiopathic orbital inflammation. Shields and colleagues [1] noted that, for the most part, orbital cellulitis, inflammatory pseudotumor, capillary hemangioma, optic nerve glioma, and fibrous dysplasia, although common causes of proptosis in children, often do not require biopsy and can be diagnosed and treated based on clinical information alone. Therefore the incidence of these entities is higher than reflected in Shields's series.

The more common malignant lesions are rhabdomyosarcoma, metastatic and secondary tumors including neuroblastoma and Ewing's sarcoma, extension of retinoblastoma, and orbital involvement by leukemia or lymphoma. If one excludes cases of orbits secondarily involved by retinoblastoma (which would be unlikely to present as proptosis), the incidence of malignant disease is only approximately 5% [1, 8]. In a series of 60 cases of orbital tumors in African children, 50% of patients were found to have Burkitt's lymphoma, reflecting the high incidence of this rare disease in that endemic area [4].

There is little value in attempting to define the absolute incidence of each of the orbital diseases that can cause proptosis in childhood. However, it is comforting to recognize that the vast majority of these cases represent benign processes amenable to treatment. Familiarity with the differential diagnosis of proptosis is necessary for appropriate consideration of all entities and for planning an appropriate, prompt, and efficient workup. Although frequently benign, many of the orbital tumors of childhood, if managed inadequately, can be associated with devastating permanent sequelae.

■ Congenital Developmental Orbital Cysts

Congenital developmental orbital cysts are benign choristomas which arise from primitive dermal elements that are pinched off during embry-

Table 1 *Incidence of Orbital Disease in Childhood*

Lesion Type	Shields [1][a]	Bullock [8][b]	Rootman [5][b]	Youssefi [2][b]	Total
No. of cases	250	121	210	62	643
Cystic lesion	130 (52.0)[c]	48 (39.7)	27 (12.9)	29 (46.7)	234 (36.4)
Inflammatory or infectious process	41 (16.4)	2 (1.7)	55 (26.2)[d]	3 (4.8)[d]	101 (15.7)
Adipose-containing lesion	17 (6.8)	11 (9.1)	7 (3.3)	2 (3.2)	37 (5.8)
Vascular lesion	17 (6.8)	21 (17.4)	49 (23.3)	9 (14.5)	96 (14.9)
Rhabdomyosarcoma	10 (4.0)	3 (2.5)	5 (2.4)	2 (3.2)	20 (3.1)
Metastatic or secondary lesion	9 (3.6)	4 (3.3)	5 (2.4)	7 (11.3)	25 (3.9)
Lacrimal lesion	6 (2.4)	3 (2.5)	2 (1.0)	1 (1.6)	9 (1.4)
Lymphoid or leukemic lesion	6 (2.4)	5 (4.1)	—	—	11 (1.7)
Glioma or meningioma	6 (2.4)	6 (5.0)	16 (7.6)	2 (3.2)	30 (4.7)
Peripheral nerve tumor	4 (1.6)	9 (7.4)	9 (4.3)	—	22 (3.4)
Fibro-osseous tumor	3 (1.2)	6 (5.0)	15 (7.1)	1 (1.6)	25 (3.9)
Histiocytic lesion	1 (0.4)	3 (2.5)	3 (1.4)	—	7 (1.1)
Hemorrhage	—	—	17 (8.1)	1 (1.6)	18 (2.8)

[a]The series of Shields's group included biopsied cases only.
[b]The Rootman, Bullock, and Youssefi series include clinically diagnosed disease as well as biopsy-proved cases.
[c]First number indicates number of patients in series who exhibited the condition; number in parens is percentage of patient population that first number represents.
[d]Includes thyroid orbitopathy.
Note: All series include patients up to age 18.

onic development along bony suture lines of the skull. Orbital dermoids represent approximately 10% of head and neck dermoids [5]. Despite their benign nature, these lesions continue to expand intermittently during life and frequently present in school-age children as a painless nodule along the anterior superolateral orbit (Fig 1). This common location, frequently anterior to the orbital septum, makes these lesions easily detectable as they expand. Henderson [9] elected not to include these as orbital tumors because they were not in the orbital cavity proper. Similarly, Grove [10] suggested that dermoids be classified as superficial (simple) or deep (complicated) lesions. The trapped epidermal tissue develops into a cyst lined

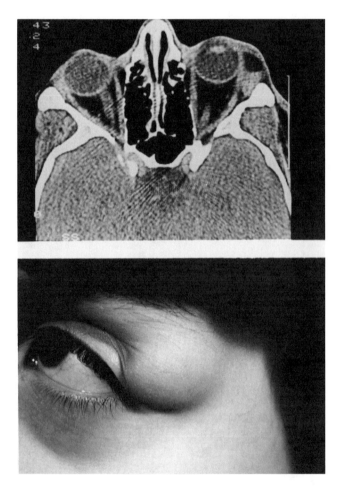

Figure 1 *(Bottom) Clinical appearance of orbital dermoid of the left orbit. (Top) Computed tomographic scan of left orbital dermoid demonstrating cystic component and molding of adjacent lateral orbital rim. (Courtesy of Dr. Richard Lisman.)*

by keratinizing epithelium and frequently attaches by a stalk to the zygo-maticofrontal, frontolacrimal, or nasofrontal suture. Histopathologically, if the cyst lining contains dermal adnexa such as hair follicles, sweat glands, or sebaceous glands (Fig 2), the cyst is considered a dermoid, and if it contains only squamous epithelium, it is considered an epidermoid.

On examination, the simple dermoid is a mass usually 1 to 2 cm in diameter, smooth and nontender. It is freely mobile under the skin and usually does not displace the eye at the time of initial presentation. Computed tomographic (CT) scanning reveals a heterogeneous, well-circumscribed lesion with a low-density lumen and, in long-standing cases, molding of the adjacent orbital bones (Fig 1). Simple excision is carried out between ages 1 and 5 to avoid accidental traumatic rupture, which can cause lipogranulomatous inflammation and scarring.

The complicated dermoid often is not identified until the teen or young adult years. These dermoids present with proptosis and can arise from any of the orbital bony sutures including the orbital apex and supe-rior orbital fissure. Occasionally, deep orbital lesions will demonstrate rim calcification on CT scanning. Characteristically, bone molding or bony de-fects, or both, are present as well. Surgical excision should be planned carefully so as to maximize complete excision without the risk of cyst rup-ture. Giant dermoids histopathologically represent dermoids with evidence of previous rupture and granulomatous inflammation [11].

Teratoma is another cystic orbital lesion that is congenital and typically presents at birth. The tumor arises from aberrant germ cells and more often occurs in the gonads, retroperitoneum, and mediastinum. Patients

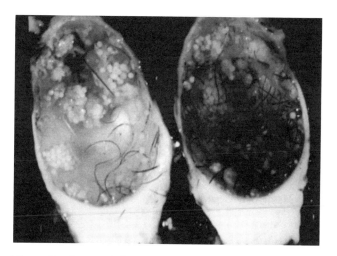

Figure 2 *Gross pathological appearance of orbital dermoid con-taining hair follicles and sebaceous material. (Courtesy of Dr. Elise Torczynski.)*

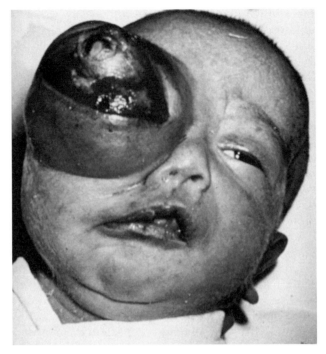

Figure 3 *Orbital teratoma of the right eye with massive proptosis. The eye can be seen on the superoanterior surface of the tumor. (Courtesy of the Armed Forces Institute of Pathology.)*

present with dramatic proptosis caused by large, reddish, cystic masses (Fig 3). The eye is usually present on the superoanterior surface of the tumor and is usually severely damaged by the tumor. Management entails exenteration as soon as possible. Heroic efforts to save the eye have proved largely unsuccessful but should be attempted whenever possible [12]. Histopathologically, the tumors are benign and consist of tissues from all three primitive germ cell layers (frequently including mucin-secreting gastrointestinal mucosa [Fig 4] [13]).

■ Vascular Tumors

Capillary Hemangioma

The capillary hemangioma is the most common vascular tumor in children; it represents approximately 60% of pediatric orbital vascular tumors, with lymphangioma and cavernous hemangioma (more typically diagnosed in adults) making up the majority of the other cases [1, 8, 9]. Capillary hemangiomas typically develop in the first month or so of life and grow

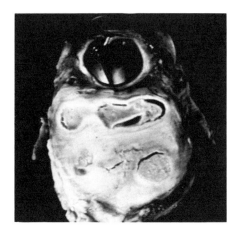

Figure 4 *Gross pathological appearance of orbital teratoma. (Courtesy of Armed Forces Institute of Pathology.)*

until age 2 or 3, at which point they begin to involute on their own. They appear as the typical "strawberry" mark and can be seen on other parts of the body. They are usually identified before they cause proptosis, but deeper lesions can mimic rhabdomyosarcoma or neuroblastoma with rapid onset of exophthalmos. Crying may cause the infantile hemangioma to enlarge temporarily, a feature not seen with rhabdomyosarcoma [9]. The lesions can be confined to the eyelid and conjunctiva anterior to the septum or involve the deeper orbital structures as well. The upper eyelid is commonly involved (Fig 5) and can induce strabismic, occlusive, and anisometropic amblyopia [14, 15]. Although these tumors are benign, they have the ability, because they are unencapsulated, to infiltrate tissues and, on CT scan, can appear as well-encapsulated or infiltrating lesions. They typically enhance with contrast material and do not demonstrate calcification. Histopathologically, these tumors are proliferations of normal-appearing endothelium arising from primitive mesenchymal elements forming small, capillarylike vascular spaces. Sometimes these capillary spaces can become ectatic, simulating cavernous type histology.

Significant morbidity can be associated with capillary hemangiomas. Locally, as mentioned earlier, they can secondarily cause amblyopia. The tumors can also be complicated by local hemorrhage, infection, ulceration, and necrosis. Occasionally, large tumors can trap platelets and induce a bleeding disorder or cause cardiac failure secondary to the low-resistance vascular mass lesion (Fig 6). These more serious complications can force surgical intervention. However, the majority of cases can be managed conservatively with observation alone if cosmetic and functional issues do not supersede. In these settings, successful involution of lesions has been reported with both systemic and intralesional steroids [16, 17] as well as the use of radiotherapy by external beam or placement of intralesional radon

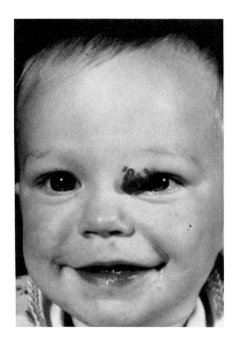

Figure 5 *Clinical appearance of capillary hemangioma involving the left upper eyelid.*

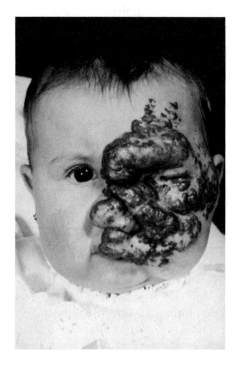

Figure 6 *Clinical appearance of large capillary hemangioma involving the left orbit.*

seeds [9]. All modes of therapy are frequently associated with rebound growth of the lesion.

Lymphangioma

Lymphangiomas represent hamartomatous growth of hemodynamically isolated lymph channels. This has been considered a particularly unusual lesion since the retroseptal orbital tissue is not believed normally to contain lymph channels. The distinction from an orbital varix has been controversial [18], and some authors have referred to the lesion as simply a *vascular hamartoma* [19]. It is likely that both arise from a similar vascular endothelial cell precursor. Most clinicians agree that the isolation of the lesion from the circulatory system distinguishes the lesion from varix, which would typically enlarge on Valsalva's maneuver. Histopathologically, the lesions consist of thin-walled vascular channels with collagenous stroma containing smooth muscles and scattered lymphoid tissue. There is frequently evidence of old hemorrhage and lymphocytes.

Clinically, lymphangiomas can be superficial (limited to conjunctiva and eyelid) or deep, or a combination of the two (Fig 7). They typically present in school-age children as a soft bluish mass most commonly in the superonasal quadrant. They can remain unchanged for long periods of time until they enlarge suddenly because of a concurrent viral illness or spontaneous intralesional hemorrhage with mass effect secondary to the so-called chocolate cyst. Children with recurrent bouts of orbital cellulitis associated with viral illnesses should be suspected to have lymphangiomas. They can be associated with similar vascular anomalies of the nasopharynx and oropharynx, which can bleed spontaneously. On CT scan, the lesions may appear as low-density cystic lesions with enhancement of the border with contrast injection or as diffusely infiltrative, unencapsulated masses (Fig 7).

The clinician must be cautious in managing these patients. In infants, tumor shrinkage can occasionally be achieved with radon seed implantation [9]. Frequently, cosmetic concerns become so great to the parents that a surgical excision is attempted. In this setting, only incomplete excision can be accomplished, and it is more difficult if the upper eyelid is involved. Advantages and successful tumor destruction have been reported with the adjuvant use of cryotherapy or the carbon dioxide laser at the time of dissection [20].

■ Acute Orbital Inflammatory Syndrome (Pseudotumor)

The now less-accepted term, *pseudotumor*, refers to a nonneoplastic, inflammatory mass lesion of the orbit currently referred to as *acute orbital*

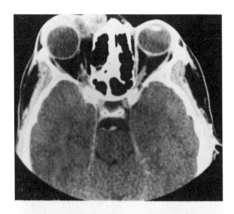

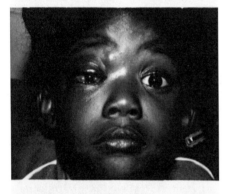

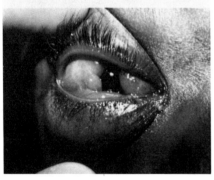

Figure 7 *(Middle, bottom) Clinical appearance of lymphangioma of the right eye with conjunctival and orbital involvement. (Top) Computed tomographic scan of lymphangioma demonstrating low-density mass of the anterior orbit.*

inflammatory syndrome. As with other inflammatory conditions, patients present with the rapid onset of pain and congestion. Because this process can frequently be associated with abrupt onset of mass effect, it may be difficult to distinguish these patients from those with aggressive malignant tumors or an infectious process.

Since this is a relatively rare disease, clinical suspicion must be high to make the diagnosis. Children often present with a history of abrupt onset (occurring over a period of days) of pain, proptosis, conjunctival chemosis and injection, and soft-tissue swelling around the eye. Unlike adult pseudotumor, there may be an antecedent history of trauma in a significant number of patients, and the disease is frequently bilateral (45% of pediatric cases are bilateral at some time during the course of the illness) [21]. Bilaterality in adult patients should suggest an underlying systemic etiology.

There is usually no complaint of decreased visual acuity. Mottow and Jakobiec [21] found that nearly 90% of patients presented with better than 20/40 vision. The most commonly reported symptoms in that series were swelling (93%), pain (69%), and ptosis (42%). Other reported symptoms included proptosis, palpable mass (most commonly in the superolateral or midsuperior orbital rim), photophobia, diplopia, pain on eye movement, erythema, and warmth (Figs 8, 9). Swelling is most prominent early in the day, and the most common location for the mass lesion is superiorly. Unlike the disease in adults, pediatric orbital inflammatory disease is associated with intraocular inflammation (iritis) in one-fourth of the cases [21]. Also, the disease can be associated with peripheral eosinophilia in children [22]. Cerebrospinal fluid pleocytosis and elevated sedimentation rate have also been noted [5].

Mottow and Jakobiec [21] further divided the patients into three clinical patterns. The first group presented with a single unilateral attack. These cases were likely to demonstrate persistent proptosis and motility disturbances despite treatment. The second group had multiple unilateral attacks. Although half of these patients had residual exophthalmos, none

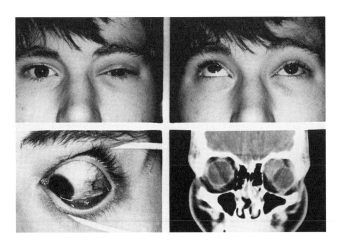

Figure 8 *(Top) Clinical appearance of acute orbital inflammatory syndrome with ptosis and restricted motility. (Bottom left) Congested episcleral blood vessels in same patient with acute orbital inflammatory syndrome. (Bottom right) Computed tomographic scan of discrete superomedial orbital mass.*

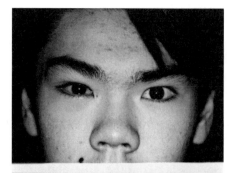

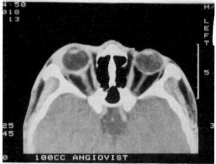

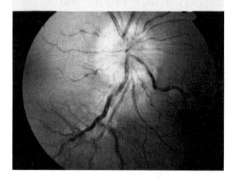

Figure 9 *(Top) Clinical appearance of acute orbital inflammatory syndrome with conjunctival injection and chemosis. (Middle) Computed tomographic scan shows posterior scleral thickening and obscuration of optic nerve-globe junction. (Bottom) Fundoscopic examination shows disc edema in acute orbital inflammatory syndrome. (Courtesy of Dr. Deborah Jacobs.)*

had persistent extraocular motility defects. The most severe category were those patients with multiple bilateral attacks. They were the most likely to have associated iritis and papillitis and were also the most likely to have visual loss and permanent proptosis. Of the patients with iritis, 7 of 8 had bilateral disease and 5 of 8 went on to have visual defects. A subset of patients were identified with contiguous inflammation in the cavernous sinus and marked ophthalmoplegia; they were believed to have a form of the Tolosa-Hunt syndrome. Patients who had biopsies were more likely to suffer serious residua. Proptosis and motility disturbances occurred more frequently and were more severe in the biopsied patients. These sequelae may be less likely with the perioperative use of high-dose steroids.

The CT picture is typically one of diffuse anterior orbital inflammation adjacent to the globe with evidence of scleral and choroidal thickening. Occasionally, a discrete mass is seen (Fig 8). Classically, this will obscure the junction of the optic nerve to the globe and obscure the nerve margin for a variable amount into the posterior orbit (Fig 9). Both CT scan and B-scan ultrasonography may show enlargement of Tenon's space and of the extraocular muscles.

Histopathologically, the lesion typically consists of nonspecific polymorphic lymphocytic and plasmacytic infiltrate with eosinophilia. Frequently, polymorphonuclear leukocytes and macrophages are present as well. The lesions can appear diffusely cellular, suggestive of lymphoma, or may have well-defined germinal centers. There is frequently associated capillary proliferation and prominent fibrosis.

The treatment of acute idiopathic orbital inflammatory syndrome is accomplished most successfully with oral prednisone. Patients started on 60 to 80 mg prednisone daily can be expected to demonstrate a dramatic response with reduction of proptosis and improvement of impaired motility. In fact, prompt resolution of signs and symptoms can be used as a diagnostic test since malignant tumors would not be expected to change dramatically (although they may improve slightly). Poor response to steroid therapy should push the clinician to biopsy. Therapy is continued and tapered over a 2- to 3-month period and reinstituted if disease recurs. Radiotherapy has been of questionable benefit and is reserved for the most recalcitrant cases.

■ Rhabdomyosarcoma

Rhabdomyosarcoma is the most common primary orbital malignancy in children and the most common soft-tissue malignancy of childhood. However, it accounts for only a small proportion of orbital space-occupying lesions. Because of dramatic improvement in survival of patients treated promptly with appropriate chemotherapy and radiotherapy, this entity must always be considered in the differential diagnosis of acute proptosis in childhood, so that biopsy and histological diagnosis can be accomplished as soon as possible.

The tumor most commonly occurs in the first decade of life, with an average age of 7 years at time of presentation and with 90% of patients presenting before age 16 [5, 23, 24]. The cases of rhabdomyosarcoma can be further divided into bimodal age peaks depending on histology (as discussed later), with the embryonal and alveolar subtypes presenting in childhood and the pleomorphic type presenting more commonly in adults.

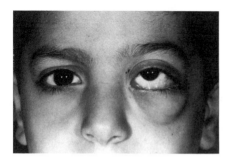

Figure 10 *Proptosis and globe displacement from orbital rhabdomyosarcoma arising in the left inferior orbit. (Courtesy of Dr. Peter Rubin.)*

Clinical Features

The clinical presentation, as is true of many of the lesions already discussed, is that of rapidly progressive exophthalmos developing over days to weeks (Fig 10). In children, the symptoms are frequently attributed to a misleading and insignificant history of inadvertent trauma. There are some discrepancies among the various series concerning the most common tumor site. Some found the superonasal orbit to be the most common location [25–27], but Jones and co-workers [23] found 50% to be retrobulbar, 25% superior, and 12% inferior orbit. Other common findings at presentation are a palpable mass and ptosis, which occur in roughly one-third of patients. Subsequent to the onset of proptosis, the children frequently develop swelling and injection of the overlying skin. The skin is not hot which, along with the absence of fever, helps differentiate these cases from orbital cellulitis.

CT scan typically reveals a poorly defined mass of homogeneous density [28]. There are often areas of adjacent bony destruction and spread of tumor into the paranasal sinuses. There is no significant enhancement with intravenous contrast material. CT scan has been used to perform guided needle biopsy of the tumor [29].

Histological Features and Tumor Staging

The tumor arises from rests of primitive mesenchymal cells in the orbit. Histologically, the tumors can be divided into three main types; embryonal, alveolar, and pleomorphic, each of which behaves differently clinically. The most common type in the pediatric population is the *embryonal* type, responsible for approximately two-thirds of cases. These tumors are composed of a loose meshwork of spindle-shaped rhabdomyoblasts with eosinophilic cytoplasm and elongated central nuclei. Because of the lack of differentiation, cross-striations are not seen. Electron microscopy can be helpful and may identify actin and myosin filaments in various stages of sarcomere formation. The botryoid variant of the embryonal rhabdomyosarcoma occurs when the tumor grows in an unrestricted fashion next to a mucosal surface. The tumor takes on a polypoid form with a dense submucosal layer. This tumor occurs primarily in the pelvis and does not occur in the orbit.

The *alveolar* histological pattern consists of poorly differentiated cells arranged in groups along fibrovascular septa separating alveolar spaces, thus resembling the alveoli of the lung. The alveolar spaces frequently contain free-floating cells attached by thin processes to the adjacent septa and seemingly participate in their formation. This is the second most common tumor type, occurring more frequently in the inferior orbit and having the worst prognosis [30].

The third type, the *pleomorphic* rhabdomyosarcoma, occurs primarily in adults. The cells are larger than the alveolar and embryonal subtypes and have granular cytoplasm containing glycogen. Differentiation from other sarcomas can be difficult.

Great advances have been made in the treatment of orbital rhabdomyosarcoma in the past two decades with the availability of newer chemotherapeutic agents and radiotherapy. Prior to this, the disease was almost uniformly fatal, with the only available means of treatment being an attempt at complete surgical excision. The survival in localized orbital rhabdomyosarcoma is now more than 90% at 5 years [31]. The survival time is intimately dependent on the staging and location of the disease at time of diagnosis as well as the histopathological type of tumor (the alveolar type has the worst prognosis).

At the time of initial diagnosis, a prompt workup for metastatic disease should begin and include chest x-ray, liver function tests, bone marrow biopsy, lumbar puncture, and skeletal survey. The staging of the disease as set forth by the Intergroup Rhabdomyosarcoma Study [32] is presented in Table 2.

The majority of orbital tumors fit into groups 1 and 2 of the Intergroup's staging, and patients with orbital disease have the best prognosis compared with the other common primary sites [33]. The more common sites of metastatic orbital rhabdomyosarcoma are to the lung and bones. Unlike the embryonal type seen elsewhere in the body, which frequently metastasizes to regional lymph nodes, orbital disease rarely involves the lymphatics (likely reflecting the absence of lymphatic channels in the orbit).

Table 2 *Staging of Rhabdomyosarcoma*

Group 1	Localized disease, completely resected
Group 2	Regional disease, with or without lymph nodes involved, grossly resected
Group 3	Incomplete resection or biopsy with gross residual disease
Group 4	Distant metastases (lung, bone marrow, and brain)

Source: Adapted from Maurer et al [32].

Management

Although the disease in the orbit is most commonly localized, the management of choice is not complete exenteration but rather biopsy followed by radiation and chemotherapy [34, 35]. At the time of biopsy, the largest amount of tumor that can be safely resected is taken. Subsequent to this, a combination of radiation and chemotherapy is given. If residual disease in the orbit is microscopical, a total of 4,000 rads is used; in gross residual disease or regional disease, doses up to 5,000 to 6,000 rads are required. Systemic adjuvant chemotherapy with vincristine, actinomycin, and cyclophosphamide is given subsequently. Protocols vary according to the extent of disease and treatment center. The Intergroup Rhabdomyosarcoma Study has shown that in group 3 cases with gross residual disease after surgery, a 6-week course of systemic chemotherapy is efficacious prior to radiation [36]. A significant number of patients undergoing chemotherapy show tumor shrinkage similar to that seen with radiation.

In summary, in rhabdomyosarcoma localized to the orbit and treated with chemotherapy and radiation, survival at 5 years is greater than 90%. Patients with group 3 disease drop to approximately a 35% survival rate at 5 years. Survivors of the alveolar type are unusual, and recurrent disease is nearly always fatal [31, 37]. Unfortunately, side effects from local radiation are not rare. In one series of 50 patients, 90% developed cataracts [38]. Other common problems included corneal scarring, enophthalmos, lacrimal stenosis, and facial asymmetry. There also appears to be an increased incidence of secondary leukemias in patients treated with the combined radiation and chemotherapy regimen [38, 39].

■ Metastatic Orbital Tumors

Metastatic orbital tumors in children are very different from the disease that occurs in adults. Metastatic disease to the eye and its adnexa in children almost exclusively involves the orbit. Metastatic disease to the uvea is extremely uncommon. Also, metastases commonly do not arise from carcinomas, as in adults, but from sarcomas. The more common sources of metastatic disease to the orbit are neuroblastoma and Ewing's sarcoma. Neuroblastoma is second only to rhabdomyosarcoma as the most frequent malignant tumor of the orbit occurring in children. Medulloblastoma and Wilms' tumor metastasize to the orbit less frequently [27, 40–42]. Musarella and co-workers [42] found that 20% of children with neuroblastoma had ocular involvement, with three-fourths having proptosis or ecchymoses. The typical presentation for children with neuroblastoma is that of rapidly expanding exophthalmos with eyelid ecchymoses. Bilateral disease is common. Frequently, the temporal orbit is involved with a lytic bone lesion (Fig 11). The most common site of primary tumor is the adrenal

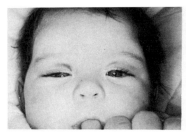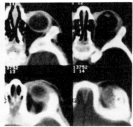

Figure 11 *(Left) Clinical appearance of bilateral orbital ecchymoses in a baby with metastatic neuroblastoma. (Right) Computed tomographic scan of metastatic neuroblastoma with lytic bone lesions. (Courtesy of Dr. John Woog.)*

gland for cases with orbital involvement. It is unclear whether the metastases arise in the orbital soft tissue or in the bone, with contiguous spread. Metastatic neuroblastoma is a disease of infants, with 90% of cases occurring before age 5; the prognosis is best in children younger than 1 year. Horner's syndrome occurs commonly, and neuroblastoma is also associated with a paraneoplastic syndrome of opsoclonus and myoclonus.

Metastatic Ewing's sarcoma is a disease of the second decade and can present as a sudden onset of proptosis due to a hemorrhagic metastasis from the long bones. The disease has also been seen to arise primarily in the soft tissues or bone of the orbit [5]. Albert and colleagues [40] found the disease to be unilateral in all 12 of their patients. The pathological findings are usually undifferentiated and, as in neuroblastoma, the prognosis is poor despite combined radiotherapy and chemotherapy.

The orbit is more commonly involved by leukemia in children than it is in adults. Rootman [5] found that in his series of orbital tumors, leukemia was the cause of acute proptosis in children in 11% of the malignant cases. Granulocytic sarcoma or the extramedullary form of acute myeloblastic leukemia can present initially as an orbital mass [43]. The average age of presentation is 7, and the disease can be bilateral. This condition can be successfully managed with chemotherapy prior to development of systemic disease. In children, lymphomas infrequently involve the orbit.

Histiocytosis X includes three disorders: Hand-Schüller-Christian disease, Letterer-Siwe disease, and eosinophilic granuloma. The name comes from the lesion's unknown etiology and the common presence of histiocytes. Histiocytosis X does not represent a true malignancy but, more likely, an abnormal immune response. One case occurs per 80 cases of acute leukemia in children [5]. The entity is more common in children, and 10% will have ophthalmic manifestations.

The lesions are believed to represent abnormal accumulations of histiocytes of the dendritic or Langerhans cell type. These cells are typically from

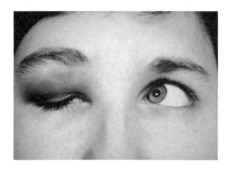

Figure 12 *Clinical appearance of eosinophilic granuloma of the right superolateral orbit with soft tissue growth.*

the epidermis and can be recognized by the characteristic racquet-shaped cytoplasmic granules (Birbeck granules) seen on electron microscopy. The cells are involved by a surrounding granulomatous infiltrate with numerous granulocytes, particularly eosinophils. The lesions frequently involve medullary bone but can have systemic dissemination with multiple organ involvement.

The classical description is that systemic disease with visceral involvement is termed *Letterer-Siwe disease,* multifocal bone disease is called *Hand-Schüller-Christian disease,* and single bone lesions are called *eosinophilic granuloma.* Prognosis is related to age, with younger children having a worse prognosis (60% mortality in children younger than 2 years). The disease of the orbit typically involves the superolateral orbit with bony lysis and soft-tissue growth (Fig 12) [44]. Treatment includes low-dose radiotherapy, chemotherapy, and steroids. Orbital disease often responds to local curettage.

■ Fibro-Osseous Tumors

Fibro-osseous tumors take many forms and include fibrous dysplasia, osteomas, giant-cell lesions, and ossifying fibroma. The etiology is uncertain. The most common is fibrous dysplasia, a condition that develops almost exclusively in the first two decades of life. In this condition, normal bone is replaced by immature bone and osteoid in a fibrous matrix [27, 45]. The disease can be localized to the orbit or throughout the body. If multiple lesions are associated with endocrine abnormalities (including precocious puberty) and skin pigmentation, the condition is called *Albright's syndrome.* In Rootman's series [5], fibro-osseous tumors represented one-third of bone tumors. Since the frontal bone is most frequently involved, children often present with proptosis and downward displacement of the globe. Pain is common. If the ethmoids and sphenoids become involved, narrowing of the optic canal may compromise optic nerve function and necessitate optic canal decompression (Fig 13). There may be associated cranial nerve palsies and elevation of intracranial pressure. Radiographic

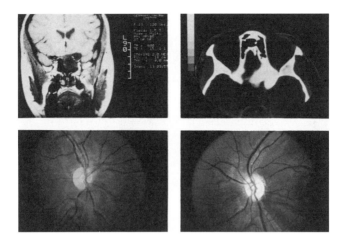

Figure 13 *(Top left) Magnetic resonance image of fibrous dyspla-sia showing growth of sphenoid bone. (Top right) Computed tomo-graphic scan of fibrous dysplasia of the sphenoid bone showing pro-liferation of bone around optic canal. (Bottom) Appearance of optic nerves in same patient with optic atrophy of the left optic nerve sec-ondary to compression by fibrous dysplasia of the optic canal. (Cour-tesy of Drs. Myron Yanoff and Martha Lean.)*

studies show either homogeneous sclerotic expansion of bone or alternat-ing light and dark areas (pagetoid growth). Therapy is aimed at local surgi-cal debulking and decompression of the optic nerve when it is compro-mised. The lesion may represent an arrest in the normal maturation of bone [27]. Ossifying fibroma may represent a more aggressive form of fibrous dysplasia and appears more well-demarcated from normal bone than is fibrous dysplasia. Histopathologically, the tumor consists of spicules of bone in a vascularized stroma. Often bone spicules are difficult to distin-guish from psammoma bodies, thus making distinction from meningioma difficult. Therapy is aimed at complete excision.

Osteomas are benign tumors that arise in the paranasal sinuses, most commonly the frontal sinus [5]. Some believe that these occur secondarily in patients who have had orbital trauma or sinus infections. Others believe that they represent a developmental lesion occurring at the site of fusion of membranous and cartilagenous bone. Common presenting signs include sinus congestion and proptosis. The lesion represents compact bone (with-out fibrovascular stroma) and is managed by simple excision.

■ References

1. Shields JA, Bakewell B, Augsburger JJ, et al. Space-occupying orbital masses in children: a review of 250 consecutive biopsies. Ophthalmology 1986;93:379–384

2. Youssefi B. Orbital tumors in children: a clinical study of 62 cases. J Pediatr Ophthalmol 1969;6:177–181
3. Eldrup-Jørgensen P, Fledelius H. Orbital tumours in infancy: an analysis of Danish cases from 1943–1962. Acta Ophthalmol (Copenh) 1975;53:887–893
4. Templeton AC. Orbital tumours in African children. Br J Ophthalmol 1971;55: 254–261
5. Rootman J. Diseases of the orbit: a multidisciplinary approach. Philadelphia: Lippincott, 1988
6. Porterfield JF. Orbital tumors in children: a report on 214 cases. Int Ophthalmol Clin 1962;2(2):319–335
7. MacCarty CS, Brown DN. Orbital tumors in children. Clin Neurosurg 1964;11: 76–93
8. Bullock JD. Orbital tumors in childhood. Ophthalmology 1986;93:379–384
9. Henderson JW. Orbital tumors, ed 2. New York: Thieme Stratton, 1980
10. Grove AS Jr. Orbital disorders: diagnosis and management. In: McCord CD Jr, ed. Oculoplastic surgery. New York: Raven Press, 1981:274
11. Grove AS Jr. Giant dermoid cysts of the orbit. Ophthalmology 1979;86:1513–1520
12. Chang DF, Dallow RL, Walton DS. Congenital orbital teratoma: report of a case with visual preservation. J Pediatr Ophthalmol 1980;17:88–95
13. Ide CH, Davis WE, Black SPW. Orbital teratoma. Arch Ophthalmol 1978;96:2093–2096
14. Haik BG, Jakobiec FA, Ellsworth RM, Jones IS. Capillary hemangioma of the lids and orbit: an analysis of the clinical features and therapeutic results in 101 cases. Ophthalmology 1979;86:760–789
15. Robb RM. Refractive errors associated with hemangiomas of the eyelids and orbit in infancy. Am J Ophthalmol 1977;83:52–58
16. Kushner BJ. Intralesional corticosteroid injection for infantile adnexal hemangioma. Am J Ophthalmol 1982;93:496–506
17. Brown BZ, Huffaker G. Local injection of steroids for juvenile hemangiomas which disturb the visual axis. Ophthalmic Surg 1982;13:630–633
18. Wright JE. Orbital vascular anomalies. Trans Am Acad Ophthalmol Otolaryngol 1974;78:OP606–616
19. Jakobiec FA, Jones IS. Vascular tumors, malformations and degenerations. In: Jones IS, Jakobiec FA, eds. Diseases of the orbit. Hagerstown, MD: Harper & Row, 1979:269–308
20. Kennerdell JS, Maroon JC, Garrity JA, Abla AA. Surgical management of orbital lymphangioma with the carbon dioxide laser. Am J Ophthalmol 1986;102:308–314
21. Mottow LS, Jakobiec FA. Idiopathic inflammatory orbital pseudotumor in childhood: clinical characteristics. Arch Ophthalmol 1978;96:1410–1417
22. Mottow-Lippa L, Jakobiec FA, Smith M. Idiopathic inflammatory orbital pseudotumor in childhood: II. Results of diagnostic tests and biopsies. Ophthalmology 1981;88:565–574
23. Jones IS, Reese AB, Krout J. Orbital rhabdomyosarcoma: an analysis of sixty-two cases. Trans Am Ophthalmol Soc 1965;63:223–255
24. Spaeth EB, Cleveland AF. Rhabdomyosarcoma in infancy and childhood. Am J Ophthalmol 1962;53:463–466
25. Fledelius H. Embryonal sarcoma of the orbit: a clinical review of 19 Danish cases. Acta Ophthalmol (Copenh) 1976;54:693–703
26. Frayer WC, Enterline HT. Embryonal rhabdomyosarcoma of the orbit in children and young adults. Arch Ophthalmol 1959;62:203–210
27. Jakobiec FA. Orbit. In: Spencer WH, ed. Ophthalmic pathology: an atlas and textbook, ed 3. Philadelphia: Saunders, 1986
28. Vade A, Armstrong D. Orbital rhabdomyosarcoma in childhood. Radiol Clin North Am 1987;25:701–714

29. Czerniak B, Woyke S, Daniel B, et al. Diagnosis of orbital tumors by aspiration biopsy guided by computerized tomography. Cancer 1984;54:2385–2389
30. Enzinger FM, Shiraki M. Alveolar rhabdomyosarcoma: an analysis of 110 cases. Cancer 1969;24:18–31
31. Wharam M, Beltangady M, Hays D, et al. Localized orbital rhabdomyosarcomas: an interim report of the Intergroup Rhabdomyosarcoma Study committee. Ophthalmology 1987;94:251–254
32. Maurer HM, Moon T, Donaldson M, et al. The Intergroup Rhabdomyosarcoma Study: a preliminary report. Cancer 1977;40:2015–2026
33. Kingston JE, McElwain TJ, Malpas JS. Childhood rhabdomyosarcoma: experience of the Children's Solid Tumour Group. Br J Cancer 1983;48:195–207
34. Hays DM. The management of rhabdomyosarcoma in children and young adults. World J Surg 1980;4:15–28
35. Sagerman RH, Tretter P, Ellsworth RM. The treatment of orbital rhabdomyosarcoma of children with primary radiation therapy. Am J Roentgenol Radium Ther Nucl Med 1972;114:31–34
36. Maurer HM. Rhabdomyosarcoma in childhood and adolescence. Curr Probl Cancer 1978;2(9):1–36
37. Grosfeld JL, Weber TR, Weetman RM, Baehner RL. Rhabdomyosarcoma in childhood: analysis of survival in 98 cases. J Pediatr Surg 1983;18:141–146
38. Heyn R, Ragab A, Raney RB Jr, et al. Late effects of therapy in orbital rhabdomyosarcoma in children: a report from the Intergroup Rhabdomyosarcoma Study. Cancer 1986;57:1738–1743
39. Meyers PA, Ghavimi F. Secondary acute non-lymphoblastic leukemia (ANLL) following treatment of childhood rhabdomyosarcoma (Abstract). Proc Am Soc Clin Oncol 1983;2:77
40. Albert DM, Rubenstein RA, Scheie HG. Tumor metastasis to the eye: II. Clinical study in infants and children. Am J Ophthalmol 1967;63:727–732
41. Fratkin JD, Purcell JJ, Krachmer JH, Taylor JC. Wilms' tumor metastatic to the orbit. JAMA 1977;238:1841–1842
42. Musarella MA, Chen HSL, DeBoer G, Gallie BL. Ocular involvement in neuroblastoma: prognostic implications. Ophthalmology 1984;91:936–940
43. Davis JL, Parke DW II, Font RL. Granulocytic sarcoma of the orbit: a clinicopathologic study. Ophthalmology 1985;92:1758–1762
44. Baghdassarian SA, Shammas HF. Eosinophilic granuloma of the orbit. Ann Ophthalmol 1977;9:1247–1250
45. Moore AT, Buncic JR, Munro IR. Fibrous dysplasia of orbit in childhood. Ophthalmology 1985;92:1250–1251

Optic Nerve Tumors of Childhood: A Decision-Analytical Approach to Their Diagnosis

Leonard A. Levin, M.D., Ph.D.
Frederick A. Jakobiec, M.D.

The optimal diagnosis of optic nerve tumors of childhood is difficult. Although gliomas make up the majority of these tumors, the importance of distinguishing them from the less common meningioma is sometimes underestimated. Meningiomas may be much more ominous in children than in adults, and thus accurate diagnosis and appropriate management of optic nerve masses can determine morbidity and even mortality from these tumors. This chapter reviews the clinical, ultrasonographic, and radiological features of pediatric optic nerve tumors and formulates a data base that can be used for a probabilistic decision-analytical approach to their optimal diagnosis. Coupled with current knowledge of the relative risks and benefits of the modalities available for treating these tumors, a step-by-step approach to their diagnosis and management is outlined.

Children, like adults, are subject to a wide variety of tumors of the optic nerve (Table 1); gliomas and meningiomas make up the vast majority. By far the most frequent tumor is the optic nerve glioma, with meningioma running a close second. Since pediatric optic nerve meningiomas are usually more aggressive than gliomas (and more aggressive than adult optic nerve meningiomas), we will focus on the distinctive features of these two tumors. On the other hand, a child with a concurrent systemic malignancy or inflammatory disease, or orbital evidence of same, should be studied with respect to the broader range of diagnoses shown in Table 1. For example, clinical evidence of an optic neuropathy in a patient with leukemia and an optic nerve mass on computed tomography (CT) scanning should be considered leukemic infiltration of the nerve until proved otherwise.

Table 1 *Differential Diagnosis of Pediatric Optic Nerve Lesions*

Glioma
Meningioma
Schwannoma
Metastasis
Leukemia
Teratoma
Inflammation (pseudotumor)
Sarcoid
Juvenile xanthogranuloma
Medulloepithelioma (diktyoma)
Hemangioblastoma

■ Optic Nerve Gliomas

Prevalence

Optic nerve gliomas are predominantly tumors of childhood. In a review of the literature, Alvord and Lofton [1] noted that 510 of 623 patients with optic nerve or chiasmal gliomas (82%) were younger than 20 years. Although an uncommon childhood malignancy, these tumors may represent a frequent cause of optic nerve dysfunction in the young. Among 218 cases of childhood optic atrophy, Repka and Miller [2] found 27 patients (12%) had optic nerve or chiasmal tumors, all of which were gliomas. They are uncommon with respect to other orbital neoplasms; Henderson [3] reported 19 optic nerve gliomas (2.5%) in a series of 764 orbital tumors of adults and children.

It is well known that patients with neurofibromatosis are predisposed to optic gliomas, with many harboring tumors that are clinically inactive. Lewis and colleagues [4] studied 217 patients with neurofibromatosis, finding 33 (15%) with CT-proved optic nerve or chiasmal gliomas, of which 22 (10%) were asymptomatic. The mean age of these patients was 16 years, with the asymptomatic patients tending to be younger. Patients with chiasmal gliomas also tended to be younger (mean age, 6 years) than those with optic nerve gliomas (mean age, 21 years).

The prevalence of optic gliomas is difficult to estimate. Certain figures are known: The prevalence of neurofibromatosis is approximately 1 in 3,000 [4], 5% of patients with neurofibromatosis have symptomatic optic nerve or chiasmal gliomas and, in several studies [5, 6], the proportion of patients with optic nerve or chiasmal glioma who have neurofibromatosis ranges from 20 to 58%. From these data, the prevalence of optic glioma in the pediatric population can be calculated to be from 1 in 15,000 to 1 in 83,000.* This range is in accord with the overall *incidence* observed by Arkhangelski [7] of approximately 1 in 100,000 patients.

$$*\left(\frac{1}{3,000} \times 5\% \times \frac{100\% - 20\%}{20\%}\right) \text{ to } \left(\frac{1}{3,000} \times 5\% \times \frac{100\% - 58\%}{58\%}\right)$$

Pathological Features

Gliomas of the optic nerve are, for the most part, low-grade, pilocytic astrocytomas, although more malignant astrocytomas have been reported, usually in adults [8]. Optic nerve gliomas may invade through the pia and arachnoid and may grow in the subdural space [9], although this is more likely when the disease is associated with neurofibromatosis [10]. There is much controversy in the literature regarding whether these tumors are true neoplasms or are actually hamartomas, based on their slow growth. Perhaps the best answer lies in the macroscopical behavior of these tumors, not in their microscopic character. Alvord and Lofton [1] point out that most patients are not followed long enough to ensure lack of progression and that statistical methods (linearity with log-log plotting) suggest that both optic nerve and chiasmal gliomas are progressive over the very long term. The work of these investigators is analyzed below. It is also worth noting that reactive hyperplasia of the arachnoid in response to the neoplastic astrocytes may account for the occasional misdiagnosis of a glioma as a meningioma [11]. In 14 optic nerve gliomas examined histopathologically by Wright and co-workers [12], 7 (50%) had prominent arachnoid hyperplasia.

Prognosis

The prognosis of glioma of the optic nerve is considerably better than that of chiasmal glioma. Because of the infrequency of these tumors, there has been controversy over the type of treatment and even over whether treatment is necessary. Alvord and Lofton [1] reviewed 623 cases of optic glioma from 85 reports in the literature. In 155, the glioma involved the nerve only and, in 468, the chiasm also. The following summary and calculations derived from their work relates only to patients younger than 20 years.

Of the patients with glioma of the nerve, those who had no treatment had a 71% progression rate (with 5% mortality) over an extended follow-up period. Radiotherapy had an effect only when the dose exceeded a certain level. Those patients treated with an unspecified radiation dose had a 51% recurrence or progression rate, with 7% mortality, whereas none of the patients treated with more than 4,500 rads (45 Gy) of radiation died or had progression or recurrence. In contrast, those treated with complete excision of the tumor had a 14% recurrence rate, with none dying, in a follow-up of up to 20 years. Of those treated with complete excision, 12% of the patients without neurofibromatosis had recurrence, compared with 30% of the patients with neurofibromatosis. The authors emphasized that there were no recurrences in any of the patients with an optic nerve glioma that was completely excised and whose cut end was found microscopically to be free of tumor.

In the pediatric patients with chiasmal glioma without concurrent hydrocephalus who were not treated or who were given less than 4,500 rads of radiation, 56% had recurrence or progression, with 35% dying, over the next 20 years. Those with chiasmal glioma without hydrocephalus who were given 4,500 rads or more of radiation had a 61% recurrence or progression rate, 32% dying, and those treated with chemotherapy had a 51% recurrence or progression rate, with none dying over a 6-year follow-up.

Pediatric patients with chiasmal glioma with hydrocephalus generally fared much worse but were more responsive to radiation. Of those untreated, 74% had recurrence or progression, with 57% dying. When treated with less than 4,500 rads, 90% had recurrence or progression, with 60% dying. When treated with more than 4,500 rads of radiation, 49% had recurrence or progression, with a 29% mortality.

In summary, the only clearly advantageous treatment for optic nerve gliomas appears to be complete excision. Radiotherapy of greater than 4,500 rads prevents recurrence but presumably also results in some amount of radiation-induced changes in local ocular and cerebral structures. Irradiation with more than 4,500 rads may be beneficial for chiasmal gliomas in patients with hydrocephalus but may not be in those without hydrocephalus, although Flickinger and associates [13] suggest that radiation with 4,500 rads or greater may benefit patients with chiasmal glioma without hydrocephalus.

■ Optic Nerve Meningiomas

Prevalence

It is extremely difficult to estimate the prevalence of optic nerve meningiomas, which are most unusual in children. An imprecise estimate may be calculated using the data of Henderson [3], who found 3 pediatric optic nerve meningiomas and 19 pediatric optic nerve gliomas in his study of 764 orbital tumors. Given the range of prevalences for gliomas, as calculated previously, one may estimate the prevalence of pediatric optic nerve meningioma as between 1 in 95,000 and 1 in 525,000.* Even this may be an overestimation, since most other studies have found far fewer optic nerve meningiomas than optic nerve gliomas in their patient populations.

Like gliomas of the optic nerve, optic nerve meningiomas are associated with neurofibromatosis. Although the tumors are too infrequent to study statistically, in Walsh's [15] series of 7 children with optic nerve meningioma, 2 (29%) had evidence of neurofibromatosis. In the study of Karp and colleagues [16], 3 of 10 patients (30%) younger than 20 with

---

$*\left(\dfrac{1}{15,000} \times \dfrac{3}{19}\right)$ to $\left(\dfrac{1}{83,000} \times \dfrac{3}{19}\right)$

optic nerve meningioma had neurofibromatosis, and a fourth had a single café-au-lait spot.

Pathological Features

Optic nerve meningiomas are histologically either meningothelial or transitional and virtually never angioblastic or fibroblastic. Psammoma bodies are common. Unlike gliomas of the optic nerve, the meningiomas invade the dura and can fill the orbit. There have been reports of intra-ocular extension of optic nerve meningiomas [14, 17]. As mentioned previously, arachnoid hyperplasia in an optic nerve glioma may be confused with meningioma.

Prognosis

Meningioma of the optic nerve, although much more common in adults, is generally more aggressive in the pediatric population [15]. Karp and co-workers [16] studied 25 cases of optic nerve sheath meningioma, primarily from the Armed Forces Institute of Pathology (AFIP) collection, which may have a bias toward younger patients due to the consultative nature of many of their cases. When diagnosed, 10 patients (40%) were younger than 20 years; 6 (24%) were younger than 10 years. Three of the 10 patients under 20 had neurofibromatosis, 5 had recurrence of their orbital disease, and 3 had intracranial extension. None of the older patients had either recurrence of the primary tumor or intracranial extension.

The figures of Karp and colleagues [16] are relatively high, and it has been suggested that several of the patients from this study with presumed meningioma actually had optic nerve glioma, with reactive arachnoid hyperplasia simulating meningioma [11]. However, others have also found optic nerve meningioma in the pediatric age group to be more common and more malignant than clinical experience would predict. Wright and associates [18] reported 50 patients with optic nerve sheath meningiomas, 6 (12%) of whom were 20 years or younger, with 1 (2%) younger than 10 years. Of the 6 patients, 3 were originally misdiagnosed as having optic nerve glioma on the basis of CT scanning; one was 10 and the others were 20 years old. Four of the 6 patients younger than 20 (67%) developed intracranial extension, compared with 13 of the 44 patients older than 20 (30%). As mentioned previously, Henderson [3] described 3 patients younger than 20 (14%) in his series of 22 patients with primary orbital meningioma. All 3 pediatric patients (100%) had either postoperative residual tumor or required multiple operations for tumor removal, compared with 5 of the 19 adult patients (26%). Finally, Walsh [15] described 7 pediatric patients with optic nerve meningioma, 4 (57%) of whom had recurrent or progressive disease.

■ Diagnosis

The preceding review should serve to emphasize the importance of distinguishing optic nerve meningiomas from optic nerve gliomas. Meningiomas have a much more threatening course in children compared with what is generally seen in adults. Therefore, correct diagnosis of these less common lesions has important implications for prognosis. What follows is a discussion, in a decision-analytical context, of the data available for making the best possible diagnosis.

History and Physical Examination

In children, optic nerve tumors may present with decreased visual acuity, strabismus, optic atrophy, obscurations of vision, proptosis, or other symptoms. Unlike other orbital tumors, the proptosis associated with tumors of the optic nerve is usually disproportionately low compared with the acuity deficit. An optic nerve mass or enlargement of the optic canal may be seen on a radiographic study done for another reason. Certain signs and symptoms, some of which have been proposed to help distinguish meningiomas from gliomas, may be utilized.

Visual Acuity The literature is not helpful in deciding whether presenting visual acuity is worse in pediatric glioma or meningioma. In the study by Rush and colleagues [5] of 25 histopathologically verified cases of optic nerve glioma with vision recorded, 20 (80%) had visual acuity worse than 20/200, whereas in the study by Jakobiec and co-workers [10] of clinical and CT evaluation in the diagnosis of optic nerve gliomas and meningiomas, 10 of 15 patients (67%) younger than 20 years with optic nerve glioma had visual acuity of counting fingers or worse. In their 2 pediatric meningioma cases, the acuity is not stated, but in their adult meningioma cases, only 12 of 44 patients (27%) had acuity worse than counting fingers. Wright and associates [12] described 31 patients with optic nerve glioma, 11 (35%) of whom had acuities worse than 20/200, and 5 (16%) with vision of 20/40 or better. Grossly similar proportions were seen in an accompanying study of 50 patients with optic nerve meningioma [18]; 30 (60%) had visual acuity of 20/200 or worse, whereas 10 (20%) had acuity of 20/30 or better. They did not stratify the acuity of their pediatric cases, and thus it is impossible to say whether children with optic nerve meningioma have similar acuity to those with gliomas. In summary, there is a suggestion that (mostly adult) meningioma presents with better visual acuity than (mostly pediatric) glioma, but that may merely reflect the fact that adults are more likely to come to medical attention for minimal acuity changes than are children.

Proptosis Jakobiec and colleagues [10] reported proptosis ranging from 1 to 10 mm (mean, 2 mm; median, 2 mm) in patients with optic nerve glioma, and 0 to 7.5 mm (mean, 3.3 mm; median, 2 mm) in patients with optic nerve meningioma. These values are grossly similar, given the reliability of this measurement.

In Walsh's [15] report of 7 patients with childhood optic nerve meningioma, proptosis of 0, 0, 2, 3.5, and 5 mm were measured; in one patient, proptosis was stated but not measured, and in another the presence of proptosis was unclear. The mean of 2.1 mm and median of 2 mm of proptosis are remarkably similar to those described for the gliomas of Jakobiec's group and correlate with the mean of 3.3 and median of 2 described by Wright and co-workers [18] for mostly adult meningiomas, but these data contrast with Henderson's [3] older series of meningiomas, in which the mean of proptosis was 7 mm.

It appears that the presence and degree of proptosis are of little value in distinguishing childhood optic nerve meningioma from glioma.

Optociliary Shunt Vessels Optociliary (or, more properly, retinociliary) shunt vessels are often a sign of chronic compression of an optic nerve, presumably secondary to central retinal vein compression. Jakobiec and colleagues [10] found that 10 of 47 patients (21%) with optic nerve meningioma had optociliary shunt vessels, compared with 1 of 22 patients (5%) with optic nerve glioma. Wright and co-workers [18] saw shunt vessels in 12 of 50 patients (24%) with meningioma and in 1 of 31 patients (3%) with glioma [12]. Adding these cases together, approximately 23% of patients with optic nerve meningioma have shunt vessels versus 4% of those with optic nerve glioma. Since these studies did not identify which patients with shunt vessels were in the pediatric age group, the disproportion may reflect only the relatively greater chronicity of meningiomas in an adult, compared with gliomas in children.

Presence of Neurofibromatosis As discussed previously, approximately 20 to 60% of patients with optic nerve glioma have neurofibromatosis. The figures for childhood optic nerve meningioma are unclear but in two studies were 28% and 30% [15, 16]. The overlap of these two sets of figures precludes making a distinction based on the presence of neurofibromatosis, although the use of molecular genetics to distinguish different forms of the disease may make this possible in the future.

Ultrasonography

A-scan ultrasonography can be used to study the intraorbital optic nerve. Gans and associates [19] examined 59 optic nerve lesions and 73 normal nerves. All gliomas, but only 7% of meningiomas, were of low

Table 2 *Ultrasonographic Diagnosis of Optic Nerve Tumors*

Test	No. (%) of Gliomas	No. (%) of Meningiomas
Nerve diameter > 2× control	3/4 (75)	13/15 (87)
Positive 30-degree test		
Anterior	2/2 (100)	3/10 (30)
Posterior	0/2 (0)	3/12 (25)
Both	0/2 (0)	1/9 (11)
Reflectivity		
Low	4/4 (100)	1/15 (7)
Medium	0/4 (0)	12/15 (80)
High	0/4 (0)	2/15 (13)

Source: Data from Gans et al [19].

reflectivity (Table 2). The values for the other measurements they reported are either too small or too similar to discriminate between gliomas and meningiomas.

Computed Tomography

The contributions of CT to the diagnosis of optic nerve tumors have been manifold. Peyster and colleagues [20] studied 9 intraorbital meningiomas with high-resolution CT. Eight (89%) had diffuse thickening of the nerve, with 2 showing apparent focal fusiform expansion. The remaining lesion (11%) had segmental thickening. None had calcification. A tramtrack appearance was noted in 8 of 9 (89%). These investigators also described 1 optic nerve glioma, which was fusiform.

Jakobiec and co-workers [10] studied 22 patients with optic nerve glioma and 47 with optic nerve meningioma using high-resolution CT. They found that a fusiform appearance, especially with a kink, was unique to the gliomas, whereas calcification was unique to the meningiomas (Table 3). Diffuse expansion of the nerve was seen in both types, although certain focally expansile patterns were seen only in meningiomas.

Rothfus and associates [21] studied 10 patients with optic nerve glioma and 19 with meningioma. Three patients (30%) with glioma had fusiform expansion, compared with 8 (42%) with meningioma. However, none of the glioma fusiform expansions had central lucencies, whereas 7 of the 8 (88%) with meningioma demonstrated these. Four of the 10 patients (40%) with glioma had a tubular expansion, compared with 7 (37%) of the meningioma patients. This is probably similar to the "diffusely enlarged with narrow expansion" category of Jakobiec and colleagues [10]. Again, none of the glioma patients had a central lucency, whereas 6 of the 7 meningioma patients (86%) did. This central lucency is identical to the tram-track sign. Finally, in 3 of the glioma patients (30%) there was an excrescent appearance to the optic nerve, none of which showed central lucency,

Table 3 *Computed Tomographic Diagnosis of Optic Nerve Tumors*

Pattern	No. (%) of Gliomas	No. (%) of Meningiomas
Fusiform	19/22 (86)	0
With kink	7/22 (32)	0
With cyst	2/22 (9)	0
Narrow expansion	3/22 (14)	11/47 (23)
Apical expansion	0	16/47 (34)
Anterior expansion	0	2/47 (4)
Irregular expansion	0	7/47 (15)
Calcification	0	10/47 (21)
Orbital replacement	0	1/47 (2)

Source: Data from Jakobiec et al [10].

compared with 4 of the meningioma patients (21%), all of which had central lucency.

Johns and colleagues [22] studied 225 patients with orbital tumors, 3 of whom had an optic nerve meningioma. All 3 had a fusiform nerve, which is relatively unusual for meningioma, and all had a central lucency (tram-track sign). Interestingly, the authors observed in all 3 a perineural enhancement with contrast, which they attributed to subarachnoid spread of tumor.

Clearly, the CT appearance of the tumor is one of the most useful methods for distinguishing optic nerve glioma from optic nerve meningioma.

Magnetic Resonance Imaging

Magnetic resonance imaging (MRI) has not been as well studied as CT in the diagnosis of optic nerve lesions. The disadvantages of MRI in discriminating optic nerve meningiomas from gliomas are that calcification is not imaged, since it does not contain protons, and that the tram-track sign of meningioma is usually not appreciated owing to the isointensity of the nerve and the tumor [23]. However, more recent work using fat-suppression sequences* has demonstrated an ability to image optic nerve meningiomas more accurately [24]. In this study of 6 optic nerve meningiomas, only 3 were visualized with MRI alone, with 1 appearing as a diffuse enlargement of the nerve, 1 as an apical fusiform enlargement, and 1 as a questionable abnormality. After gadolinium enhancement and the use of fat suppression sequences, all 6 nerve meningiomas were clearly seen as a high-signal intensity (tumor) surrounding a lower-signal intensity (nerve). Three gliomas that were imaged demonstrated diffuse isointense enlargement of the nerve in 1 patient with diffuse thickening. Gadolinium, fat suppression, or both, failed to change the appearance of the lesion.

---

*Fat suppression sequences are specific sequences of radiofrequency pulses that are pre-applied, so as to maximize the signal from water and minimize that from fat.

■ Decision-Analytical Model

Test Sensitivities and Specificities

The major clinical and radiographic criteria for distinguishing optic nerve gliomas from optic nerve meningiomas are summarized in Table 4. In addition to the raw frequency rates (of occurrence of the particular item in gliomas and meningiomas), the sensitivity and specificity of the item as a test for either glioma or meningioma are given. The equivalent values for the tumor *not* specified can be calculated as:

$$\text{Sensitivity}_{\text{glioma}} = 100\% - \text{specificity}_{\text{meningioma}}$$

$$\text{Specificity}_{\text{glioma}} = 100\% - \text{sensitivity}_{\text{meningioma}}$$

These data assume that the two tumors are the only serious possibilities in the differential diagnosis. In the presence of clinical evidence of other pathological processes, the sensitivities and specificities listed in Table 4 are inaccurate. All 0% and 100% figures were replaced with 1% and 99% values, respectively, to reflect the fact that although a test appeared completely sensitive or specific, these data were often based on small numbers of patients.

In Table 4, entries followed by an asterisk indicate that the test may be of use in discriminating gliomas from meningiomas. From this information, Bayes's theorem may be used to calculate the probability of having a glioma or meningioma, given the result of a specified test and the prior probability of having one or the other tumor. Since the incidence of optic nerve meningiomas in children is small, it is difficult to estimate its relative frequency with respect to gliomas. A rough figure may be calculated from the study of Henderson [3], in which 3 pediatric meningiomas and 19 gliomas were seen, and the studies of Wright and colleagues [12, 18], in which 3 pediatric meningiomas and 31 gliomas, most of which were in young patients, were seen. Taken together, there was a ratio of 6 meningiomas to approximately 50 gliomas, or 1:8.3.

Table 5 is the result of applying Bayes's theorem using each test alone. It allows one to estimate the relative probability of a meningioma or glioma, assuming a clinical or radiological sign is present (test positive) or absent (test negative). These figures are based on the sensitivities and specificities from Table 4, which are estimates derived from the literature and sometimes based on small studies.

If it is desired to use more than one test in succession, the formula of Bayes described in the following sections may be employed, using the probability from Table 4 as the pretest probability and simply plugging in the appropriate sensitivity and specificity.

Table 4 *Sensitivities and Specificities of Tests for Optic Nerve Glioma and Meningioma*

Test	Incidence in Glioma (%)	Incidence in Meningioma (%)	Sensitivity (%)	Specificity (%)
Acuity better than 20/40	16	20 (?)	Poor	Poor
Acuity worse than finger counting	35–67	27–50	Poor	Poor
Proptosis >2 mm	50	50	Poor	Poor
Optociliary shunt vessels*	4	23	23 (meningioma)	96 (meningioma)
Associated neurofibromatosis	20–60	28–30	Poor	Poor
Ultrasonography: mid- or high-intensity echo*	1	93	93 (meningioma)	99 (meningioma)
CT: calcification*	1	18	18 (meningioma)	99 (meningioma)
CT: fusiform*	56	14	56 (glioma)	86 (glioma)
CT: fusiform kink*	32	1	32 (glioma)	99 (glioma)
CT: diffuse expansion	22	35	Poor	Poor
CT: diffuse and focal expansion*	1	48	48 (meningioma)	99 (meningioma)
CT: central lucency*	7	91	91 (meningioma)	93 (meningioma)
MRI	?	?	?	?
MRI: fat suppression*	1	99	99 (meningioma)	99 (meningioma)

CT = computed tomography; MRI = magnetic resonance imaging.
*May be useful in discriminating gliomas from meningiomas.

Table 5 *Probabilities of Glioma and Meningioma Given Single Test Results*

Test	Probability of Glioma: Test Positive (%)	Probability of Meningioma: Test Positive (%)	Probability of Glioma: Test Negative (%)	Probability of Meningioma: Test Negative (%)
Optociliary shunt vessels	59	41	91	9
Ultrasonography: mid- or high-intensity echo	8	92	99	1
CT				
Calcification	32	68	91	9
Fusiform	97	3	81	19
Fusiform kink	99	1	85	15
Diffuse and focal expansion	15	85	94	6
Central lucency	39	61	99	1
MRI: tram-track with fat suppression	8	92	99	1

CT = computed tomography; MRI = magnetic resonance imaging.

Example *What is the probability of meningioma in a pediatric patient with optociliary shunt vessels and a central lucency in a diffusely enlarged nerve on CT scanning?*

From Table 5, one can see that the probability (P) of meningioma in a patient with optociliary shunt vessels is 41%. From Table 4, the sensitivity and specificity for meningioma if there is lucency on the CT scan are 91% and 93%, respectively. Since

$$P_{posttest} = \frac{P_{pretest} \times sensitivity}{P_{pretest} \times sensitivity + (1 - P_{pretest}) \times (1 - specificity)}$$

then

$$P_{meningioma} = \frac{0.41 \times 0.91}{0.41 \times 0.91 + [(1 - 0.41) \times (1 - 0.93)]} = 0.90 \, (90\%)$$

Thus, by using two separate pieces of information, the diagnostic likelihood of the patient having an optic nerve meningioma is greatly increased. Several caveats are in order. First, the data items used in this method must be independent. For example, it would be incorrect to use information about a central lucency in an optic nerve mass from both CT and MRI scanning, since statistically these two techniques are dependent, or correlated. Second, some of the data items reflect studies in the literature using small numbers of patients. For example, the 99% sensitivity and specificity for detecting a tram-track sign with fat-suppressed MRI is based on only 6 patients. If the authors' seventh patient with that sign turned out to have a glioma, the specificity would drop to approximately 86%. In other words, the data in the tables should be used only as a rough guide. Third, this entire analysis has been restricted to the two most common pediatric optic nerve tumors. Clearly, signs or symptoms consistent with other rarer lesions must be sought (e.g., the presence of another malignancy that could be metastatic to the nerve, or an orbital inflammatory process).

Choice of Treatment

Wright and colleagues [12] have proposed using a period of observation to decide on treatment of pediatric optic nerve malignancies. In patients with good visual acuity, these authors advocate biopsy if there are clinical and radiographic grounds for the presence of meningioma, with removal of the tumor if it is a biopsy-proved meningioma but observation if it is a glioma. If the tumor progresses (Wright's "active" group) or if the acuity is poor, they advocate biopsy and removal of the nerve if meningioma is present or vision is lost. If the chiasm is involved with glioma, the authors suggest biopsy, possibly followed by debulking or radiotherapy, or both [12].

A variation on Wright's plan of management of these tumors may be formulated using the data from the reports discussed previously. First, a diagnosis of meningioma should be attempted, using clinical data, CT scanning, and even ultrasonography in difficult cases. Gadolinium-enhanced and fat-suppressed MRI may be of use. If the tumor is likely to be a meningioma (a conservative threshold of 10 to 20% probability), biopsy and possible removal of the tumor if it proves to be a meningioma are advised. If the visual acuity is good, there is no evidence of chiasmal involvement, and the tumor is assuredly a glioma based on diagnostic studies, then Wright's suggestion for a period of observation should be used. If there is any progression or if visual acuity is poor, removal of the tumor is advocated, given Alvord and Lofton's [1] finding that 71% of optic nerve gliomas progressed and 5% of patients died when the tumor was not completely excised. If the chiasm is involved, based on clinical and radiographic findings or from evidence at surgery, biopsy and at least 4,500 rads of radiation in 180-rad fractions are advocated [13], although this is controversial.

■ Appendix: Decision Analysis

The techniques described in this section aid in deciding on the optimal way to diagnose a disease and in arriving at an optimal treatment plan. A more detailed description may be found in Chang [25].

Probabilities

Diagnosis may be thought of as a process in which several possible diagnoses (the *differential diagnosis*) are sifted through until a single diagnosis is chosen. More specifically, the end point is achieved when the *probability* of one of the diagnoses is high enough (reaches a *diagnostic threshold*) to satisfy the clinician's desire for diagnostic certainty. This end point may never be reached; in fact, many patients go through several rounds of medical testing without a single, final diagnosis ever being chosen. Alternatively, the diagnostic threshold may be so low that relatively few studies need be performed before a satisfactory diagnosis is made. Nonetheless, this model of diagnosis as a process of assigning probabilities to the various diagnoses in the differential, and choosing the one with the highest probability, is intuitively similar to what clinicians do every day.

How does one arrive at these final probabilities? To answer this, it is important to distinguish several uses of the term *probability*. First, the probability of the disease before any examination or testing is performed is called the *pretest* (or *a priori* or *prior*) *probability*. In cases where patients are randomly drawn from the population, this is identical to the prevalence of the disease. More commonly, however, patients are referred (or self-referred) based on symptoms or previous examination and testing. In these cases, the pretest probability is usually much higher than the disease prevalence. For example, the likelihood that a patient seen in the office for a red, painful eye has acute angle closure is obviously much higher than that of a patient seen for a routine checkup. The probability of angle closure in the latter, healthy patient is equivalent to the prevalence of angle closure in the entire population, most of whom have no ocular symptoms. The pretest probability may also depend on the particular demographic subgroup to which the patient belongs. For example, a teenager is much less likely to have a cataract than is a nonagenarian, and a man is far more likely to have congenital red-green dyschromatopsia than is a woman.

How can the probability of a disease be increased or decreased from the pretest, or starting, probability? This is achieved by testing. Here the word *test* is used broadly to represent not only laboratory and radiographic investigations but also elements in the history taking and clinical examination. For example, the patient with the red, painful eye can undergo the test of applanation tonometry to determine intraocular pressure. If the pressure is very high, the probability of acute angle closure is greater. If the pressure is low, the probability of acute angle closure is less. This probability of the disease after testing is called the *posttest* (or *a posteriori* or *posterior*) *probability*.

This transformation from pretest to posttest probability via testing may be repeated indefinitely. The posttest probability after one test becomes the pretest probability for the next test. For example, assume the pressure of the patient with the red, painful eye is 65 mm by applanation. Therefore, the posttest probability of angle closure is higher, say 0.95 (95%). If Goldmann gonioscopy is then performed and no angle structures are visible, the current pretest probability of 0.95 rises to 0.99 or higher. If, on the other hand, the angle is open to the ciliary body band, the posttest probability may approach zero.

Sensitivity and Specificity

Some tests do not aid in diagnosis. In the language we have used, some tests do not measurably change the posttest from the pretest probability. For example, the probability of congenital red-green dyschromatopsia is neither more nor less likely if the patient has ultrasonographic evidence of an increased globe axial length. A test such as this is an example of the posttest probability perfectly reflecting the pretest probability. Other tests are so accurate that they can be considered gold standards; the posttest probability is dramatically altered by the testing. For example, an enucleated globe showing pathological evidence of retinoblastoma represents a test (enucleation and histological examination) with high cost (surgery and loss of the eye), but one that is virtually completely decisive (raising the posttest probability to 1.0, or 100%).

Fortunately, there are ways of quantifying the ability of tests to adjust the probabilities of various diagnoses. The *sensitivity* of a test is the proportion of patients with a disease who have a positive result on the test. For example, an applanation tension greater than 30 mm Hg is a highly sensitive test for acute angle closure, since almost all patients with angle closure will have an intraocular pressure greater than that. In this case, the number 30 is important. If only patients with intraocular pressures greater than 80 were chosen, the test would be much less sensitive, since there are many patients with angle closure who have pressures of less than 80 mm Hg. This dependence of the sensitivity on a *discrimination parameter* is common for many tests. There are ways to choose these parameters to optimize the diagnosis procedure, but these will not be discussed here.

Although certainly patients with acute angle closure will have an intraocular pressure of greater than 30 mm Hg, making applanation tonometry a sensitive test for the disease, it can be recognized intuitively that this is a poor test overall because most patients with intraocular pressures in excess of 30 mm Hg do not have acute angle closure, but rather some other cause for their ocular hypertension. Tests such as this are not *specific*. The specificity of a test is the proportion of patients who *do not* have the disease who test negative. With a highly specific test, virtually all the patients without the disease should test negative, and only a few patients without the disease should test positive. Thus, using 30 mm Hg as a discrimination parameter for angle closure makes for a nonspecific test, since a high proportion of patients who do not have angle closure will test positive (e.g., open-angle glaucoma).

Bayes's Theorem

Given the sensitivity and specificity of a test and the pretest probability of a disease, how is the posttest probability determined? Fortunately, there is a simple formula, developed by Bayes, that relates these various quantities. Briefly, the posttest probability of the disease if the test (T) is positive is equal to the pretest probability multiplied by the probability of the test being positive if the patient has the disease (D) (the sensitivity) and divided by the overall probability of the test being positive (whether or not the patient has the disease). More precisely,

$$P(D|T^+) = \frac{P(D) \times P(T^+|D)}{P(T^+)}$$

where the "|" symbol may be translated as "given," so that $P(D|T^+)$ means "the probability of the disease, given that the test is positive." It turns out that $P(T^+|D)$ is identical to the sensitivity, whereas $P(T^+)$ can be expressed in terms of the sensitivity and specificity, so that the formula may be written thus:

$$P_{posttest} = \frac{P_{pretest} \times sensitivity}{(P_{pretest} \times sensitivity) + [(1 - P_{pretest}) \times (1 - specificity)]}$$

This formula is the basis for the decision-analytical approach to the diagnosis of pediatric optic nerve tumors described in the text.

■ References

1. Alvord EC Jr, Lofton S. Gliomas of the optic nerve or chiasm: outcome by patient's age, tumor site, and treatment. J Neurosurg 1988;68:85–98
2. Repka MX, Miller NR. Optic atrophy in children. Am J Ophthalmol 1988;106:191–193
3. Henderson JW. Orbital tumors. New York: Thieme-Stratton, 1980:472–496
4. Lewis RA, Gerson LP, Axelson KA, et al. Von Recklinghausen neurofibromatosis: II. Incidence of optic gliomata. Ophthalmology 1984;91:929–935
5. Rush JA, Younge BR, Campbell RJ, MacCarty CS. Optic glioma: long-term follow-up of 85 histologically verified cases. Ophthalmology 1982;89:1213–1219
6. Hoyt WF, Baghdassarian SA. Optic glioma of childhood: natural history and rationale for conservative management. Br J Ophthalmol 1969;53:793–798
7. Arkhangelski VN. Neoplasm of the optic nerve. Ophthalmologica 1966;151:260–271
8. Hoyt WF, Meshel LG, Lessel S, et al. Malignant optic glioma of adulthood. Brain 1973;96:121–132
9. Eggers H, Jakobiec FA, Jones IS. Tumors of the optic nerve. Doc Ophthalmol 1976;41:43–128
10. Jakobiec FA, Depot MJ, Kennerdell JS, et al. Combined clinical and computed tomographic diagnosis of orbital glioma and meningioma. Ophthalmology 1984;91:137–155
11. Cooling RJ, Wright JE. Arachnoid hyperplasia in optic nerve glioma: confusion with orbital meningioma. Br J Ophthalmol 1979;63:596–599
12. Wright JE, McNab AA, McDonald WI. Optic nerve glioma and the management of optic nerve tumours in the young. Br J Ophthalmol 1989;73:967–974
13. Flickinger JC, Torres C, Deutsch M. Management of low-grade gliomas of the optic nerve and chiasm. Cancer 1988;61:635–642
14. Henderson JW, Campbell RJ. Primary intraorbital meningioma with intraocular extension. Mayo Clin Proc 1977;52:504–508
15. Walsh FB. Meningiomas, primary within the orbit and optic canal. In: Smith JL, ed. Neuro-ophthalmology symposium of the University of Miami and the Bascom Palmer Eye Institute, vol 5. St Louis: Mosby, 1970:240–266
16. Karp LA, Zimmerman LE, Borit A, Spencer W. Primary intraorbital meningiomas. Arch Ophthalmol 1974;91:24–28
17. Cibis GW, Whittaker CK, Wood WE. Intraocular extension of optic nerve meningioma in a case of neurofibromatosis. Arch Ophthalmol 1985;103:404–406
18. Wright JE, McNab AA, McDonald WI. Primary optic nerve sheath meningioma. Br J Ophthalmol 1989;73:960–966

19. Gans MS, Byrne SF, Glaser JS. Standardized A-scan echography in optic nerve disease. Arch Ophthalmol 1987;105:1232–1236
20. Peyster RG, Hoover ED, Hershey BL, Haskin ME. High-resolution CT of lesions of the optic nerve. AJR 1983;140:869–874
21. Rothfus WE, Curtin HD, Slamovits TL, Kennerdell JS. Optic nerve/sheath enlargement: a differential approach based on high-resolution CT morphology. Radiology 1984;150:409–415
22. Johns TT, Citrin CM, Black J, Sherman JL. CT evaluation of perineural orbital lesions: evaluation of the "tram-track" sign. AJNR 1984;5:587–590
23. Elster AD. Cranial magnetic resonance imaging. New York: Churchill Livingstone, 1988:360–364
24. Hendrix LE, Kneeland JB, Haughton VM, et al. MR imaging of optic nerve lesions: value of gadopentetate dimeglumine and fat-suppression technique. AJNR 1990; 11:749–754
25. Chang PJ. Bayesian analysis revisited: a radiologist's survival guide. AJR 1989; 152:721–727

Controversies in Ophthalmology
Frederick A. Jakobiec, M.D., Section Editor

Immunosuppressive Drugs in the Management of Progressive, Corticosteroid-Resistant Uveitis Associated with Juvenile Rheumatoid Arthritis

Ramzi K. Hemady, M.D.
John C. Baer, M.D.
C. Stephen Foster, M.D.

■ Background

Juvenile rheumatoid arthritis (JRA) affects an estimated 60,000 to 200,000 children in the United States; 60% of these suffer from the pauci-articular form of the disease [1]. Sight-threatening uveitis develops in 10 to 50% of children with this subset of JRA [1]. Conventional therapy of JRA-associated uveitis has typically consisted of mydriatics and corticosteroids. Poorly controlled inflammation and prolonged corticosteroid therapy, however, lead to secondary cataracts in 28 to 30% and glaucoma in 14 to 22% of these patients. Management of such complications usually necessitates surgical intervention, the results of which are often poor.

Despite excellent efforts on the part of ophthalmologists and rheumatologists alike, roughly 12% of patients progress to blindness from complications of JRA-associated uveitis and corticosteroid therapy [2]. Efforts to develop corticosteroid-sparing yet effective nonsteroidal antiinflammatory drug (NSAID) strategies to control uveitis activity have had limited success. This prompted us to evaluate the efficacy and safety of immunosuppressive alternatives for corticosteroids in the treatment of JRA-associated uveitis.

The role of immunosuppressive drugs in the management of JRA-associated uveitis recalcitrant to conventional therapy (mydriatics, corticosteroids) is undefined. Since JRA is relatively uncommon, patients are young (pediatric age group), and the systemic disease is usually mild (requiring only conservative therapy), randomized, controlled clinical trials that assess the efficacy and safety of immunosuppressive therapy for uveitis in this setting are lacking. Our data suggest a beneficial therapeutic role for immunosuppressive drugs in selected patients with corticosteroid-resistant JRA-associated uveitis.

■ Patients and Methods

Twenty-six patients with JRA-associated uveitis were seen by one of us (CSF) in the Immunology Service of the Massachusetts Eye and Ear Infirmary between January 1977 and September 1989 and form the basis of this report. All patients were referred by their rheumatologists, pediatricians, or primary ophthalmologists; subsequent follow-up was performed in close conjunction with the referring physician. All 26 patients satisfied the criteria for the diagnosis of JRA—namely, the onset of arthritis involving one or more joints before the age of 16 and lasting 3 or more consecutive months [1]. Other possible diagnoses were excluded where appropriate.

Patient sex, age at onset of uveitis, duration of uveitis, type of joint involvement, and previous systemic and ocular management were determined through a detailed questionnaire completed by each patient, a careful review of systems, and communications with referring physicians.

At each examination, visual acuity was determined, and slit-lamp and ophthalmoscopic examinations were performed. Uveitis activity, synechiae and cataract formation, presence of band keratopathy, intraocular pressure, and status of the retina were recorded. Active uveitis was defined as the presence of inflammatory cells in the anterior chamber or vitreous. Treatment (conventional or immunosuppressive) was considered successful if inflammation was eliminated or reduced to the point (less than 1+ cells in the aqueous or vitreous) that vision-threatening complications (e.g., synechiae formation, macular edema) were avoided without relapse and without major drug-induced side effects, through the end of the follow-up period. Laboratory workup included antinuclear antibody, HLA-B27 typing, and rheumatoid factor on all patients. Other laboratory tests were performed as indicated.

Chi-square and unpaired Student's t-test were used for statistical analysis of the differences between the treatment groups.

■ Immunosuppressive Therapy

Immunosuppressive therapy was initiated if ocular inflammatory activity persisted despite therapy with mydriatics, topical, periocular, or systemic corticosteroids, and systemic NSAIDs. During immunosuppressive therapy, patients continued their previous medications; these were modified according to therapeutic response and patient tolerance. Prior to initiation of immunosuppressive therapy, patients and their parents were educated about the possible undesirable side effects and the necessity for close monitoring. Eight patients were treated with immunosuppressive drugs. Since no single immunosuppressive drug has proved superior for the control of JRA-associated uveitis, methotrexate, azathioprine, and chlorambucil were used in selected patients. Methotrexate (5 to 15 mg once weekly) was used in 3 patients, azathioprine (1 to 2 mg/kg/day) in 3, a combination of methotrexate and azathioprine in 1, and chlorambucil (0.1 mg/kg/day up to a maximum daily dose of 12 mg) in 2, one of whom had failed to respond to azathioprine. Complete blood cell counts with platelet levels and white cell differentials, serum creatinine and blood urea nitrogen assessment, and urinalysis were obtained before starting immunosuppressive therapy and then weekly until drug dosage, disease activity, and hematological parameters were stabilized. After stabilization, monitoring every 2 weeks was performed longitudinally. Liver function tests (serum transaminase, alkaline phosphatase) were similarly monitored in patients receiving methotrexate.

■ Results

Twenty-six patients (44 eyes) with JRA-associated uveitis were seen in our Immunology Service over a 13-year period. Follow-up ranged from 3 to 156 months. Therapeutic management is presented in Table 1. Inflammation in 18 patients (69%, 31 eyes) responded to conventional (nonimmunosuppressive) management: In 4 patients, topical corticosteroids and mydriatics were sufficient; transseptal injections of corticosteroids were additionally required in 12 (average of three injections per patient), systemically administered corticosteroids in 10, and NSAIDs in 13 patients. Two of the 18 patients required therapy with a combination of corticosteroid and mydriatic eye drops, transseptal corticosteroid injections, and systemically administered corticosteroids and NSAIDs.

Inflammation in the remaining 8 patients (patients 3, 8, 9, 10, 12, 15, 18, and 22 in Table 1) (31%, 13 eyes) failed to respond to the preceding therapeutic measures. Therefore, immunosuppressive drugs were used in these individuals. Specific indications for immunosuppressive therapy were as follows: All 8 patients had persistent 2 to 3+ inflammatory cells in the anterior chamber despite maximum tolerated conventional therapy; 6 developed progressively worsening cataracts; 2 developed persistent maculopathy; 2 developed disc edema while on maximum conventional therapy; and 1 developed glaucoma that was increasingly resistant to medical therapy. Successful abolition of inflammation was achieved in 6 of the 8 patients (75%) treated with immunosuppressive drugs (patients 8, 9, 12, 15, 18, and 22). Anterior chamber inflammatory reaction resolved 3 weeks to

Table 1 *Management of JRA-Associated Uveitis*

Patient No.	Management	Outcome
1	Topical CS	Controlled
2	Topical and systemic CS	Controlled
3	Topical, local, systemic CS, NSAID, AZA, MTX	Failed
4	Topical CS, NSAID	Controlled
5	Topical and local CS, NSAID	Controlled
6	Topical and systemic CS, NSAID	Controlled
7	Topical, local, systemic CS, NSAID	Controlled
8	Topical, local, systemic CS, NSAID, MTX	Controlled
9	Topical, local, systemic CS, NSAID, Ch	Controlled
10	Topical CS, NSAID, MTX	Failed
11	Topical CS, NSAID	Controlled
12	Topical, local, systemic CS, NSAID, AZA, Ch	Controlled
13	Topical and local CS, NSAID	Controlled
14	Topical, local, systemic NSAID	Controlled
15	Topical, local CS, NSAID, MTX	Controlled
16	Topical and local CS, NSAID	Controlled
17	Topical CS, NSAID	Controlled
18	Topical, local, systemic CS, AZA	Controlled
19	Topical CS	Controlled
20	Topical CS, NSAID	Controlled
21	Topical and local CS, NSAID	Controlled
22	Topical CS, NSAID, AZA	Controlled
23	Topical CS	Controlled
24	Topical CS, NSAID	Controlled
25	Topical and systemic CS	Controlled
26	Topical CS	Controlled

JRA = juvenile rheumatoid arthritis; CS = corticosteroids; NSAID = nonsteroidal antiinflammatory drug; AZA = azathioprine; MTX = methotrexate; Ch = chlorambucil.

3 months after initiation of immunosuppressive therapy in all 6 responders (mean, 5.8 weeks). Cataract progression was arrested in all responders. In patients 9 and 12, disc edema resolved 3 weeks and 2 months after initiation of immunosuppressive therapy, respectively. Macular edema resolved in patient 12 within 3 months after starting immunosuppressive therapy, whereas patient 22 developed a macular cyst that remained unchanged after immunosuppressive therapy. Glaucoma in patient 18 was controlled without surgical intervention. Visual acuities before and after immunosuppressive therapy are presented in Table 2.

Inflammation was controlled in 2 of 3 patients treated with methotrexate, 2 of 3 patients treated with azathioprine, and 2 patients treated with chlorambucil; inflammation in 1 of the latter 2 patients had not responded to azathioprine. Ocular inflammation failed to respond in a patient treated with a combination of azathioprine and methotrexate. Two patients treated with azathioprine complained of transient nausea and vomiting. No other

Table 2 *Visual Acuity*

Patient No.	Pretreatment Acuity		Posttreatment Acuity*	
	OD	OS	OD	OS
3	20/100	20/25	20/60	20/25
8	HM	20/40	CF	20/40
9	20/200	20/400	20/30	20/30
10	20/40	20/20	20/200	20/20
12	20/80	20/300	20/40	20/300
15	20/25	20/50	20/20	20/40
18	20/100	CF	20/40	20/200
22	20/400	20/300	20/200	20/80

OD = oculus dexter (right eye); OS = oculus sinister (left eye); HM = hand motions; CF = counting fingers.
*Visual acuity at last visit.

Table 3 *Adverse Effects of Immunosuppressive Therapy*

Adverse Effect	Drug		
	AZA (n = 3)	MTX (n = 3)	CHLM (n = 2)
Nausea	2	0	0
Alopecia	0	0	0
Hematopoiesis	0	0	0
Hepatitis	0	0	0
Malignancy	0	0	0
Sterility or menstrual dysfunction	0	0	0

AZA = azathioprine; MTX = methotrexate; CHLM = chlorambucil.

subjective or objective adverse effects of immunosuppressive therapy were encountered (Table 3).

Duration of immunosuppressive therapy was 2 to 12 months (mean, 6.4 months). In 2 patients without significant recurrence of ocular inflammation over a follow-up period of 10 years and 3 months, chlorambucil was withdrawn 2 and 8 months after initiation of immunosuppressive therapy, respectively. In the remaining patients, immunosuppressive therapy was maintained until the last recorded examination. Follow-up after initiation of immunosuppressive therapy ranged from 12 to 156 months (mean, 28 months).

Data concerning patient age at diagnosis of uveitis, ocular complications (iridocyclitis, vitreous cells, retinitis, disc and macular edema, cataract, band keratopathy, glaucoma, synechiae, surgery) (Figs 1, 2), number of joints involved, patient sex, antinuclear antibody titers, and HLA-B27 typing were collected and analyzed in order to identify risk factors that might

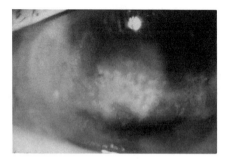

Figure 1 *Band keratopathy in a patient with juvenile rheumatoid arthritis–associated uveitis.*

predict the need for immunosuppressive therapy (Tables 4, 5). Presence of inflammatory cells in the vitreous on presentation was the only factor significantly more common (p = .001) in patients requiring immunosuppressive therapy: Vitreous cells were present in 7 of 13 eyes requiring immunosuppressive therapy (5 of these responded to therapy) and in 4 of 31 eyes not requiring immunosuppressive therapy.

■ Case Reports

Patient 12

A 21-year-old woman with a history of JRA-associated uveitis in both eyes since age 12 was referred with a flare-up of iridocyclitis. The patient had developed secondary cataracts and dense vitreous haze and had had bilateral intracapsular cataract extraction (without intraocular lens implantation) and vitrectomy 5 years previously. Medications at the time of our first evaluation were sulindac (Clinoril) and topical prednisolone acetate 1% (which she was taking erratically).

Examination disclosed visual acuities of 20/300 in the right eye and 1/200 in the left eye, 2 + cells in each anterior chamber, and bilateral disc and retinal edema. In January 1987, prednisone was begun, 100 mg/day

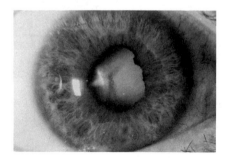

Figure 2 *Cataract and posterior synechiae in a patient with juvenile rheumatoid arthritis–associated uveitis.*

Table 4 *Patient Characteristics*

Characteristic	No. (%) of Patients Treated with Immunosuppressives* (n = 8)	No. (%) of Patients Treated Conventionally (n = 18)
Age at onset of uveitis (mean ± SEM)	12.6 ± 5.2	9.7 ± 6.7
Female	7 (88)	15 (83)
ANA-positive	6 (75)	14 (78)
HLA-B27-positive	1 (13)	2 (11)
Pauciarticular onset	8 (100)	18 (100)
Cataract extraction done	5 (63)	9 (50)

SEM = standard error of the mean; ANA = antinuclear antibody.
*Two-tailed, unpaired Student's *t*-test was used to analyze the difference between ages; chi-squared analysis was used to determine the difference between the remaining patient characteristics studied. No statistically significant difference was found between the treatment groups.

Table 5 *Ocular Manifestations*

Manifestation	No. (%) of Patients Treated with Immunosuppressives[a] (n = 13)	No. (%) of Patients Treated Conventionally (n = 31)
Iridocyclitis	13 (100)	31 (100)
Vitritis[b]	7 (54)	4 (13)
Cataract	11 (85)	22 (71)
Band keratopathy	6 (46)	19 (61)
Synechiae	7 (54)	19 (61)
Glaucoma	2 (15)	9 (29)
Disc edema	2 (15)	2 (7)
Macular edema	2 (15)	5 (16)

[a]Chi-squared analysis was used to determine the statistical difference between the treatment groups.
[b]Difference was statistically significant ($p = .001$).

per os. Improvement to 1+ cells in the anterior chamber with a decrease in the disc edema occurred over the next 2 months. Two transseptal injections of methylprednisolone acetate and triamcinolone diacetate were administered during this period. In March 1987, azathioprine (150 mg/day) was started after obtaining the appropriate laboratory studies and patient consent. Nausea necessitated reduction of azathioprine to 125 mg/day. Two months later, inflammation had improved, but disc edema and anterior uveitis recurred in August 1987; these did not improve after increasing azathioprine to 200 mg/day. In November 1988, azathioprine was withdrawn, and chlorambucil (Leukeran), 12 mg/day, was begun. One month later, inflammation had subsided. The eyes remained inflammation-free over the next 6 months. Prednisone and chlorambucil were tapered and eventually discontinued in June 1989. One year later, mild anterior uveitis without disc edema recurred and responded promptly to topical corticosteroids. The eyes have remained free of inflammation, and visual acuities at the time of the last examination were 20/30 in the right eye and 20/200 in the left eye.

Patient 22

A 16-year-old girl with JRA-associated iridocyclitis since age 6 was referred in October 1988 with refractory anterior uveitis. Treatment consisted of atropine sulfate 1% twice daily in each eye, prednisolone acetate 1% every 3 hours in both eyes, piroxicam (Feldene), 20 mg/day per os, and flurbiprofen sodium 0.03% (Ocufen) twice daily in each eye. Management in the past had included systemic corticosteroids, with limited therapeutic response. The patient had developed secondary cataracts in both eyes and had undergone intracapsular cataract extraction without intraocular lens implantation 3 and 4 years previously in the right and left eyes, respectively.

Examination on presentation to us revealed visual acuities of 20/400 in the right eye and 20/320 in the left eye, 2+ cells and 3+ flare in the anterior chamber, and 3+ cells in the vitreous cavity of both eyes. In October 1988, azathioprine (Imuran), 150 mg/day, was begun after the appropriate laboratory investigations and patient consent had been obtained. The patient experienced transient nausea that resolved within 1 week. In December 1988, trace cells were found in the anterior chamber and vitreous cavity. In February 1989, vitrectomy was performed in the left eye to reduce vitreous haze. One month later, the eyes were still quiet and vision had improved from 20/400 to 20/80. In January 1990, azathioprine was decreased to 100 mg/day. Recurrence of uveitis necessitated resumption of the previous dose of azathioprine in February 1990. After 6 months of anterior chamber and vitreous cavity quiescence, azathioprine was tapered to 100 mg/day, which was again followed by recurrence of uveitis that responded to increasing azathioprine to 150 mg/day. Laboratory parameters have remained stable throughout the treatment period, and visual acuities at last examination were 20/300 in the right eye and 20/80 in the left eye.

■ Discussion

JRA and its associated uveitis is a disease of presumed autoimmune etiology. Investigators have demonstrated the presence of anti-T-cell (possibly T-suppressor cell) antibodies [3–5], hyperimmunoglobulinemia [6–9], and hypercomplementemia [7, 10] in the sera of patients with active JRA. Synovial tissue and fluid may contain IgG complexes [7, 11, 12]. Other researchers have demonstrated a humoral immune response to S antigen [13] and reactivity of sera with retinal tissue [14, 15] in children with JRA and uveitis. Immunoreactivity against collagen has been implicated in the immunopathogenesis of uveitis and arthritis in patients with JRA [2]. Elevated IgM, IgA, IgE, and antinuclear antibody have been demonstrated in the aqueous humor of patients with JRA [16], and antinuclear antibody positivity is a well-recognized risk factor for the development of JRA-associated uveitis [1, 16, 17]. Plasma cells have been described in the iris and ciliary body [18–20].

Mydriatics, topical, periocular, and systemic corticosteroids, and NSAIDs have long been the mainstay of therapy for JRA-associated uveitis [2, 21, 22]. Uveitis in certain patients may, however, remain refractory to these therapeutic measures, leading to progressive deterioration of ocular function. In addition, adverse effects of corticosteroids are many and common and are similar in children and adults, with iatrogenic Cushing's syndrome and cataract being the most common [23–25]. Also, systemically administered corticosteroids in children may lead to stunted growth (especially if the daily dose exceeds 3 to 5 mg). Topical corticosteroid administration may lead to glaucoma, cataract development, or increased susceptibility to ocular infection. Uveitis not responding to topical corticosteroids often tends not to respond to corticosteroids administered systemically [26]. Immunosuppressive therapy offers an alternative mode of treatment (especially attractive considering the immune-mediated etiology previously discussed) for patients in whom ocular inflammation has not responded to therapy with corticosteroids or in patients who have developed unacceptable adverse effects of corticosteroid therapy.

Few published data on immunosuppressive therapy for JRA-associated uveitis exist. Most reports describe the results of retrospective, uncontrolled clinical trials in a few selected patients. Wong [27] reported improvement in 1 patient with "childhood uveitis" treated with a combination of methotrexate and cyclophosphamide. Lazar and colleagues [28] used methotrexate to treat 1 patient with Still's disease and associated uveitis, with encouraging results. Mehra and co-workers [29] reported a favorable response in 1 patient with JRA-associated uveitis treated with chlorambucil (2 mg/day) for 9 months. No adverse effects were reported. Godfrey and colleagues [30] reported "intermediate" results in 1 such patient treated with chlorambucil, and Kanski [31] reported encouraging results in 5 of 6 patients treated with this drug. Palmer and associates [32] also reported their experience using chlorambucil to treat 6 patients with anterior uveitis associated with JRA. The lowest dose used was 2 mg/day and the highest dose was 6 mg/day. Long-term beneficial results were achieved in 4 eyes of

2 patients, with "intermediate results" in 1 eye of another patient. Serious adverse side effects (herpes zoster and ovarian failure) occurred in 2 patients [32]. It is unclear whether these were the same patients included in Kanski's earlier report [31]. Two patients were treated with a combination of cyclophosphamide and azathioprine by Key and Kimura [33], without significant therapeutic response (dosage was not specified).

We now report a favorable outcome in 6 of 8 patients treated with immunosuppressive drugs. This relatively large number of patients requiring immunosuppressive therapy probably reflects the referral nature of our practice. All patients had been unresponsive to corticosteroid therapy. No serious adverse effects of immunosuppressive therapy were encountered. This confirms several recent reports that suggest that low-dose methotrexate treatment (used for 6 months to 4 years) may be safe in children with JRA [34, 35]. We would caution, however, that the potential to develop serious adverse effects from immunosuppressive therapy is very real, and therefore the use of such drugs in caring for patients with ocular inflammation must be restricted to individuals who, by virtue of training and experience, possess intimate knowledge of the properties of immunosuppressive drugs and special expertise in their use. Even expert chemotherapists may not avoid serious adverse effects. Chlorambucil, for example, has been associated with the development of acute leukemia in patients with JRA and may lead to chromosomal damage that is dose-dependent and cumulative [36, 37]. The potential for infertility may also be of concern when using this drug in children.

Our data indicate that the presence of inflammatory cells in the vitreous cavity on presentation was associated with a need for immunosuppressive therapy to control ocular inflammation. Cells in the vitreous cavity may reflect active vitritis. Alternatively, inflammatory cells in the vitreous could be a passive phenomenon representing spillover of inflammatory cells from the anterior chamber. Vitreous cells, however, did not preclude success of immunosuppressive therapy: Five of 7 (74%) eyes with cells in the vitreous responded to treatment.

In conclusion, our data suggest that immunosuppressive therapy in patients with JRA and progressive, corticosteroid-resistant uveitis can be effective and safe in controlling inflammation if carefully (and judiciously) administered and closely supervised. A controlled, randomized, prospective, masked clinical trial with long-term follow-up of patients that compares corticosteroids with immunosuppressives in the treatment of JRA-associated ocular inflammation may be a logical extension of these observations. Such a study would be logistically difficult and would require the participation of many large referral centers.

This work was supported in part by the Susan M. Hilles Fund.

■ References

1. Singsen BH. Pediatric rheumatic diseases. In: Schumacher HR Jr, ed. Primer on the rheumatic diseases, ed 9. Atlanta: Arthritis Foundation, 1988:160–164

2. Rosenberg AM. Uveitis associated with juvenile rheumatoid arthritis. Semin Arthritis Rheum 1987;16:158–173

3. Strelkauskas AJ, Callery RT, McDowell J, et al. Direct evidence for loss of human suppressor cell during active autoimmune disease. Proc Natl Acad Sci USA 1978;75:5150–5154

4. Morimoto C, Reinherz EL, Borel Y, et al. Autoantibody to an immunoregulatory inducer population in patients with juvenile rheumatoid arthritis. J Clin Invest 1981;67:753–761

5. Barron KS, Lewis DE, Brewer EJ, et al. Cytotoxic anti-T cell antibodies in children with juvenile rheumatoid arthritis. Arthritis Rheum 1984;27:1272–1280

6. Bluestone R, Goldberg LS, Katz RM, et al. Juvenile rheumatoid arthritis: a serologic survey of 200 consecutive patients. J Pediatr 1970;77:98–102

7. Bianci NE, Panush RS, Stillman JS, Schur PH. Immunologic studies of juvenile rheumatoid arthritis. Arthritis Rheum 1971;14:685–696

8. Bianci NE, Dobkin LW, Schur PH. Immunological properties of isolated IgG and IgM anti-gamma-globulins (rheumatoid factors). Clin Exp Immunol 1974;17:91–101

9. Rudnicki RD, Ruderman M, Scull E, et al. Clinical features and serologic abnormalities in juvenile rheumatoid arthritis. Arthritis Rheum 1974;17:1007–1015

10. Wedgewood RJP, Janeway CA. Serum complement in children with "collagen diseases." Pediatrics 1953;6:569–580

11. Munthe E. Complexes of IgG and IgG rheumatoid factors in synovial tissues of juvenile rheumatoid arthritis. Scand J Rheumatol 1972;1:153–160

12. Hedberg H. The depressed synovial complement activity in adult and juvenile rheumatoid arthritis. Acta Rheum Scand 1964;10:109–127

13. Petty RE, Hunt DW, Rollins DF. Autoimmunity to retinal antigen (S) in juvenile rheumatoid arthritis (JRA) with uveitis (U). Arthritis Rheum 1984;(suppl)27:S41

14. Petty RE, Hunt DWC, Rollins DF. Immunity to two ocular antigens in juvenile rheumatoid arthritis and uveitis. Arthritis Rheum 1986;(suppl)29:S24

15. Uchiyama RC, Osborn TG, Moore TL. Indirect immunofluorescence studies on human eye tissue using sera from juvenile rheumatoid arthritis patients with iridocyclitis. Arthritis Rheum 1986;(suppl)29:S67

16. Rahi AHS, Kanski JJ, Fielder A. Immunoglobulins and antinuclear antibodies in aqueous humor from patients with juvenile "rheumatoid" arthritis (Still's disease). Trans Ophthalmol Soc UK 1977;97:217–222

17. Schaller JG, Johnson GD, Holborow EJ, et al. The association of antinuclear antibodies with the chronic iridocyclitis of juvenile rheumatoid arthritis (Still's disease). Arthritis Rheum 1974;17:409–416

18. Sabates R, Smith T, Apple D. Ocular histopathology in juvenile rheumatoid arthritis. Ann Ophthalmol 1979;11:733–737

19. Godfrey WA, Lindsley CB, Cuppage FE. Localization of IgM in plasma cells in the iris of a patient with iridocyclitis and juvenile rheumatoid arthritis. Arthritis Rheum 1981;24:1195–1198

20. Merriam JC, Chylack LT, Albert DM. Early-onset pauciarticular juvenile rheumatoid arthritis: a histopathologic study. Arch Ophthalmol 1983;101:1085–1092

21. Chylack LT, Bienfang DC, Bellows R, Stillman JS. Ocular manifestations of juvenile rheumatoid arthritis. Am J Ophthalmol 1975;79:1026–1033

22. Kanski JJ. Juvenile arthritis and uveitis. Surv Ophthalmol 1990;34:253–267

23. Schaller JG. Corticosteroids in juvenile rheumatoid arthritis. Arthritis Rheum 1977;20:537–543

24. Chylack LT. The ocular manifestations of juvenile rheumatoid arthritis. Arthritis Rheum 1977;20:217–223
25. Wolf MD, Lichter PR, Ragsdale CG. Prognostic factors in the uveitis of juvenile rheumatoid arthritis. Ophthalmology 1987;94:1242–1248
26. Kanski JJ, Shun-Shin GA. Systemic uveitis syndromes in childhood: an analysis of 340 cases. Ophthalmology 1984;91:1247–1252
27. Wong VG. Methotrexate treatment of uveal disease. Am J Med Sci 1966;251: 239–241
28. Lazar M, Weiner MJ, Leopold IH. Treatment of uveitis with methotrexate. Am J Ophthalmol 1969;67:383–387
29. Mehra R, Moor TL, Catalano JD, et al. Chlorambucil in the treatment of iridocyclitis in juvenile rheumatoid arthritis. J Rheumatol 1981;8:141–144
30. Godfrey WA, Epstein WV, O'Conner GR, et al. The use of chlorambucil in intractable idiopathic uveitis. Am J Ophthalmol 1974;78:415–428
31. Kanski JJ. Care of children with anterior uveitis. Trans Ophthalmol Soc UK 1981;101:387–390
32. Palmer RG, Kanski JJ, Ansell BM. Chlorambucil in the treatment of intractable uveitis associated with juvenile chronic arthritis. J Rheumatol 1985;12:967–970
33. Key SN, Kimura SJ. Iridocyclitis associated with juvenile rheumatoid arthritis. Am J Ophthalmol 1975;80:425–429
34. Speckmaier M, Findeisen J, Woo P, et al. Low-dose methotrexate in systemic onset juvenile rheumatoid arthritis. Clin Exp Rheumatol 1989;7:647–650
35. Wallace CA, Bleyer WA, Sherry DD, et al. Toxicity and serum levels of methotrexate in children with juvenile rheumatoid arthritis. Arthritis Rheum 1989;32: 677–681
36. Palmer RG, Ansell BM. Acute leukemia related to chlorambucil therapy for juvenile chronic arthritis. Clin Exp Rheumatol 1984;2:81–83
37. Palmer RG, Dore CJ, Denman AM. Chlorambucil induced chromosome damage to human leukocytes is dose dependent and cumulative. Lancet 1984;1:246

Index

U.S. Postal Service Statement of Ownership, Management and Circulation (required by 39 U.S.C. 3685). 1A. Title of publication: INTERNATIONAL OPHTHALMOLOGY CLINICS. 1B. Publication no.: 00208167. 2. Date of filing: October 1, 1991. 3. Frequency of issue: quarterly. 3A. No. of issues published annually: 4. 3B. Annual subscription price: $81.00. 4. Complete mailing address of known office of publication (street, city, county, state and ZIP code) (not printers): 34 Beacon Street, Boston, Suffolk County, Massachusetts 02108-1493. 5. Complete mailing address of the headquarters or general business offices of the publishers (not printers): 34 Beacon Street, Boston, Suffolk County, Massachusetts 02108-1493. 6. Full names and complete mailing address of publisher, editor, and managing editor (this item *must not* be blank): Publisher (name and complete mailing address): Little, Brown and Company, Inc., 34 Beacon Street, Boston, Massachusetts 02108-1493. Editor (name and complete mailing address): Gilbert Smolin, MD, and Mitchell Friedlaender, MD, 931 West San Bruno Avenue, San Bruno, CA 94066. Managing Editor (name and complete mailing address): Sherri Frank, Little, Brown and Company, 34 Beacon Street, Boston, Massachusetts 02108-1493. 7. Owner (If owned by a corporation, its name and address must be stated and also immediately thereunder the names and addresses of stockholders owning or holding 1 percent or more of total amount of stock. If not owned by a corporation, the names and addresses of the individual owners must be given. If owned by a partnership or other unincorporated firm, its name and address, as well as that of each individual must be given. If the publication is published by a nonprofit organization, its name and address must be stated.) (Item must be completed): Full name: Little, Brown and Company (Incorporated). Complete mailing address: 34 Beacon Street, Boston, Massachusetts 02108-1493; The Time Inc. Book Company, Rockefeller Center, New York, New York 10020, which is a wholly owned subsidiary of Time Warner Inc., Rockefeller Center, New York, NY 10020. To the best of Time Warner's knowledge, the names and addresses of stockholders owning or holding one percent or more of the stock of Time Warner Inc. are as follows: Time Warner Inc., Common Stock (as of 8/23/91 unless otherwise indicated); *The Capital Group, Inc., 333 South Hope Street, Los Angeles, CA 90071 (as of December 31, 1989); *The Depository Trust Company, P.O. Box 20, Bowling Green Station, New York, NY 10274; The Henry Luce Foundation, Inc., 111 West 50th Street, New York, NY 10020; *Pitt & Co., % Bankers Trust Co., 16 Wall Street, New York, NY 10005; *SIOR & Co., % Bankers Trust Co., Box 704 Church Street Station, New York, NY 10015; Salomon Bros., 55 Water Street, New York, NY 10041; *The Equitable Life Assurance Society of the United States, 787 Seventh Avenue, New York, NY 10019. Time Warner Inc., Series C 8¾% Convertible Exchangeable Preferred Stock (as of 9/12/91 unless otherwise indicated): BHC Communications Inc., 600 Madison Avenue, New York, NY 10022-1615; Chris Craft Television Inc., 600 Madison Avenue, New York, NY 10022-1615; United Television Inc., 8501 Wilshire Blvd., Suite 340, Beverly Hills, CA 90211-3119; Time Warner Inc., Series D 11% Convertible Exchangeable Preferred Stock (as of 9/12/91); BHC Communications Inc., 600 Madison Avenue, New York, NY 10022-1615; Chris Craft Television Inc., 600 Madison Avenue, New York, NY 10022-1615; United Television Inc., 8501 Wilshire Blvd., Suite 340, Beverly Hills, CA 90211-3119; *The Depository Trust Company, P.O. Box 20, Bowling Green Station, New York, NY 10274-0020; ¯Security Pacific National Bank, custodian as of April 16, 1991, for John R. Garamendi cons. Executive Life Insurance Company, P.O. Box 2140, Pasadena, CA 91102; *¯Fayez Sarofim & Co., 2907 Two Houston Center, Houston, TX 77010 (as of 12-31-90); ⁺Eagle Asset Management Inc., 880 Carillon Parkway, P.O. Box 10520, St. Petersburg, FL 33733-0520 (as of 12-31-90). (*Held for the account of one or more security holders; ¯Series C Preferred Stock only; ⁺Series D Preferred Stock only.) 8. Known bondholders, mortgagees, and other security holders owning or holding 1 percent or more of total amount of bonds, mortgages or other securities (if there are none, so state): *The Depository Trust Company, P.O. Box 20, Bowling Green Station, New York, NY 10274 (as of 9/13/91; *Held for the account of one or more security holders.) 9. For completion by nonprofit organizations authorized to mail at special rates (Section 423.12, DMM only). The purpose, function, and nonprofit status of this organization and the exempt status for Federal income tax purposes (Check one): (1) Has not changed during preceding 12 months; (2) Has changed during preceding 12 months (If changed, publisher must submit explanation of change with this statement.): None. 10. Extent and nature of circulation: A. Total no. copies (net press run): average no. copies each issue during preceding 12 months, 3295; actual no. copies of single issue published nearest to filing date, 3308. B. Paid circulation: 1. Sales through dealers and carriers, street vendors and counter sales: average no. copies each issue during preceding 12 months, 58; actual no. copies of single issue published nearest to filing date, 57. 2. Mail subscription: average no. copies each issue during preceding 12 months, 2067; actual no. copies of single issue published nearest to filing date, 2005. C. Total paid circulation (sum of 10B1 and 10B2): average no. copies each issue during preceding 12 months, 2125; actual no. copies of single issue published nearest to filing date, 2062. D. Free distribution by mail, carrier or other means, samples, complimentary, and other free copies: average no. copies each issue during preceding 12 months, 138; actual no. copies of single issue published nearest to filing date, 93. E. Total distribution (sum of C and D): average no. copies each issue during preceding 12 months, 2263; actual no. copies of single issue published nearest to filing date, 2155. F. Copies not distributed: 1. Office use, left over, unaccounted, spoiled after printing: average no. copies each issue during preceding 12 months, 1032; actual no. copies of single issue published nearest to filing date, 1153. 2. Return from news agents: average no. copies each issue during preceding 12 months, none; actual no. copies of single issue published nearest to filing date, none. G. Total (sum of E, F1 and 2—should equal net press run shown in A): average no. copies each issue during preceding 12 months, 3295; actual no. copies of single issue published nearest to filing date, 3308. H. I certify that the statements made by me above are correct and complete. Signature and title of editor, publisher, business manager, or owner: Christine Finn, Business Manager.

Future Issues

Volume 32, 1992

Spring (No. 2)

RETINAL AND VITREAL SURGERY
Joseph Olk, M.D., Guest Editor

Summer (No. 3)

ORBITAL DISEASE
John Shore, M.D., Guest Editor

Fall (No. 4)

COMPLICATIONS IN OPHTHALMIC SURGERY